BIRD DISEASES

ISBN 0-87666-950-X

Distributed in the U.S.A by T.F.H. Publications, Inc., 211 West Sylvania Avenue, P.O. Box 27, Neptune City, N.J. 07753; in England by Bailliere Tindall, 7/8 Henrietta Street, London WC2E 8QE; in Canada to the book store and library trade by Clarke, Irwin & Company, Clarwin House, 791 St. Clair Avenue West, Toronto 10, Ontario; in Canada to the pet trade by Rolf C. Hagen Ltd., 3225 Sartelon Street, Montreal 382, Quebec.

BIRD DISEASES

AN INTRODUCTION TO THE STUDY OF BIRDS IN HEALTH AND DISEASE

L. ARNALL
B.V.Sc. M.R.C.V.S

Revised and augmented by

I. F. KEYMER
Ph.D. F.R.C.V.S. M.R.C. Path F.I. Biol

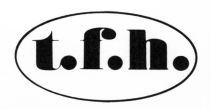

Contents

5

ACKNOWLEDGEMENTS

Although the conception of this book was relatively painless, its later gestation became more and more difficult. To Dr Ian Keymer therefore, whose assistance in editing and ornithological experience enabled the work to come to fruition, I give my heartfelt thanks.

He has further added a section on the "Classification of Birds and Host List of Important Diseases", compiled a list of species mentioned in the text and made numerous additions, including coloured plates. His enthusiasm and relentless perseverence have made the book more valuable, while his wife, Janet, has provided some excellent drawings. Initials in the chapter heading indicate which of us has been primarily responsible for that section.

For his sympathetic encouragement during the early years of the book, I should like to acknowledge the kindness of the late Professor G. Wright, then Dean of Liverpool University School of Veterinary Science. To my head of department at that time, Mr A. C. Shuttleworth, I offer thanks for his sympathy to indulge my avian interest.

To Mr Oliver Graham-Jones, I offer my appreciation for stimulation and for reading through the preliminary manuscript. Professor A. S. King gave valuable help in the Anatomy and Physiology section, especially with the respiratory system. I am also indebted to Dr David K. Blackmore for his encouragement, practical help and certain irreplaceable illustrations and to Professor A. Ferguson who read much of the final manuscript and made many useful suggestions. I should also like to thank the following:

Mr Hugh P. Harding and Dr John M. K. Mackay whose enthusiasm, detailed pathological knowledge and discussion of my clinical cases enkindled and sustained my early interest in cagebirds; this was later continued by Drs John Mc. C. Howell, John Ishmail and Duncan Allan under Professor David L. Hughes.

Messrs George Weston, T. Dennett and G. Dibley for specimen preparation and photography of interesting pathological materials. Mr Wilfred Lee and staff of the Central Medical Photographic Department of the University of Liverpool for their studies of the classical cagebird diseases.

Mr G. S. Walton for his great kindness, and computer-like retrieval of "inaccessible" knowledge—later continued by Mr G. Dibley who assisted the editor. Mrs Margaret L. Petrak for her enthusiasm and stimulating correspondence.

The Veterinary Record and Journal of Small Animal Practice for permission to reproduce plates and diagrams from my earlier publications and those of colleagues recognised above: the Library of the Royal College of Veterinary Surgeons, London, in particular the librarian, Miss B. Horder; the Harold Cohen Library of the University of Liverpool, the Picton Reference Library at Liverpool and the library of the Zoological Society of London for facilities.

The many veterinary surgeons in private practice for referring challenging cases and outbreak problems to me in the past 15 years. To the several ladies who have typed drafts of sections of the book; and in particular to Miss R. Benson, who prepared the typescript for publication—some of it several times over.

Since this is not a book for specialists, the writer has not attempted to name every author of the published articles which underlie its information. Apologies are therefore due to many colleagues and friends whose names may not appear in the list of authorities.

Finally, I offer grateful thanks to my wife for her understanding and support in the anxious and not infrequently frustrating periods in bringing this work to press.

L. Arnall.

INTRODUCTION

This book is a practical guide to all who have a real interest in birds. It is, we think, the first that has been written in this way: to unfold a general view of this large subject and be useful both to the layman and the professional veterinarian.

Books on cage birds frequently include chapters on hygiene and disease, but more often than not these are too brief and inaccurate. They do not for example help the bird-keeper to understand why his valuable parrot shows a disinclination to go on living, why his cock canary refuses to sing any more, or why his budgerigar has suddenly taken to drinking excessive quantities of water.

Whether you keep one or two birds as pets in an apartment, or whether you have an aviary and are spurred by the ambition to breed rare species and gain prizes in shows, this book should help you to maintain healthy stock. It will also be valuable to commercial breeders, bird curators in zoological gardens, dealers and pet shop owners—as well as to the veterinarian who is not a specialist and only treats birds occasionally.

The book deals mainly with the cage birds most commonly kept. These are the budgerigar and other psittacines, the canary, and other passerines under the general name of "hardbills". Diseases of game birds and waterfowl are included; but they are not covered in such detail since this information is readily to hand in books dealing with poultry. The diseases of pigeons are included, as well as those of birds of prey and the host of other species kept in captivity, especially in zoos.

This volume is not intended to encourage the bird-keeper to be his own vet. Its purpose is to help him to keep his stock healthy, to prevent disease, and to recognise it if it does occur. The emphasis throughout is therefore on prevention and diagnosis. Suitable treatments are suggested so that there can be a common body of knowledge shared between the owner and the veterinarian. In most cases, however, it is only the qualified practitioner who can decide which drug to use and by which route, the dosage, and for how long it should be given. Incorrect dosages can do more harm than good and may be fatal.

It will be controversial, but chapters are included on anaesthesia and operations. This has been done for completeness, *not* to promote the practice of "do-it-yourself" surgery. Only in exceptional circumstances should an unqualified person attempt even the simplest operation on a bird because the results may well be disastrous, ending in suffering and death. Nevertheless the elements of the subject are included so that the bird-keeper can have some knowledge of the operations that it is possible to carry out. The information may also act as a guide in emergencies, especially in those parts of the world where veterinarians are not easy to contact.

Similarly, a chapter has been included which deals with *post-mortem* techniques. It is not suggested at all that a bird keeper should set himself up as a pathologist. This is a skilled discipline and the handling of birds' carcases can be dangerous to humans and to other stock. Nevertheless, it is more constructive to slit open a bird which has just died in order to see if there are any gross abnormalities, than simply to dispose of the carcase and hope for no more deaths. If such a necropsy indicates that death probably resulted from disease rather than injury, then it is wise to take advice.

The reader is introduced to diseases by an outline of the bird's anatomy, physiology and biochemistry. A glossary of the necessary scientific terms is also included. Another, and very important feature of the book is its tables. These contain a wealth of information that has never before been gathered together in this convenient form. They cover such matters as: the vital statistics of many birds—their heart-beat and respiratory rates, body temperatures; anaesthetics, dosages and precautions; antibiotic drugs; fungicidal drugs; parasiticidal substances; disinfectants; hormones and nutritional additives. A list of the scientific names of birds mentioned in the text has also been included. Lastly, to help the reader, the contents of some chapters have been designed to overlap a little. This will assist in tracking down specific points; cross references are given when the topic is dealt with in detail elsewhere.

Veterinary and medical students spend two or three years learning about health before they are taught about disease. It is important, therefore, to read first those parts of the book which deal with the normal and healthy bird. You will then become familiar with the organs and processes of a bird's body which will enable you to make the best possible use of the information on diseases.

PART ONE: **THE NORMAL BIRD**

HEALTH AND HEREDITY

Health

Everyone understands the general meaning of health, but it is not easy to define the state precisely. Dictionaries give varying definitions: "a soundness of body" or "a normal condition of body with all parts functioning well", whilst one authority merely states that it is "an absence of disease".

The diagnosis of disease in all live animals, but especially in birds, is particularly difficult compared with man. A sick person is able to describe his symptoms to the doctor, but the veterinarian relies entirely upon his powers of observation and those of the patient's owner. When consulting a vet. therefore, it is very important to be able to provide as much information as possible. The Appendix includes a table of the principal points of aid in diagnosis. To give the fullest information entails being fully conversant with the normal behaviour of the species, otherwise it may not be possible to recognise certain signs of sickness or unusual behaviour. Sometimes it can be very difficult to tell the difference between a healthy and a sick animal, particularly in the early stages of an illness. Veterinarians, however, are specially trained to be aware of the signs of ill-health in domestic animals and much of their knowledge can be applied to other species, including birds. Although your vet. may not have personal experience of the species of birds which you keep, he may well, with your help and his specialised knowledge, be able to diagnose the cause of sickness in your bird.

The metabolic rate or "rate of living" varies considerably among the different species of birds and determines the normal heart and respiratory rates and the body temperature, as well as physical and mental activity. Therefore, before attempting to keep any species it is essential to become familiar with its normal behaviour, including its temperament and dietary requirements. Generally speaking, healthy birds have a sleek "tight" plumage unless moulting. They are also inquisitive, bright-eyed and hold their wings close to the body. Many birds, for example, draw one leg up beneath the abdomen during sleep and tuck the bill under the wing. The appearance of the excreta varies with different species and according to the diet. Most birds, especially seed-eaters, have relatively soft but formed droppings, with a dark greenish part representing the faeces and a white portion being the urate excretion. Fruit-eating birds such as lorikeets, however, normally have wet droppings which must not be confused with diarrhoea.

The maintenance of health depends on environment, diet and heredity.

Environment is an all-embracing term which includes such factors as temperature and humidity of the air, ventilation, draughts, infections, injuries, intensity and nature of light, presence or absence of predators, and circumstances causing fear, excitement and boredom.

Diet greatly affects health, although its effects may not always be realised. A bird caged alone for example with a liberal supply of suitable food may fail to thrive because it may become excessively fat. This applies particularly to budgerigars. On the other hand recently captured birds given a well balanced but unvaried diet may waste away and die through failure to eat sufficient food. These dietetic and other nutritional problems, however, are discussed in detail later in the book.

Heredity

Heredity can be defined as "the inheritance of qualities or of diseases from the parents and previous generations". It determines such characteristics as the bird's sex, shape, size, colour, resistance to disease, muscular build and, to a great extent, its behaviour, food preferences and other activities. Many of these characteristics, however, are also modified by environment.

Genetics is the science which deals with the origin of the characteristics of the individual. It is the study of heredity and is a complicated subject which can be dealt with here only very briefly. In fact, relatively little is known about the subject in birds—with the exception of the domestic fowl and to a lesser extent the pigeon, budgerigar and canary.

All the cells which make up the body contain chromosomes within their nuclei, the number of which is the same in every cell and constant for each species. All the body chromosomes are paired, and with the exception of the sex chromosomes, are identical. The latter, occurring in the reproductive or germ cells of the sperm and ovum, carry the hereditary characteristics from one generation to the next; to explain the inheritance of sex it is customary to label them with capital letters.

Hen birds have a pair of sex chromosomes, one being an X and the other a Y chromosome in each ovum or egg, whereas cocks have a pair consisting of two X chromosomes for each sperm, this being the opposite to the situation in mammals. It is important to note that prior to fertilization the number of chromosomes in each germ cell is halved, one of each pair separating, otherwise the resultant zygote formed by the fusion of a sperm and an ovum would contain twice the number of chromosomes for that particular species. When fertilization occurs and a sperm unites with an ovum in the upper part of the oviduct, the chromosomes of each parent separate so that one X chromosome from the cock unites with one X from the hen, to produce XX (a male), or alternatively one X from the cock unites with one Y from the hen to produce XY which is a female. It can be seen, therefore, that in theory the chances of equal numbers of both sexes being produced in a brood are equal. In practice, however, this seldom occurs. The same laws of chance apply as when a coin is tossed in the air an equal number of times. Theoretically, the results should be 50 per cent "heads" and 50 per cent "tails", but this does not always happen in the short run, the chances of it doing so increasing the greater the number of tosses. In addition to statistical reasons, however, there are many others why equal numbers of both sexes are not produced.

The chromosomes, as stated previously, carry all the characteristics of the individual. Specific characters or "genes", of which there are many, are normally located in the same position on a chromosome. Geneticists have been able to produce chromosome maps for some species showing the sites of genes which represent many different physical characters such as colour of eyes, colour of body, etc. Sometimes a whole group of genes or

Parents	Pure Green GG	x	Yellow yy				Green Gy	x	Green Gy

Gy Green	**Gy** Green
Gy Green	**Gy** Green

GG Green	**Gy** Green
Gy Green	**yy** Yellow

F_1
1st filial generation

100% Green

F_2
2nd filial generation

75% Green
25% Yellow

Figure 1   Inheritance of pure green (GG) and yellow (yy) factors in budgerigars.

genetic units is involved in producing a single character such as colour. This is the case when it is not a straightforward specific colour such as the yellow of a budgerigar, but based on a variety of factors, as in the plumage colouration of a peacock. Sex chromosomes may also carry genes other than those for sex and if these genes (for certain colours for example) are confined to one type of sex chromosome, then the characters are said to be sex-linked; examples in budgerigars being albinos and the colours known as opaline and lutinos. These factors are always linked to the X and never to the Y chromosomes.

When factors such as colour are not sex-linked, they are inherited according to the Law of Mendel. Gregor Johann Mendel was a monk who lived in the 19th century and worked out the general principles of heredity by experimenting with peas. He found that in the first generation of a cross between two individuals with different characters, one of the characters alone appears —the "dominant"; the other lies latent and is called the "recessive". The dominant factor is always designated by using a capital letter, e.g. GG represents a pure green budgerigar of

any of the three shades. Gy is a green bird which is the result of crossing green and yellow, the latter factor being recessive. If GG is crossed with yy (yellow) the offspring will all be Gy. This is called by geneticists the first filial or F_1 generation. The birds will look green, but they will have inherited the yellow factor.

If a Gy is mated with a Gy, then according to the Law of Mendel, 25 per cent will be pure green, 50 per cent green inheriting yellow, and 25 per cent pure yellow.

This second generation is called the F_2 and it is impossible from the outward appearance to tell which of the green birds (representing 75 per cent) are pure green and which carry yellow genes. It is easy to see that working out the inheritance of characters in the next and subsequent generations becomes increasingly complex. In the F_3 generation for example, there are theoretically 16 possibilities, by mating GG with Gy, GG with yy, Gy with Gy and Gy with yy.

When a germ cell contains genes that produce like characters, e.g. GG or yy as illustrated above, it is said to be homozygous, whereas if it contains different characters, *e.g.* Gy, it is stated to be heterozygous.

In order to reduce the number of individuals that are heterozygous for any one pair of genes and to increase the number that are homozygous for one or other member of the gene pair, many breeders practice a system known as in-breeding. This is the mating together of individuals which are related to each other through having one or more ancestors in common. It ultimately produces uniformity of genetic constitution; but because undesirable as well as desirable characters can become concentrated in the stock, the method requires a great deal of skill in order to eliminate the undesirable characters.

Inheritance of specific characters is not always as straightforward and predictable as it may seem. Sometimes for example, a derangement of the genes occurs at the moment of fertilization when sperm and ovum unite, due to the chromosomes crossing over each other, instead of lying side by side. Any pair of chromosomes may be involved in this way, thus giving rise to unexpected characters in the resultant offspring. Occasionally the chemical nature of a gene becomes altered, resulting in a permanent change of some specific character. The process is known as mutation and the resultant individual is called a sport or mutant. Mutations, however, unlike crossing-over of chromosomes, occur very infrequently. Mutants transmit the altered character to their offspring and are usually recessive. Mutations are seldom beneficial to the species and are in fact usually harmful, sometimes even resulting in the death of the individual, in which case of course the mutation is not perpetuated. Mutations have been responsible for the development of some unusual breeds or colours of canaries and budgerigars. A well known example is the lutino budgerigar which has a pure yellow plumage and pink eyes.

When it is remembered what a vast number of characters are inherited in addition to colour (chosen here for simplicity), it will be appreciated that the study of genetics is extremely complicated and beyond the scope of this book.

SELECTED BIBLIOGRAPHY

ARMOUR, M. D. S. (1956). *Exhibition Budgerigars*. 2nd Ed. London. Iliffe. 159pp.

AUERBACH, C. (1962). *The Science of Genetics*. London. Hutchinson. 275pp

BUCKLEY, P. A. (1969). *In* Diseases of Cage and Aviary Birds, pp.3–43. Ed. Petrak, M. L. Philadelphia. Lea and Febiger.

GILL, A. K. (1951). *Cinnamon Inheritance in Canaries*. London. Iliffe. 32pp.

GILL, A. K. (1955). *New-coloured Canaries*. London. Iliffe. 103pp.

HUTT, F. B. (1964). *Animal Genetics*. New York. Ronald Press Co. 546pp.

TAYLOR, T. G. and WARNER, C. (1961). *Genetics for Budgerigar Breeders*. London. Iliffe. 129pp.

THOMSON, Sir A. Landsborough (1964). *A New Dictionary of Birds*. London and Edinburgh. Thomas Nelson. 927pp.

ANATOMY AND PHYSIOLOGY

These two subjects are so closely related that they will be discussed together. Anatomy is concerned with the structure of the body and physiology with the function of the organs.

Two branches of these subjects are biochemistry—the chemistry of the processes of life—and embryology, which is concerned with how the complex differences between species evolve from similar, single-celled eggs.

It is impossible to explain evolution in a few paragraphs, but it must be remembered that through the ages, as changes occurred in climate, the availability of water, food supply, etc., those animals which adapted most efficiently to the new conditions were those most likely to survive. Freaks or "sports" as they are called, flourish if they prove to be more successful than the normal members of the species. The majority of "sports," however, are less suited to the environment and perish without trace. These accidental variations have produced the vast variety in birds we know today. In bird-keeping, it will be noted that some species, usually the rarer types, are not suited to a wide range of temperatures, diets, and environments, whilst others can flourish in an exposed aviary on a north wall and on the most unnatural diet. It is the rare and delicate birds which are probably destined to become extinct and which represent therefore such a challenge to keep and to attempt to breed in captivity. Before acquiring such birds we should study their biology and aim to meet as many of their natural requirements as possible. A well balanced, palatable diet acceptable to the bird is particularly important and if this cannot be maintained, then the bird should not be kept.

It would be tedious and of little value to describe in detail the anatomy of each species. An appreciation, however, of a few of the variations of form and function among species is helpful in understanding the problems of disease. It is assumed that the reader possesses some general knowledge of the anatomy of vertebrates and has an idea of the function of the main organs of the body.

THE CELL

When one looks at a bird or any animal, it is difficult to realise that it is made of millions of tiny bits of living matter or cells, each entirely covered with its own membrane. The simplest complete forms of life are one-celled; that is, they are minute blobs of jelly or protoplasm enclosed in a skin. The make-up of the protoplasm within this cell, varies in different areas. There is a central nucleus or nerve centre in a contractile, clear jelly containing undigested and partly digested food and waste material, but there are no obvious divisions between the various areas. Such unicellular organisms, of which the amoeba is one, are called protozoa which simply means "first animals." Amoebae are primitive but highly successful forms of life and are numerous throughout the world, especially in fresh water. They obtain food by flowing around particles of organic material, which are totally enveloped and slowly digested. They travel in a similar way by pushing a part of themselves forward as a sort of foot (pseudo-podium), and then "pour" themselves into this foot. Simple as their structure seems, they are attracted to suitable food and moderate warmth; they avoid heat, cold, and strong light; and they generally respond to their environment as do many more advanced creatures. Some protozoa which are parasitic in animals and man, are little different from their free-living relations. *Plasmodium*, the cause of malaria, and trypanosomes, which cause the tropical sleeping sickness in man, are two important members of the group.

After protozoa, the next step in evolution was for numbers of these simple and identical cells to fuse into solid and then hollow spheres, thus producing organisms made up of some hundreds of cells. In these more advanced organisms some cells became modified and adapted for special purposes, such as conducting messages from one part of the body to another. Evolution from these simple creatures has taken millions of years and has resulted in the development of vast numbers of species, of both invertebrates such as insects, and vertebrates such as fish, amphibians, reptiles, birds and mammals. All evolutionary development has resulted in an increase in cell specialization: but all body cells are developments of the basic type of cell.

Cell specialization is bewilderingly complex; yet a few cells of very primitive types persist. White blood cells are little different from the simple amoeba and feed in a similar manner. Most white cells, however, are much less mobile than the amoebae of the duck-pond and it is the circulation of the blood which provides movement to new areas. In contrast there are nerve, muscle, bone and gland cells, all of which are very different from amoebae. Body cells also vary considerably in size, the longest being muscle and certain nerve cells, whilst the largest cell is the egg.

THE TISSUES

The body cells are arranged in an organised fashion and gathered into sheets or masses called tissues. A tissue may contain several cell types, but a unit which contains groups of various types with one overall function is called an organ.

The skin, mucous membranes, and other covering and lining tissues protect against attacks by mechanical, chemical, or microbial agents.

The skeleton helps to hold the body together; it is a mixture of different cells which make up its bone, cartilage, and fibrous tissue. In these tissues many of the cells are fixed in a large amount of protein and lifeless mineral.

Skeletal muscles, mainly associated with bones, are tissues generally gathered in parallel bundles of long, narrow cells. Because these contract on impulse from the brain, they are called voluntary muscles, although they are also known as striated muscle from their striped appearance. Involuntary muscles are automatic and are found in the intestinal or oviduct walls and some other internal organs. A short piece of intestine, detached and placed in salty water will continue to shorten and lengthen rhythmically: this automatic action comes from the alternate contraction of encircling and longitudinal muscles. Such involuntary muscle, also known as smooth muscle, is paler than skeletal muscle, and its cells are long and spindle-shaped.

20

A third type of muscle is found in the heart. Although composed of inter-linked short fibres showing the striations of voluntary muscle, its action is automatic. Heart muscle contraction (the heart rate) is governed by various factors including hormones. A conscious effort on the part of a bird or other animal cannot cause its heart to stop or restart.

Glandular tissues (such as the liver and thyroid) are in reality chemical factories. They are usually grouped into two main types, the typical glands with ducts or tubes, *e.g.* salivary glands, which are under nervous control; and the ductless glands, *e.g.* the adrenals, which are controlled by hormones. The blood and lymph systems are pipelines conveying warmth, moisture, gases, salts, food and waste materials to the appropriate parts of the body. Blood is considered to be a tissue. Lymph is a colourless, alkaline liquid which has similar functions to the blood. It has no red corpuscles and therefore does not convey oxygen. Nerve tissue is the most complex and specialized of all, both in structure and function. The most important organ in the body is the brain and this controls all the organs either directly or indirectly.

Although these cell types and tissues look and act differently from one another, they all derive from the primitive cell symbolized by the simple avian egg. They still retain many common characteristics, although there is a great degree of variation. The power of preventing damage to a threatened part is demonstrated by a rapid increase of blood to the area which carries white cells to devour the antagonist, antibodies to neutralize it and finally the walling off of the damaged part. The sensitivity of the response to damage varies with different organs. White cells and sex gland cells are very susceptible to damage by radiation, for example, while skin, bone, and brain cells are amongst the least affected.

THE EGG

The egg is very large in relation to the adult bird, but it is similar in many ways to the microscopic ovum of a

Figure 1   Structure of the avian egg. (Janet Keymer)

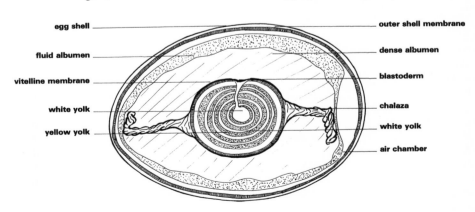

egg shell — outer shell membrane

fluid albumen — dense albumen

vitelline membrane — blastoderm

white yolk — chalaza

yellow yolk — white yolk

— air chamber

Eggs of some species commonly kept in captivity with normal clutch size (c.s.) and approximate incubation period (i.p.) in days:

1. Mute swan (*Cygnus olor*)   c.s. 5-7   i.p. 35
2. Canada goose (*Branta canadensis*)   c.s. 5-6   i.p. 28-29
3. Peafowl (*Pavo cristatus*)   c.s. 4-6   i.p. 28
4. Mallard duck (*Anas platyrhynchos*)   c.s. 10-12   i.p. 28
5. Scarlet macaw (*Ara macao*)   c.s. 3-6   i.p. 25
6. Greater sulphur crested cockatoo
   (*Kakatoe galerita*)   c.s. 2-3   i.p. 30
7. Mandarin duck (*Aix galericulata*)   c.s. 9-12   i.p. 28-30

(I.F. Keymer and T.C. Dennett, Z.S.L.)

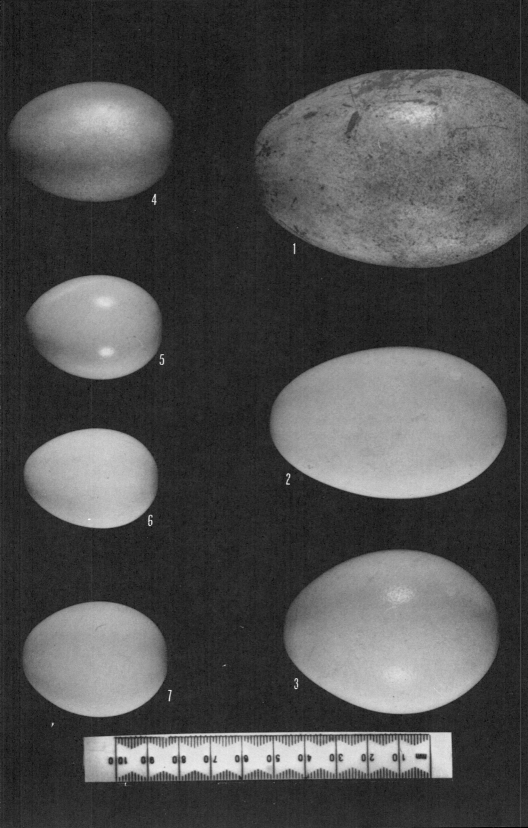

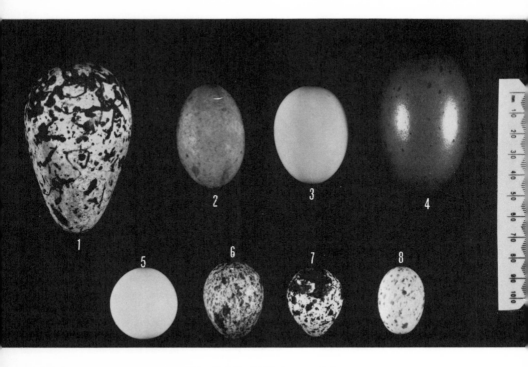

SHAPES OF EGGS. Eggs vary considerably in shape depending upon the species. Eight main types are recognised:

1. Pyriform. Auks, e.g. guillemot or common murre (*Uria aalge*).
2. Bi-conical. Grebes, e.g. great crested grebe (*Podiceps cristatus*).
3. Oval. Ducks, e.g. shoveller (*Anas clypeata*).
4. Longitudinal. Divers or loons, e.g. red-throated diver (*Gavia stellata*).
5. Spherical. Owls, e.g. little owl (*Athene noctua*).
6. Elliptical. Crows, e.g. carrion crow (*Corvus corone*).
7. Conical. Plovers, e.g. killdeer (*Charadrius vociferus*).
8. Cylindrical. Nightjars, e.g. European nightjar (*Caprimulgus europaeus*).
(I.F. Keymer and T.C. Dennett, Z.S.L.)

24

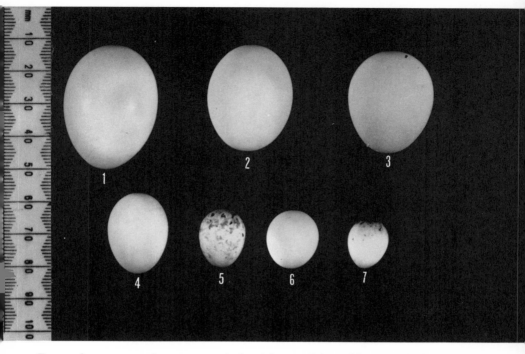

Eggs of some species commonly kept in captivity with normal clutch size
(c.s.) and approximate incubation period (i.p.) in days:

1. Domestic pigeon (*Columba livia*)   c.s. 2   i.p. 17-19
2. Yellow-backed lory (*Domicella garrula*)   c.s. 2   i.p. 25
3. Alexandrine parakeet (*Psittacula eupatria*) c.s. 3   i.p. 24-26
4. Cockatiel (*Nymphicus hollandicus*)   c.s. 4-6   i.p. 21
5. Canary (*Serinus canaria*)   c.s. 3-4   i.p. 14
6. Budgerigar (*Melopsittacus undulatus*)   c.s. 5-6   i.p. 18
7. Goldfinch (*Carduelis carduelis*)   c.s. 5-6   i.p. 12-13
(I.F. Keymer and T.C. Dennett, Z.S.L.)

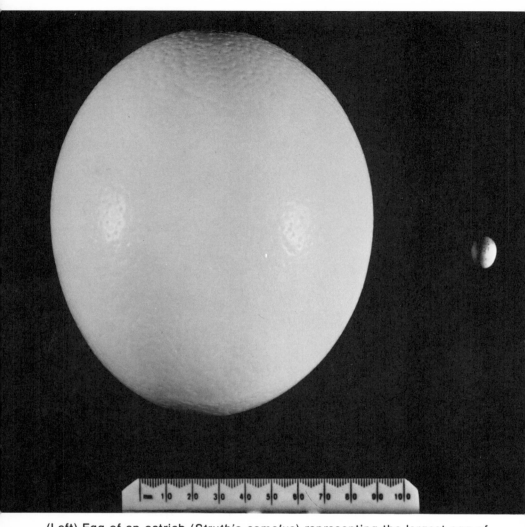

(Left) Egg of an ostrich (*Struthio camelus*) representing the largest egg of any living species of bird. Shell thickness 4.5 mm.

(Right) Egg of a goldcrest (*Regulus regulus*). This is the smallest species of British bird, and its egg is only slightly larger than the smallest eggs laid by humming birds. Shell thickness 0.2 mm. (I.F. Keymer and T.C. Dennett, Z.S.L.)

woman or other female mammal. The incubation period of the fertilized avian egg corresponds to the period of pregnancy in the mammal. The main difference is that with the mammal, nourishment of the embryo is carried by blood, whereas with birds it is derived from the egg albumen. In birds the periods of greatest stress are prior to laying, and during the feeding of the nestlings. Thus the two periods of strain on the bird's resources are separated by a pause for partial recuperation, the sitting or incubation period.

The ovum is budded off from the ovary after it has acquired its full complement of yolk layers. These are deposited in response to hormones developed and liberated from the pituitary. The ovary is also influenced by the adrenal cortex, thyroid and ovarian glandular cells. Changes occur in the yolk-laden ovum which prepare it for fertilization by a sperm whilst still in the upper part of the oviduct. Irrespective of whether or not fertilization takes place, the ovum passes down the oviduct wrapped in its transparent membrane, picking up layers of albumen or egg white, the parchment-like shell membranes, and finally the shell, (see Fig. 1).

EMBRYOLOGY

After fertilization, the ovum—now with its full complement of chromosomes—begins to grow by dividing into two, four, eight, sixteen cells, etc., until by the time the egg is laid a few hours after ovulation, a minute speck or patch of cells on one face of the yolk indicates the beginnings of the embryo. At this early stage the embryo is called a blastoderm.

If the egg is incubated, cell division proceeds at different rates in different parts of the blastoderm so that variations in size and distribution begin to appear. A slight separation becomes apparent between the surface and deeper layer of cells forming the ectoderm and endoderm or outer and inner skins. In the middle of this double sheet of cells a denser line of cells develops, visible from the surface of the yolk as a line and known as the primitive streak, (Fig. 2). From here the development is best described by surface diagrams or plans of the embryo, from the primitive groove and fold to the beginning of the organ formation, (Fig. 3). The embryo proper develops in front of the primitive groove, which then forms a tail-like extension to it, (Figs. 4 and 5). In the embryo, three layers of cells are recognizable, the ectoderm, mesoderm, and endoderm.

The ectoderm forms the covering layers of the body—the skin, feathers, horny tissues, also brain, spinal cord, retina and lens of the eye. The endoderm forms the mucous linings of the alimentary canal from oesophagus to cloaca and certain glands and tubes budded off from the alimentary tract. The mesoderm produces the greater part of the bird's body, including muscle, bones, connective tissues, blood, heart, blood vessels, and the bulk of the reproductive, genital, and respiratory tracts.

The embryo's power of internal organization with each stage of development of an organ or structure is one of the miracles of nature. Not only do the parts grow, but some—like the notocord or primitive spine, and the atavistic forerunners of the tail, kidneys, and "gills"—change in form and even completely disappear by the time the chick hatches, all in harmony with its overall development.

By about one-eighth of the way through the incubation period, all major organs can be recognized, even the stumpy limbs (Fig. 6). The embryo as a whole is approaching the appearance

27

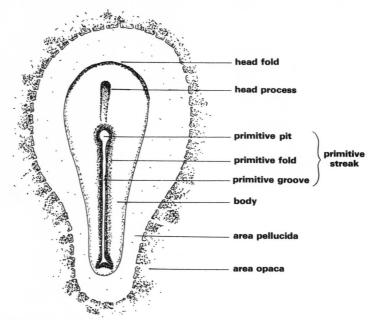

- head fold
- head process
- primitive pit
- primitive fold
- primitive groove
  } primitive streak
- body
- area pellucida
- area opaca

Figure 2 An early stage in the development of the domestic fowl chick. Approximately 18 hours after incubation. (Janet Keymer)

Figure 3 Domestic fowl, chick embryo at approximately 36 hours incubation. (Janet Keymer)

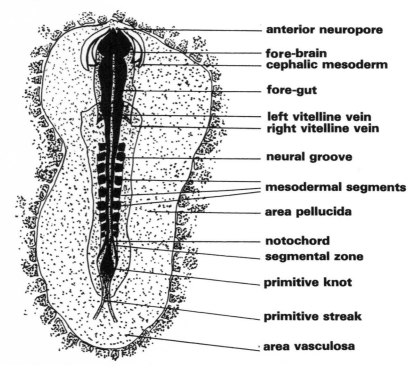

- anterior neuropore
- fore-brain
  cephalic mesoderm
- fore-gut
- left vitelline vein
  right vitelline vein
- neural groove
- mesodermal segments
- area pellucida
- notochord
  segmental zone
- primitive knot
- primitive streak
- area vasculosa

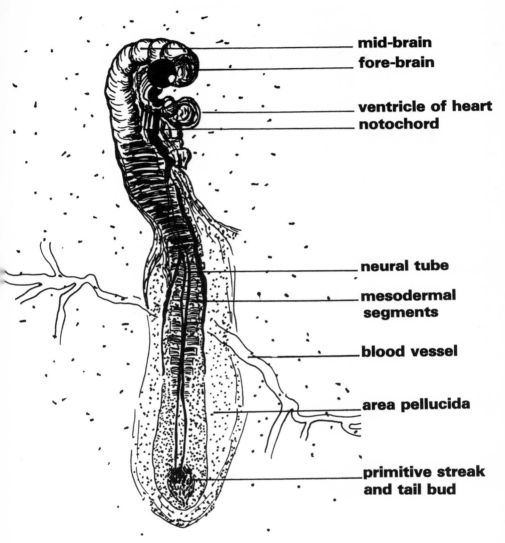

mid-brain

fore-brain

ventricle of heart

notochord

neural tube

mesodermal segments

blood vessel

area pellucida

primitive streak and tail bud

Figure 4   Domestic fowl, chick embryo at approximately 48 hours of incubation. (Janet Keymer)

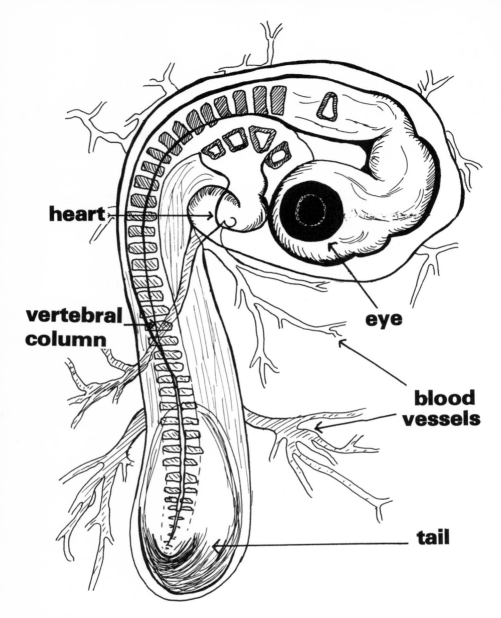

Figure 5   Domestic fowl, chick embryo at approximately 4 to 5 days of age. (Janet Keymer)

of a vertebrate. By one-quarter of the incubation period, it is recognizable as a bird, but with a massively disproportionate head. It is during development, that the organs are most susceptible to infection, dietary deficiencies and hereditary influences.

As the embryo develops, it is gradually elevated above the surface of the yolk, but becomes attached to the yolk sac by the formation of an umbilical cord connecting it with the intestine. Before hatching the yolk sac is withdrawn into the abdomen and after the bird hatches, yolk passes through the yolk stalk remnant of the umbilical cord to the intestine. This arrangement provides nourishment for the bird during the first few days of its life.

THE SURFACE ANATOMY

The main external features of birds are easy to recognize and understand. The terms used to describe them are for the most part well known. Structures which are peculiar to one or a group of birds are of special interest, and most are shown in Fig. 7.

A difficulty is that the terms used for these landmarks by anatomists differ in certain respects from those used by ornithologists or aviculturists. For

Figure 6   Domestic fowl, chick embryo at 9 days of age. (Janet Keymer)

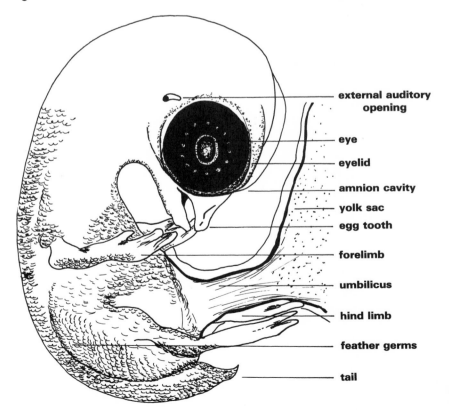

external auditory
opening

eye

eyelid

amnion cavity

yolk sac

egg tooth

forelimb

umbilicus

hind limb

feather germs

tail

31

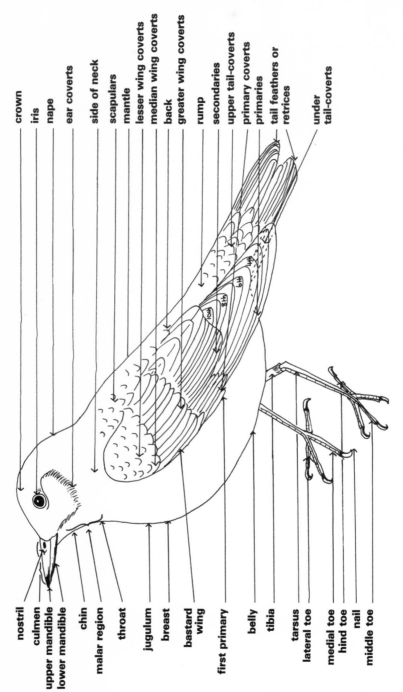

Figure 7   Topography of a typical, small, passerine bird showing the ornithological terms for various parts of the body. (Janet Keymer)

example, the terms knee, ankle, hock and tibiotarsus-tarsometatarsal joint are all synonymous, being used by the layman, the ornithologist, the veterinarian and the anatomist respectively.

The outer covering of the body is largely composed of skin. Areas where the ectodermal tissues are modified occur in the eyes, beak, cloaca, shanks and claws. Typical skin is composed of two main layers. The outer one or epidermis, is a dying layer of flattened cells covered with flakes of a protein called keratin. Feathers, scales, claws, and beak are all largely constructed of this tough inert keratin also known as horn. The second and deeper layer, the dermis, consists of cells which generate the epidermis. It contains numerous tiny blood and lymph vessels, nerve-fibre endings and usually fat. The dermis also initiates the production of special structures such as feathers and scales.

The skin and feathers are important as a protection against the elements and injury, and they also act as a barrier to disease. When large areas of skin are damaged or removed as in a severe burn, not only does infection enter readily, but shock may result from loss of heat, blood protein and minerals.

The Feathers

Various kinds of feather characterise a bird. Feathers evolved from reptilian scales and are of several types. The greater part of the plumage comprises the large wing and tail feathers and smaller-vaned covert feathers with a rigid stalk or rachis. These serve to produce an air and watertight sheath for protection and flight. Most species have long and tufted hair-like feathers called filoplumes between the larger feathers. An intermediate type, a brush-like feather occurs in waterbirds where buoyancy is required. Down feathers, the softest variety, are usually hidden under covert feathers, and have a tiny stalk at their base only. Distribution of down feathers varies considerably, being best developed in waterbirds. Other modifications occur and all types merge into one another. Primitive birds had feathers with a double shaft, the deeper or "aftershaft" (in present-day birds usually much the smaller one) being overlain by the main shaft. In some species such a structure is still present on the covert feathers, and there is no doubt it is an effective heat insulator. In pigeons and most passerine birds, however, these structures are absent or vestigial. Other specialized feathers occur for the purpose of sexual attraction or other functions, such as the extravagant tails in the birds of paradise and the whydahs. In birds of prey, where silence is essential for hunting, the soft covert feathers allow an almost noiseless flight. The colour of plumage in birds is only relevant here, insofar as it helps to understand appearance and behaviour; it may for example be influenced by the diet, or hormonal disturbances.

Outwardly, the feathers of most birds appear to be uniformly distributed, but this is not the case. In most species, feathers other than the down, grow only from definite tracts, leaving bare areas between them. Penguins, toucans, ostriches and related species, however, are exceptions. The feather tracts in most birds form a definite pattern. There is a spinal tract extending from neck to tail and a corresponding ventral tract over the thorax and abdomen. Both of these tracts have branches. Other tracts cover the wings, shoulders, thighs, legs and head.

The Normal Moult

The process of moulting, which is the normal loss and replacement of feathers, is affected by a number of factors.

The health of the feathers is dependent upon an adequate diet and a suitable environment. Feathers are constructed mainly of keratin, a protein derived from essential amino acids with the sulphur-containing members the most significant. The importance of vitamins and minerals is deduced mainly from experimental studies in poultry and other birds such as pigeons and canaries. Vitamin A, niacin, tryptophan, pantothenic acid, folic acid and iodine are all essential for the health of the feathers; deficiencies or an excess may give rise to lesions of the skin as well as the plumage.

Moulting of the different types of feathers varies depending upon age, sex, season or environment. It can be sudden, as in ducks, with most of the wing feathers being replaced in two to three weeks, during which time the bird is virtually earthbound. Alternatively it may be continuous throughout the year, with a peak in spring and early summer as in most psittacines. Passerines, including canaries, moult gradually over several months between May and December in the northern hemisphere. Most birds moult once a year, a few twice a year, and still others compromise—with primary feathers and coverts changed once, whilst the small feathers are replaced twice a year. The wing feathers in a few species are kept for two years. In most birds, nestling plumage is exchanged for the adult type at a few weeks of age. There are differences in many species between the adolescent and the sexually mature plumage. Examples are the gulls and the swans, whose young are brown or greyish and become predominantly white at maturity. There are species where the young of both sexes have female plumage—the blackbirds for example—but where the male changes at maturity.

The Skin and Its Appendages

The skin is an enveloping membrane which encloses the bird and yet permits free movement without undue wrinkling or tenseness. It is adaptable in that it can grow to cover injuries or stretch to accommodate swellings such as growths in underlying tissues. It retains body tissues, fluids and heat, and keeps out infections and foreign matter. Being covered with insulating feathers in most areas, avian skin is not a very efficient dissipator of heat. Unlike mammals, birds do not have sweat glands, and the main cooling areas for their bodies are the lungs and air sacs which lower temperature by conduction and the evaporation of water from their large surfaces.

The preen or uropygeal gland situated over the last vertebra is the only important skin modification. It is absent in the ostrich, emus, cassowaries, bustards and nightjars, as well as in some species of psittacines, woodpeckers and members of the pigeon family. This gland secretes an oily substance which was once thought to be essential to the health of the bird. However, birds from which it is removed remain surprisingly healthy with a normal bright plumage. The gland may be feathered or bare. Its functions are little understood: it was generally believed that the secretion had waterproofing qualities, but this now has been discounted, waterproofing of the plumage being due to the fine structure of the feathers. There is evidence that a high level of vitamin D is often present in the gland and it may therefore be an additional source of this vitamin.

The Head and Feet;
Special Structures

A hard, horny layer covers the jaws and feet, whilst in a few species various horn-like projections arise from the head or legs; The bony spur of the

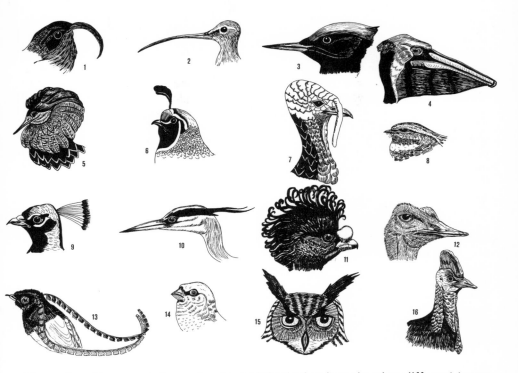

Figure 8   Representatives of various biological orders showing different types of beaks adapted for different methods of feeding. 1. White-tipped sicklebill (Passeriformes). A nectar-feeder. 2. Common curlew (Charadriiformes). Bill adapted for probing soft earth or mud. 3. Black woodpecker (Piciformes), with strong, chisel-like beak for splitting bark and wood. 4. Brown pelican (Pelicaniformes); with pouched beak for temporary retention of fish. 5. Ruff (Charadriiformes), a wader with another type of bill for probing mud. 6. Californian quail (Galliformes) and 7. Common turkey (Galliformes), both grain-eaters. Note the finger-like snood of the turkey. 8. European nightjar (Caprimulgiformes), has a very wide gape with bristles for catching insects during flight. 9. Peafowl (Galliformes), another grain-eater. 10. Great blue heron (Ardeiformes), with strong shear-like beak for piercing fish, amphibians, etc. 11. Great curassow (Galliformes), with beak adapted for feeding on buds, leaves and fruit. Note the cere. 12. Ostrich (Struthioniformes), the beak is wide and flattened, being the non-specialized type of an omnivore. 13. King of Saxony Bird of Paradise (Passeriformes), the beak is relatively simple and unspecialized. Note the long head plumes which are a secondary sexual characteristic of the males. 14. Red avadavat (Passeriformes), with typical conical-shaped beak of a small seed-eater. A so-called "hardbill." 15. Eagle owl (Strigiformes), with strong, sharp beak suitable for tearing flesh. 16. Australian cassowary (Casuraiiformes). Note the arched, bony helmet or "casque" which is believed to assist in warding off thorny twigs and to facilitate pushing through undergrowth. Long, fleshy wattles hang down either side of the neck. The bird is also omnivorous like the ostrich, but its beak is flattened laterally rather than dorso-ventrally as with the latter. (Janet Keymer)

barnyard cockerel, pheasant, and other gallinaceous birds is an example. Appendages such as the comb, wattles and other fleshy lobes ornament some birds, especially gallinaceous species—the domestic fowl, turkey, guinea fowl, pheasants and curassow (Fig. 8). These appendages are highly vascular, containing much blood, and are prone to injury, infection, and frostbite.

Structures of particular interest are the beak, cere, scales of the lower parts of the leg, and the claws. Beaks are produced by the horn-forming cells which cover the jaws. A modified area of tissue at the junction of the beak and the skin of the face produces the shiny, tough, outer layer. This special horny tissue helps to prevent splitting of the beak. When the junction between the horn and skin is damaged, a strip of defective horn is often produced; because the beak is continuously growing, this may result in it becoming distorted.

The specialised functions of the different types of beaks are discussed later (see "The Alimentary System").

The nostrils lie at various levels in the beak. In some species of diving seabirds they are enclosed. In albatrosses, however, they are open and project as horny tubes from the beak. They connect directly with slits in the roof of the mouth, known as the internal nares.

The cere is a specially modified area of skin, so called because of its waxy appearance. It forms a prominent structure in a few birds such as the budgerigar, hawks and falcons. In budgerigars its colour varies according to sex and age. The cere and nostrils in these birds offer refuge to parasites. In pigeons the name "cere" is also given to the bare area surrounding the eyes.

Scaly feet are another reminder of the reptilian ancestry of the bird. They are a tough barrier which protects the feet against rough surfaces while landing, walking or wading, (see Fig. 9).

The overlapping of the scales, can provide a home for bacteria or mites. Here these organisms multiply with a liberal supply of food in the form of dried exudates, especially if the bird is debilitated.

Claws are useful and even vital for perching, climbing, holding or tearing food, scratching and fighting. Like the beak, they are horny structures which grow continuously. Damage to the layers which generate horn produces stunted, twisted, or otherwise defective claws. These in turn, by abnormal strain on the toe joints, produce skeletal deformity which can eventually deform the entire foot and cripple the bird.

The Skeleton

The skeleton by its shape, proportions and modifications tells us a great deal about the bird's mode of life, rate of living, and even in some cases its special tendency to disease. Scientists have been able to reconstruct some of the giant prehistoric birds and reptiles from portions of fossilized skeletons. They can determine not only their shape, type of skin and diet, but even calculate internal structure and aspects of their lives.

Because the skeleton is a well-defined entity, minor differences between species and even within a species can be easily determined and measured. A similarly slight variation in soft tissue is far less appreciable: differences between species are therefore most apparent from the skeleton.

The hard but mobile skeleton serves to produce rigidity, gives protection, houses vulnerable organs, and acts as a system of levers to which the muscles are attached.

The skeleton of all vertebrates—fish, amphibians, reptiles, birds and mammals, including man—comprises two main parts; an axial skeleton which consists of the skull, vertebral column, ribs and sternum or breast bone and

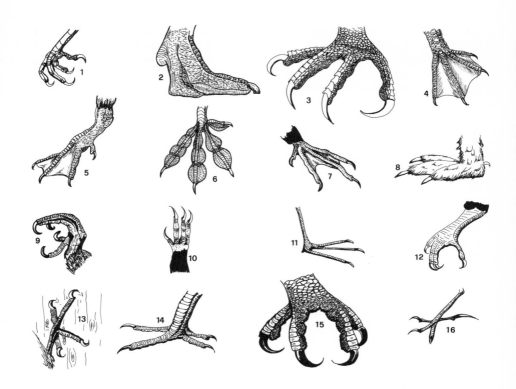

Figure 9 Feet of birds adapted for various methods of progression such as running (2 and 14), swimming (4 and 5), walking or gripping different types of surfaces (6, 7, 8, 11 and 16), gripping vertical surfaces (10 and 13), grasping prey (3, 12 and 15), and perching (1 and 9). 1. Starling (Passeriformes), typical foot of perching bird. 2. Ostrich (Struthioniformes), only two toes, the third and fourth remaining. 3. Eagle (Falconiformes), grasping talons. 4. Booby (Pelacaniformes), totipalmate, webbed foot with first digit pointing forwards on the side. 5. Duck (Anseriformes), palmate foot with only the three front toes webbed. 6. Coot (Gruiformes), foot with lobed toes. 7. Frigate bird (Pelecaniformes), foot with reduced webs. 8. Ptarmigan (Galliformes), feathered foot for walking on snow. 9. Macaw (Psittaciformes), zygodactyl foot with the fourth toe as well as the first pointing backwards. Adapted for climbing, clinging and perching. 10. Swift (Apodiformes), foot with all four toes pointing forwards and armed with sharp toes for gripping walls and rock surfaces. 11. Stilt (Charadriiformes), typical foot of a wading bird with short, hind, first digit and long slender forward pointing toes. In some species all four toes are long. 12. Kingfisher (Coraciiformes), syndactyl foot with two front toes partly joined. 13. Woodpecker (Piciformes), zygodactyl foot used for gripping tree trunks, similar to the foot of the macaw (9). 14. Roadrunner (Cuculiformes), zygodactyl foot. Unique in a ground bird. 15. Osprey (Falconiformes), foot with talons, each digit being of equal length and the foot pads armed with short, stiff spines for gripping fish. The outer fourth toe, like that of the owls, can be moved backwards to assist in grasping. 16. Lark (Passeriformes), foot of a terrestrial species with long straight claw on hind toe. (Janet Keymer)

the appendicular skeleton comprising the pectoral girdle which bears the fore-limbs or wing bones and the pelvic girdle supporting the hind limbs. The typical vertebrate arrangement of limbs, ending in a five-toed hand or foot is taken as the standard, reptiles like lizards being good examples. In fish and snakes there is little evidence of limbs, but the remnants of pectoral and pelvic girdles can be seen in the skeleton, which bears fins in the case of fish. In aquatic mammals such as whales and seals, there is also a great reduction in limb development, but in fact all limb bones are present though they are very short and contained in flippers. Man and the lower primates have a relatively unspecialized skeleton, being similar to such reptiles as lizards except for longer limbs and certain skull modifications. The horse has only the third toe remaining on each foot, and its highly specialized limbs are adapted for speed.

The skeleton of birds, (Fig. 10) has several striking differences both from the primitive reptilian type and from its more advanced mammalian relatives. The skeleton is extremely light for its bulk. It is composed of very hard, but thin-walled porcelain-like bones. Many of the commonest are hollow, with reinforcing pillars or plates of bone across the cavities where extra strength is required. The spaces are partly filled with bone marrow and partly by air cavities. In some species quite considerable air spaces are found, especially in the limb bones.

The skull includes the upper jaw or maxilla which supports the upper beak, and the lower jaw or mandible. The upper beak is perforated by the nostrils or external nares.

Immediately behind the face, two large cavities represent the orbits or eye sockets. These are separated in the middle by thin sheets of bone. In birds such as owls and hawks, the eye and optic nerve are encircled by a collar or funnel of bone. Behind the orbits, the skull widens out into the cranium which holds the brain. Suspended at each side of the posterior part of the cranium is the temporal bone in which lies the drum-like cavity of the ear, containing the organs of hearing and balance. A delicate framework of bones, the hyoid apparatus, supports the tongue and is of great importance in swallowing, breathing, and voice production.

Modifications of the head are numerous. The many differences in beaks (see under the Alimentary System) emphasise the variety of jaw shapes that may be found according to their uses. Mobility varies with the size and type of individual bones, which range from a delicate triangular lacework to a solid mass perforated by round or oval nasal spaces.

The neckbones or cervical vertebrae of birds vary from over twenty in some swans to thirteen in some passerines. The most usual number is fourteen or fifteen. Virtually all mammals—including the giraffe—possess only seven. The first cervical vertebra permits the nodding movements of the skull; it moves around the second vertebra and can rotate through almost a semi-circle. The shape of the remaining neck vertebrae permits considerable movement of the head in most birds so that they are able to look backwards and reach virtually all parts of the body with the beak. The cervical vertebrae have thick lower halves, known as the centra or bodies, which are firmly bound by ligaments to their neighbours. There is a tubular upper part called the neural arch through which runs the spinal cord. Spiky processes of bone from each vertebra are united by muscles which permit the almost unlimited movements of which the neck is capable.

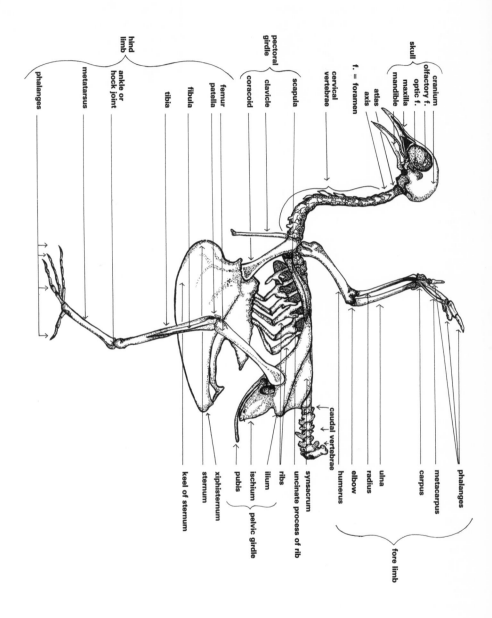

Figure 10 The skeleton of a gallinaceous bird such as the domestic fowl or a pheasant. (Janet Keymer)

39

Beyond the neck, the thoracic vertebrae form the roof of the rib cage. In some species the middle ones are fused together. In all species they are capable of little movement. Most are attached to a pair of true ribs, although the number of thoracic vertebrae and ribs varies between four and eight. Some of the anterior ribs are not attached to the breastbone or sternum. The ribs which connect with the sternum are divided into thoracic and sternal portions. The thoracic section is T-shaped, the "leg" of the T overlapping the succeeding ribs. Sternal ribs turn forward at an angle to the thoracic portion and are embedded at their lower ends into the sternum. The vertebrae immediately posterior to the thorax are mainly concealed under the pelvis. These lumbosacral or synsacral vertebrae are fused into one or two solid masses which are often fused to the pelvis. Emerging behind the pelvis, movable caudal vertebrae, from four to nine in number, precede the pygostyle which is composed of smaller, fused vertebrae and supports the tail. Primitive, extinct birds had a long reptilian type tail and much less fusion between the vertebrae.

The sternum, which is supported by the coracoids and clavicle bones of the pectoral girdle as well as the ribs, varies tremendously in proportion and development. In most non-flying birds, such as the ostrich, emu and rails, the sternum is flat or raft-like; but in the majority of birds which fly strongly it is keel-like. The area of the sternum, its notches, and projections all have some bearing on the special modifications of wing movements, but the depth of the keel is of greatest importance in establishing the size of the pectoral or breast muscles, which in turn is a measure of the power of flight.

The appendicular skeleton includes the two groups of bones of the fore and hind limbs, the wings and legs. The pectoral girdle is very different from that of mammals, in that the scapulae or shoulder blades are long and knife-like; the clavicles on each side are united to form the well-known V-shaped wishbone and a third stout pair of bones, the coracoids. These are merely a knob on each scapula in mammals, but in birds they are important and placed between the anterior thoracic vertebrae and the sternum. At the junction of the scapula and coracoid, a hole between these bones acts as a pulley over which runs the tendon of the smaller pectoral muscle for raising the wings. In the junction of scapula and coracoid is another cavity for the head of the humerus, the first bone of the wing itself. At the far end of the humerus is the elbow joint, where twin bones, the radius and ulna hinge. In birds the ulna is the larger of the two bones. The pentadactyl hand is represented by fusion of some bones and disappearance of others so that only the first (the thumb), second and third digits remain. The thumb supports the bastard wing whilst the second and third digits both carry the primary quills of the wing.

The pelvic girdle is composed of three pairs of plate-like bones, the ilia, ischia and pubes, all of which are fused in the adult bird. They form a roof to the abdomen in birds and are anchored immovably to the fused lumbosacral vertebrae. The cavity for the head of the femur or thigh bone is in approximately the middle of each plate, and a large foramen or hole in the ischium allows the passage of muscles, arteries and nerves. The kidneys lie mainly in the hollows under the ilia. The pubes are usually thin, needle-like bones, the position of which varies slightly in males and females in and out of the breeding season. The space between the pubes and the distance of each from the rear of the sternum is larger in females than males, increasing and becoming more flexible in the breeding season. It is thus a useful guide to the egg-laying potentialities of a female bird, and assists in sexing male and female adults which have similar plumage. The femur is long in land birds, but shorter in climbers and strong flyers. It articulates with the long tibiotarsus and degenerate fibula, at the stifle or knee joint. A small bone, the patella or knee cap, increases the leverage of the muscles on the front of the thigh, when straightening the stifle joint for rising or walking.

The avian hock or heel joint is a simple hinged one, and much less complicated than the group of seven or eight small bones found in mammals. A single tarsometatarsus, reduced from the five bones of the typical mammalian foot, supports the four (or in a few cases three) toes. In birds like waders, herons and storks the bone is very long. Some birds have three toes pointing forward and one backward (the first digit), whilst others have two anterior and two posterior toes, the latter being the first and fourth digits. Other modifications are a reduction to three toes in several large running birds, such as the emu, and a few diving birds. The ostrich has lost two toes in evolution, while swifts point all four toes forward. The shape of the claws, the width of the toes, and the degree of feathering or webbing, demonstrate the varying habits of birds. Since birds have no hands, the feet are very important for holding down, seizing or tearing the food.

Bone Marrow

In the middle of certain bones, notably the long, limb bones, there is a cavity with a fine bony network of struts and containing a soft substance called the marrow. This is red in colour in young birds. In adults it is red only at the end of bones, otherwise it is yellow. Red marrow is concerned mainly with the manufacture of red blood cells and to a lesser extent with certain types of white blood cells. In adult life the demand for red cells falls, so that the marrow becomes inactive and laden with fat, thus making it yellow. However, a fine network of capillary blood vessels persists, together with fibroblasts or fibrous tissue- and bone-forming cells for the repair and maintenance of bone, marrow and blood elements. In severe diseases or after repeated haemorrhage, yellow marrow may revert completely to the red type and may so damage itself that it can no longer produce blood cells; hence irreversible anaemias result, in which the number of circulating blood cells falls to dangerous levels.

Joints

Joints are vital to every movement. A well-known type is the ball-and-socket joint found in the hip and shoulder: this permits almost frictionless and therefore heat-free movement in all directions. The remaining limb joints are of the hinge-type. These allow wide, angular movement in one plane only. Rotary movement is possible between the first and second cervical vertebrae. Sliding movements with flat, curved or saddle-shaped, joint surfaces are represented by the junction of neural arches in the cervical vertebrae and contribute to movement in other joints as well. The patella forms a pulley over the lower end of the femur. Slight movements may occur between the two halves of the ribs of some species and the bodies of the vertebrae, but in these situations there are no true joint cavities and bones are united by flexible fibrocartilaginous tissue or gristle. The true joints have their opposed or articular surfaces covered with cartilage; to prevent friction, the synovial membrane around the joint secretes joint oil as a lubricant.

41

Where tendons run over large surfaces or through fibrous tubes, a synovial membrane is present to provide a similar lubricated area called a synovial bursa or sheath. Inflammation of a joint is called arthritis, and of a tendon sheath or bursa, tenosynovitis or bursitis.

Ligaments

Ligaments are the tough bands of white fibrous tissue which hold joints together, yet permit the full movement required. In some joints, where variety of movement is essential, such as the hip or shoulder, the binding action of ligaments is taken over by the more extensible but no less strong muscles. Here ligaments are absent or few in number and limited to a loose capsule and perhaps a central ligament which allows rotation.

Skeletal Muscles and Tendons

Study of the site, shape and action of individual muscles is a large subject, but for a book of this nature the general principles are important.

The muscles of the head are less well developed than in mammals, because mastication is not carried out in the mouth of birds, but in the gizzard. There are exceptions; parrots, budgerigars and other psittacines, and birds of prey all have relatively well developed jaw muscles. In psittacines they are needed for cracking nuts and seeds, and in the raptors to assist in tearing flesh from bones.

The pectoral muscles which lie against the sternum, are in two layers. The smaller and deeper ones become fibrous tendons which pass through the pulley between the coracoid and scapular bones to elevate the wings. The more powerful superficial pectorals are inserted directly into the free ends of the humeri to produce the down-beat of the wings. To spread the wings for flight,

there are groups of muscles over the back and behind the humeri which extend the elbows, while muscles on the front of the radius and ulna extend the manus, or hand. The quill feathers pass through muscle-operated fibrous bands to be pivoted over the posterior aspect of the ulnar and metacarpal bones. When the bird is frightened, the bastard wing, with the aid of a small muscle can be lifted for defence or to obtain purchase on the ground to escape.

Not all birds are adapted for flying. Some, such as parrots, climb a great deal in captivity and fly little, even if given the opportunity. Large birds such as the ostrich rely on running to elude enemies and have degenerate wings but powerful legs. Smaller landbirds, like crakes, quails and other game birds, seldom use their rather small wings, relying on camouflage, skulking or running for escape. The humming birds spend a great deal of time in the air, can fly backwards, and even feed on the wing. Other species, such as many seabirds and vultures, have proportionately large wing spans and conserve energy by gliding with very economical movements of the wings. These and many other differences are dealt with fully in ornithological works.

The intercostal and abdominal muscles play a significant part in respiration whilst at rest, but in flight and struggling, the pectorals probably have the greater influence in the volume variations of the lungs, airsacs and body-cavity. The diaphragm is absent in birds but in mammals it is a complete sheet of muscle and tendon separating the thoracic and abdominal cavities.

In the hind limbs, thigh movement is governed by several muscles arising from the pelvis. Those from the ilia are concerned mainly with drawing the thigh forward, those from the ischial region with extending it backwards and to a lesser extent sideways. Muscles

42

from the lower edge of the pelvis serve to pull the thigh towards the midline of the body. A strong muscle stretches from the femur to the pygostyle to draw the latter downward in flight. The muscles running in front of the femur pull on the patella which, fastened by tendon only to the tibiotarsus, extend the stifle joint. An interesting muscle running obliquely down the front of the femur and called the ambiens, becomes a tendon over the outer face of the stifle, and then a muscle, before it runs over the back of the hock again in tendon form to flex or close the claws. Crouching movement of the upper limb is thus accompanied by automatic gripping movements of the digits, and is of great value to perching birds. The muscles of the back of the thigh may extend the thigh and either flex or extend the stifle joint depending on where their lower end is inserted. Muscles behind the tibio-tarsus are essentially extensors of the hock and flexors of the toes and foot. These movements do not require much power and are thus operated by insignificant muscles. The leg just above the hock is slim in all birds, because muscles have been largely replaced here by tendons which do not fatigue.

THE ALIMENTARY SYSTEM

Most birds possess a relatively short and simple alimentary canal, the degree to which each portion is developed reflecting the types of food eaten by the different species.

The basic parts of the gut to be described are common to all birds. A typical avian tract is shown in Fig. 11. No teeth are present and the palate is entirely hard, stretching from near the tip of the beak to the back of the throat and forming a roof to the mouth

and pharynx. A central slit in the palate forms the inner opening of the nostrils and allows air to cross the pharynx into the larynx and trachea. Behind this palatal slit is the opening from the two eustachian tubes each of which leads to the middle ear. Tiny punctures in the hard palate mark the entry of the ducts from the salivary gland. Solid food is taken into the mouth by the beak which scoops it up by quick movements of the head. It is then thrown into the pharynx while the tongue is held well down into the lower mandible. Most birds cannot suck (pigeons being exceptions) and water has to be spooned up by the beak or tongue and allowed to trickle down to the pharynx with the head raised. Swallowing can then occur, often aided by rapid raising and lowering of the tongue.

The structure of beak and tongue is widely modified according to the diet and habits of the bird, although types of feet, size of breast muscles, eyes, wing-body ratio and other factors may tell us more about its habits and activity. Beaks vary considerably in shape and include the short, conical beak of seed-eaters; the massive, curved, nutcracking parrot type; the hooked, tearing beak of the carnivorous hawks and eagles; the relatively slender and long insectivorous type; the long, pointed fish-jabbing type of some large fish eaters; the mud-filtering type of the duck family, and the curved, slender types used for sucking nectar seen in sunbirds and hummingbirds (Figs. 8 and 12). Some highly modified beaks such as the latter are so specialized that they are almost useless for any other type of food other than that for which they were evolved.

The tongue also varies in shape and mobility. It may be as long as two-thirds of the body in the wryneck or so small as to be scarcely, noticeable. In

43

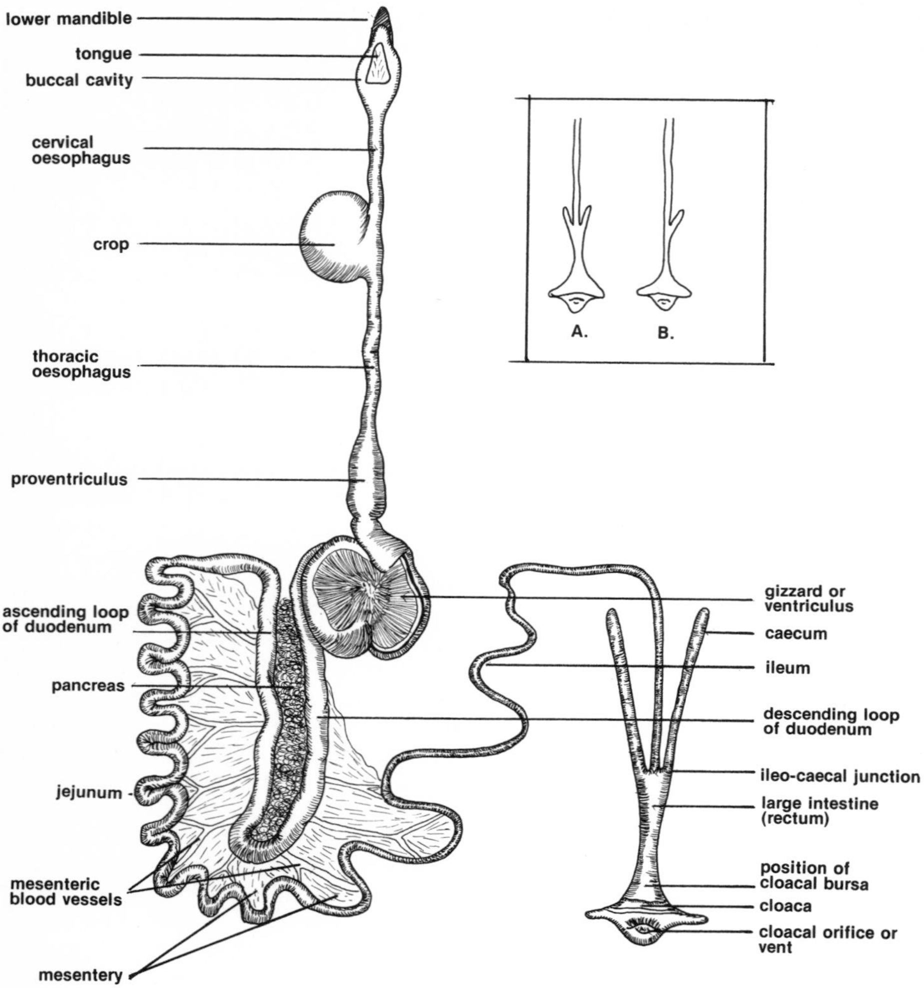
lower mandible
tongue
buccal cavity
cervical oesophagus
crop
thoracic oesophagus
proventriculus
ascending loop of duodenum
pancreas
jejunum
mesenteric blood vessels
mesentery
A.
B.
gizzard or ventriculus
caecum
ileum
descending loop of duodenum
ileo-caecal junction
large intestine (rectum)
position of cloacal bursa
cloaca
cloacal orifice or vent

Figure 11 Alimentary tract of a typical gallinaceous bird, e.g., a pheasant, partridge or quail. Note the two well developed caeca. Inset A = Lower intestinal tract of a typical small passerine bird showing two poorly developed caeca. Inset B = Lower intestinal tract of a bird such as an egret or heron with only one poorly developed caecum. (Janet Keymer)

the budgerigar it is a stumpy, fleshy structure with a great range of movement, capable of rolling a seed into any position to investigate or crack it. The tongues of birds have been adapted to probe, sieve, brush, or rasp, and they may be cylindrical, rectangular, spoon-shaped, leaf-shaped, flat, cupped, grooved, tubular, or forked.

The mouth cavity is poorly supplied with taste buds, food is passed down the oesophagus or gullet by the squeezing action of peristaltic contractions. On the right side in the lower part of the neck of many species, the oesophagus, widens into a single or double pouch known as the crop. This diverticulum is an expandable structure, and when full it usually extends into the midline of the throat or slightly to the left.

The crop is not developed to the same extent in all birds. In fact, in a number of small passerine birds and many flesh-eaters, it is absent or rudimentary. In others, for example the hoatzin, it is large and muscular. In most of the more common species of birds—the parrots, the gallinaceous species, the pigeons and many finches—the crop is large and still obvious even when empty. In some species the crop is noticeable only when it contains food. In a few species—pigeons for example when breeding—a nourishing material is produced by rupture of the surface cells of the crop lining. This so-called "crop milk" is vital for rearing the young.

Posterior to the crop, the lower oesophagus passes between the ribs, continues below the trachea and widens into the true glandular stomach, known as the proventriculus or forestomach. Here hydrochloric acid and digestive enzymes start the main softening-up process which is the first active stage of digestion, the action of swallowed saliva in the crop having done little except hydrate certain foods.

The proventriculus is usually a slightly thickened and spindle-shaped structure which varies comparatively little in different birds, because all foods require a degree of chemical digestion. In some species such as fish eaters, proventricular secretions can digest bone, whereas owls regurgitate bone and fur as pellets.

The proventriculus of the budgerigar can produce a similar substance to the crop milk of the pigeon, when the hen is rearing young.

The gizzard, muscular stomach, or ventriculus, follows immediately after the forestomach and varies greatly in development.

In one member of the tanager family the gizzard is represented by a tiny nodule at the junction of the proventriculus and small intestine. In hummingbirds, sunbirds and other honey and fruit eaters, the gizzard is also a small, poorly developed organ. In seed-eaters, however, it is highly developed, with thick, cup-like masses of muscle on either side, whilst the lining is tough and horny. Other birds have an intermediate gizzard, less specialized and less muscular, but often quite large.

After the gizzard, the first part of the intestine is a U-shaped bend called the duodenum which envelopes the pancreas. A muscular valve or sphincter separates the gizzard from the duodenum. The duodenum is usually in the form of one long strip of tissue filling the space between the two arms of the duodenal loop. The shape can vary considerably: in some birds it is partially or completely divided into three lobes which reflect its embryonic origin from three buds of tissue. Two or three fine ducts drain pancreatic secretions into the duodenum. The pancreas produces groups of digestive enzymes which are capable of digesting the three main food constituents, carbohydrates, proteins and fats. These enzymes are very powerful and are the most vital factors in the whole digestive process. So active are they that if the pancreas is even slightly damaged, the enzymes, normally stored in an inactive state, are activated and can rapidly digest the pancreas itself. Pancreatic enzymes cannot act in the presence of strong acid, such as that produced in the proventriculus, so the duodenum secretes antacids or alkalis, enabling digestion to proceed. The pancreatic duct pours its secretions into the gut where the main food constituents are digested, aided by bile introduced from the liver. The bile emulsifies the fats and oils into fine particles, greatly increasing their digestion and later absorption. The pancreas also produces the very important hormone known as insulin, the functions of which are discussed later in this Chapter.

The small intestine is a coiled tube of fairly uniform diameter, being generally about twice the overall length of the bird. It is usually longer in seed- than in meat-eaters, although many fish-eaters such as penguins and auks have long and narrow guts. In the small intestine further digestion takes place, the broken down protein, starch and cellulose being converted into amino-acids and sugars. The fats are partly absorbed as microscopic droplets in emulsion and partly converted to organic or fatty acids.

Where the small intestine (ileum) joins the large intestine at the junction with the caeca, there are two ileo-caecal valves. The caeca are represented by two, blind, hollow tubes or protuberances in most species, although in a few birds such as egrets and herons only one very small caecum is present. The caeca or blind guts are very long in grouse and most other gallinaceous birds, very small in pigeons and most passerines, and absent in some members of the orders Coraciiformes, Piciformes and Psittaciformes e.g. budgerigars and some parrots. Caeca are usually dispensable organs, but where they are well developed some digestion undoubtedly goes on. Bacteria which abound in the caeca may also play a part in digestion or even in the manufacture of vitamins.

Beyond the caeca, the gut becomes a straight, wide tube forming the large intestine and the rectum, terminating in the cloaca. The large intestine in nearly all species (the ostrich being an exception) is short. Water and soluble food substances are absorbed from the rectum into the bloodstream. The cloaca which at first glance appears to be a dilatation of the gut, has a threefold use and comprises three chambers. The coprodaeum, is a temporary store for the faeces, which at that stage are semi-solid in consistency. The urodaeum, holds the semi-fluid, white "urine", whilst the third—which can be turned inside out for the purposes of mating—is the proctodaeum, anus or vent. In the female the oviduct, and in the male the vasa deferentia open into the urodaeum and also the two ureters from the kidneys. A sac-like diverticulum of the proctodaeum, called the Bursa of Fabricius, is believed to have a glandular function associated with growth; it contains lymphoid tissue and assists in repelling infections by producing antibodies.

This brief account of the anatomy and physiology of the alimentary tract indicates how its variations are related to different diets and may help readers understand more clearly the underlying principles of avian nutrition.

Many birds have the choice of suitable foods "fixed in their brains" not only through their inherited instinct, but also as an acquired "imprint" learned very early in life from the parent bird. Budgerigars are a case in point: they will readily accept canary seeds and millets but will refuse other seed, even if the acceptable seeds have been reduced until the birds are at the point of starvation. If nestlings are fed the unfamiliar seeds by hand, however, then a wider range of seeds is acceptable to them when adult.

The various modifications of the alimentary tracts may be major factors clearly limiting the choice of food. A typical nectar or fruit-eating bird has a simple type of tract, which can, however, cope with small insects and grubs. In carnivorous birds, a relatively large, glandular proventriculus is needed to allow large pieces of flesh to be digested, and skin, fur, bones and other less digestible material to be temporarily retained before they are regurgitated. Regurgitation from the crop is of course an essential to the feeding of young in many seabirds and some other species. In scavengers like vultures and members of the crow family, the gut is a particularly versatile organ and in a few species appears to be resistant to putrefying substances and some microorganisms. Primarily seed-eating birds with a large crop and highly developed muscular gizzard, can ingest large amounts of seed when this food is in abundance and retain it until the next food source is found. Seed-eaters cannot expect to find seed all the year round in temperate climates and great seasonal variation of the diet occurs; berries, roots, insects, grubs, etc., are gladly taken at other times. Carnivores normally have a much less variable food supply. Nectar-feeders, which are confined to the tropics, would starve in the North American or European winters because they are largely dependent upon nectar.

The Liver

The liver is a large glandular, structure with about a dozen vital activities. These include the manufacture, storage and distribution of food supplies, i.e., carbohydrate, fat, protein, vitamins and minerals; disposal of waste products, including worn-out blood cells; pro-duction of bile; manufacture of blood proteins; and control of blood coagulation. All this is carried out in an organ which represents between one-twentieth and one-fiftieth of the total body weight of the bird. The liver is situated in the rear part of the chest cavity behind and below the heart and lungs; it lies in the middle, with the proventriculus, gizzard, and part of the small intestine more or less between its two lobes. In most species it consists of two large lobes and is a uniform, dark mahogany colour when healthy. The gall bladder when present, is partly embedded in the liver, usually under the right lobe and acts as a temporary store of bile. It is absent in pigeons and most psittacines. Above the liver lie the two kidneys and either the ovary or testes, while below it are situated the duodenum and pancreas. The liver lobes are attached at the front by a ligament beside which the large blood vessels pass to and from the heart. The lobes are loosely joined by folds of the serous membranes, known as the peritoneum, to neighbouring abdominal organs, thus restricting excessive movement. Blood carries absorbed nutrient from the gut through the portal veins and the liver substance. It continues back through the heart via the hepatic portal vein, and finally reaches the great posterior vena cava, which collects blood from the entire bird except the head, neck and lungs.

The Respiratory System

The bird's mechanism of breathing and the structure of its respiratory system are unique among vertebrate animals. There are marked differences between avian and mammalian respiration.

Firstly, there is no muscular diaphragm in birds to separate the abdominal from the thoracic organs. If this structure was absent in mammals, the stomach, intestines and liver would enter the chest and collapse the lungs; yet birds can perform great athletic feats without it, like flying steeply upwards, and also covering thousands of miles during migrations. Above all, birds can perform hard work at altitudes of 20,000 feet or more, heights at which mammals become moribund through lack of oxygen. In birds, the inspired air passes not only through the lungs but also through a complex system of air spaces. Respiratory rates vary greatly in different species (see Table).

A basic knowledge of the structure and function of the avian respiratory system is important in the understanding and use of volatile anaesthetics.

Inhaled air enters the external nares or nostrils. These are situated in the base of the beak or sometimes in a waxy area just above and behind it called the cere. (The petrels have flexible tubes for nostrils, whilst in gannets the external nares are blocked, the respiration being oral by means of special structures at the angle of the beak.) After passing through the nasal cavity, which is richly supplied with blood vessels and warms and moistens it, the inspired air, crosses the mouth cavity, emerging from the internal nares which are a long slit in the palate or roof of the mouth. The air then crosses the mouth cavity called the choana and passes into the glottis, the slit-like but dilatable opening into the larynx. The larynx of birds has no vocal chords, although the glottal opening may slightly modify the volume of the voice as well as control the flow of air in and out of the larynx. The larynx is a chamber made of cartilage and is situated between the "arms" or cornua of the hyoid bone. It opens into the windpipe or trachea, an incompressible tube of cartilage rings and elastic tissue lined by mucous membrane which is continuous with that of the mouth. In most birds, the trachea is a long pipe extending down the neck beside the gullet and ending a short distance inside the chest, where it branches into two smaller and narrower tubes called the primary bronchi. In cross-section it is rounded or oval. In such species as cranes and various waterfowl, portions of the trachea are kinked, dilated or coiled.

The Syrinx

The syrinx or voice box is generally situated at the end of the trachea where it divides into the two primary bronchi. It is formed by modification of the cartilaginous rings which are ossified in many species to form the tympanum. The incomplete rings in this zone are completed by a transparent membrane, capable of vibration when air is drawn across it. The tension on this membrane is altered by several delicate muscles, whose development varies enormously in different species.

There are three main types of voice box in birds, these being classified according to their site: tracheal, bronchial and tracheo-bronchial, the latter being the most common and the typical type as seen in passerine birds. In nightjars, cuckoos and the oilbird, the syrinx is the bronchial type and has no sound-producing structures, these being found in the bronchi in the form of expanded lateral membranes. A few passerine birds have a tracheal syrinx which is formed in the region of the last six rings of the trachea, the organ in this area having purely membranous walls. Birds possessing this structure have very loud voices, vocalization being accompanied by swelling of the throat. They are all from the Americas.

The Bronchi and Air Sacs

The trachea branches out into two bronchi, which run through the lung substance and open directly into the

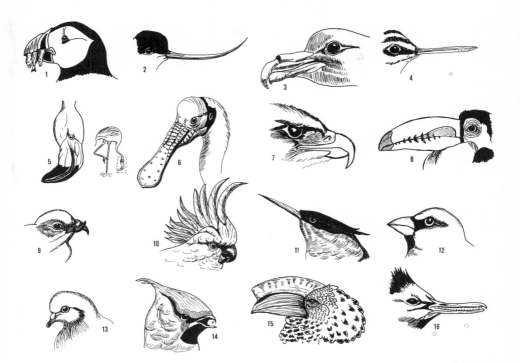

Figure 12   Representatives of various biological orders showing different types of beaks adapted for different methods of feeding. 1. Puffin (Charadriiformes). The beak is adapted for catching and holding fish. 2. Avocet (Charadriiformes), with bill designed for catching food with shallow side-to-side sweeping movements. 3. Giant fulmar (Procellariiformes). Note the tubular nostrils which may be related to the excretion of excess salt by the nasal gland of these birds. 4. Common snipe (Charadriiformes). Bill with sensitive tip for probing mud. 5. Greater flamingo (Ciconiiformes). The beak is curved to aid in sifting mainly microscopic forms of animal and plant life in the mud at the bottom of shallow water. 6. Roseate spoonbill (Ciconiiformes), with a differently shaped bill used for a similar purpose to that of the flamingos. 7. Golden eagle (Falconiformes). The strong, sharp beak is specially designed for tearing flesh. 8. Sulphur-breasted toucan (Piciformes). The long but very light bill is thought to assist these heavy birds to reach fruit at the ends of slender branches while the birds perch farther inward nearer the trunk. 9. Crossbill (Passeriformes). The bill is adapted for prising open the seeds of pine cones. 10. Sulphur-crested cockatoo (Psittaciformes), with typical strong beak for feeding on large, hard seeds and nuts. 11. Herran's thornbill (Apodiformes), with beak adapted for probing into flowers and leaves in search of small insects. 12. Hawfinch (Passeriformes), a typical seed-eating finch or "hardbill." 13. Stock dove (Columbiformes). Note the cere above the beak. Pigeons, doves and 14. Bohemian waxwing (Passeriformes), eat berries, buds and small fruits as well as seeds. 15. Silvery-cheeked hornbill (Coraciformes), a fruit-eater like a toucan with a large but light bill. 16. Red-breasted merganser (Anseriformes). The beak of this duck has a serrated edge to facilitate catching and holding fish. (Janet Keymer)

abdominal air sacs. The air sacs are transparent, membranous sacs. They vary in number and extent in different species but are basically 12 in number, (Fig. 13). There are two abdominal, two posterior and two anterior thoracic, two cervical and two pairs of interclavicular air sacs. In most birds, the interclavicular air sacs fuse into a single middle sac, reducing the total number to nine. In many species, the interclavicular air sacs communicate with air spaces in the humeri, shoulder girdle, ribs and sternum. Other air spaces are usually found in the femur, pelvis and even the vertebral column, whilst in some species they extend into most of the bones of wings and legs.

The air sacs are a valuable and unique feature of birds. They serve to lighten the body, but their most important function is to act as bellows to ventilate the lungs. Generally speaking, the posterior air sacs contain fresher air than the anterior sacs. Recent research has shown that they receive relatively fresh air from the trachea during inspiration, and that during expiration they pass this through the lungs, along the 20 or more secondary bronchi to their branches and thence to the network of air capillaries where oxygen and carbon dioxide are exchanged. The rôle of the anterior sacs is to withdraw the stale air from the lungs during inspiration and then to expel it through the trachea during the next expiration. Thus the air passes constantly through the lungs from back to front, giving oxygen to the blood and removing carbon dioxide. The filling of the air sacs during inspiration is caused by enlargement of the rib cage and abdominal cavity: on expiration, the capacity of the thorax and abdomen is reduced and this forces air from the air sacs into the trachea.

At rest, quiet respiration is carried out solely by gentle intercostal and abdominal muscle movements, whilst in flight the powerful pectoral muscles may have a function—but the mechanism of breathing during flight, is poorly understood. A non-respiratory function of the interclavicular air sac is its excessive development as a secondary sexual characteristic, e.g., in pouter pigeons and some gallinaceous and passerine birds. In such species the sac can be blown up voluntarily to a very large size.

THE URINARY TRACT OR EXCRETORY SYSTEM

The similarity to amphibians and reptiles is evident from the position, shape and primitive microscopic structure of the kidneys. They are long, roughly rectangular, reddish-brown masses, running back from the lungs on either side of the spine, (Fig. 14). They form slightly bulging lobes which are embedded in recesses on the undersurface of the pelvic girdle. Compared with those of mammals, the kidneys of birds are relatively large, and they are not divided into a dark outer cortex and inner medulla.

A straight tube or ureter arises from the lower surface of the posterior lobe of each kidney, running backward and emptying into the second compartment of the cloaca on its upper surface. In the ureters, the "urine" is quite watery, but water is reabsorbed in the urodaeum, leaving the solid mass of urates which forms the white portion of the droppings.

The elimination of protein waste by-products differs in principle from that of mammals. Because birds are essentially flying creatures, some bodily functions have been specially developed to reduce their weight. The excretion of nitrogen waste products for example, is carried out in birds in such a manner that it is not necessary to store urine. The

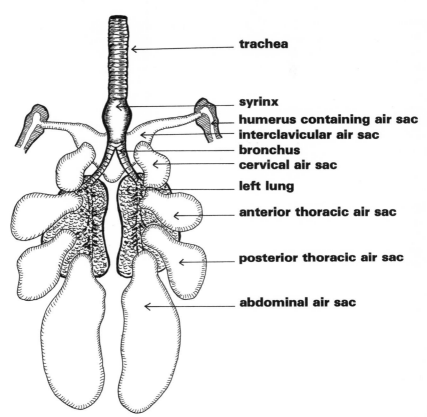

Figure 13   The respiratory system of a typical bird. (Janet Keymer)

"urine" of birds is a pasty, semi-fluid material composed of poorly soluble uric acid and related compounds together with a little water and mucus.

At rest, perhaps a tenth of the kidney tissue is in use. During strenuous activity or disease, the proportion may be increased several times. Birds can actually exist on about one quarter of their total kidney substance and still remain heathy.

The blood supply to the kidneys varies according to the general rate of blood flow and the amount of waste to be excreted, both of which depend on the various activities of the body.

The kidneys function by direct filtering of fluid from the blood. All liquids and colloids—that is, protein—of smaller size than the molecule of the blood pigment haemoglobin, can just pass through the pores of the filter. Blood proteins are thus normally retained, but in disease these too can pass through the filter. If all fluid filtered were passed out as urine this would involve a large wastage of valuable water and dissolved foodstuffs such as sugars and minerals. To counteract this, at least ninety per cent of the water is reabsorbed in the long system of tiny tubules which connect the filter with the

51

ureters. Useful substances such as sugars are almost entirely absorbed, whereas waste products such as uric acid and urates are not absorbed, several being actively excreted from the tissue fluid. Thus a "caste" system of differential excretion occurs. This may vary with the concentration of substances in the blood with hormonal influence and with kidney activity, but it is basically fixed for any single substance. This excretion rate is known as the renal clearance of a given chemical. Even foreign substances such as drugs have a renal clearance all their own and knowledge of this characteristic plays an important part in the choice of drugs used for treatment.

THE REPRODUCTIVE OR GENITAL SYSTEM

The Male. The male bird possesses two testes or testicles of roughly equal size (Fig. 14). They are ovoid in shape, vary considerably in colour, but are usually whitish. They are situated side by side and slightly apart in the dorsal part of the body cavity near the anterior ends of the kidneys. There is great seasonal variation in the size of the testes, whilst in immature birds they are often too small to see with the naked eye. They are largely made up of coiled tubes in which the tadpole-like spermatozoa are produced. The sperms mature in a ridge on the upper and inner face of the testis called the epididymis. From here a wavy tube and temporary store, known as the vas deferens, carries the sperms when required to its opening on a little hump in the lining of the urodaeum which is a section of the cloaca. In some birds, such as ducks and the ostrich, the hump or papilla is developed into a grooved penis. It is interesting to note that the testes do not descend into a pouch or scrotum in birds as they do in

mammals, where they are kept at a temperature lower than that of the body. In common with their reptilian ancestors, the body temperature of birds fluctuates; it is believed that when it falls at night, sperm production can then proceed. Sperm-generating cells exist in quite young chicks, but only produce sperm when puberty is reached.

The testes also produce a chemical messenger or hormone, known as testosterone, in addition to spermatozoa. This hormone, manufactured by small groups of glandular cells dotted about between the sperm-producing tubules, passes directly into the bloodstream and reaches all parts of the body. Testosterone generates and maintains the secondary sexual characteristics, such as the typical male head and body shape of a particular species, its posture, voice, plumage and colour. It is also responsible for the increase in size of the fleshy wattles and cere of some species.

The sperm and testosterone output depends upon secretions coming from the pituitary gland in the form of two other hormones. The output of the pituitary gland is dependent on the bird's age, nutrition, and the number of hours of daylight: this last factor determines the seasons for breeding. Testes are inactive in the winter months, being very small and containing no developed sperms. In spring, the size of the testes increases many times. In the house sparrow the enlargement is from a pinhead to as much as 1.25 cm., or about a fifty-fold increase.

Removal of the testes results in gradual loss of most of the secondary sexual characteristics, and produces a neuter bird. In appearance, neuters or capons as they are called in domestic fowls, are intermediate between males and females. They tend to be more placid, put more weight on their basically masculine bone structure, and show none of the seasonal sexual behaviour patterns. Injection or implantation with the female hormone into a normal male has a similar effect, although some male characteristics may still remain. This process of chemical caponization using the female hormone is used to speed the fattening of poultry for the table, whilst eliminating the objectionable early morning crowing and fighting. Injection or implantation of the male hormone into a surgically caponized bird restores all the external signs of masculinity, even resulting in the "treading" or attempted mating of females, although of course fertilisation is impossible. In a normal male such injections may produce an abnormal assertiveness, a tendency to mate several females, and even tread males.

The Female. The adult female has only one active gonad, the left, (see Fig. 14), the right gonad is usually rudimentary. This gonad is called the ovary. Sometimes hawks possess paired ovaries but only a left oviduct, but this is very unusual in other birds. The ovary develops from a tiny granular mass, as seen in the young female chick, into a bunch of different-sized cyst-like structures or follicles which contain the ova or undeveloped eggs at puberty. This in the wild state generally coincides with spring. The ovary lies under the anterior end of the left kidney. Its component follicles are loosely attached to one another by connective tissue. The ovary produces female hormones or oestrogens in addition to its primary function to make ova—the eggs or female germ cells. Oestrogens stimulate the female characteristics of plumage, colour and voice. The ovary, like the testes, decreases in size in winter when the hours of daylight are short, and then enlarges again when the lengthening days of spring stimulate the pituitary gland.

As the ova enlarge, they form grape-like clusters, rupture from their follicles and drop into the funnel-shaped opening or infundibulum of the oviduct. Intermittent contractions of the oviduct similar to those which occur in the intestine, propel the ovum which is now an egg yolk, down the oviduct. Its progress is also facilitated by the presence of cilia lining the inside of the oviduct. In its slow, spasmodic journey the yolk gathers up layer after layer of coverings which form the "white" or albumen, and finally the skin or egg membranes. During the last part of its journey, the egg receives the minerals which form the shell. It is at this stage that the pigments are deposited which give the characteristic colours and markings to the shells of many species.

The presence of oestrogens in the adolescent bird is essential for the widening of the pelvic outlet to enable eggs to be passed, this being one of the numerous adjustments which the female must make in order to prepare for egg-laying. At this time, calcium, magnesium, and phosphates are also withdrawn from the bones. The intestine, liver and pancreas must digest and temporarily store vastly increased amounts of proteins, sugars, fats, vitamins and minerals. After a brief respite during incubation of the eggs, the female must feed the young. The pigeon and budgerigar produce highly concentrated crop or stomach milk respectively for this; in others, regurgitated or partly digested food is given. The growth rate of pigeon and budgerigar chicks is phenomenal; they increase as much as six-fold in size in the first three weeks of age. By five to six weeks, when nestlings are about to leave the nest, the youngsters of many species are almost as large as their parents.

Feeding the young places a considerable strain on the parent birds, which usually lose weight during the rearing period.

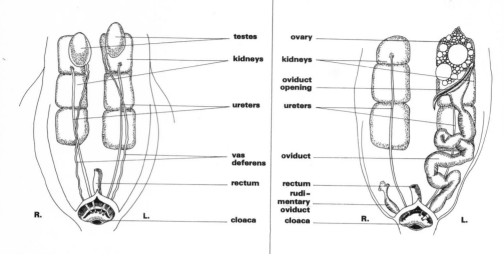

testes	ovary
kidneys	kidneys
	oviduct opening
ureters	ureters
vas deferens	oviduct
rectum	rectum
	rudi-mentary oviduct
cloaca	cloaca

R.   L.   R.   L.

Figure 14   Typical urinogenital tract of a male and a female bird. R = right side. L = left side. (Janet Keymer)

Figure 15   Greatly magnified types of red blood cells (A-G) of a gallinaceous bird such as the domestic fowl. A. = Erythroblast, the earliest form. B.-F. = Progressive stages of developing erythrocytes, so-called polychromatic erythrocytes. G. = Mature erythrocyte or red blood corpuscle. H. = Typical thrombocyte which assists in blood clotting. (Janet Keymer)

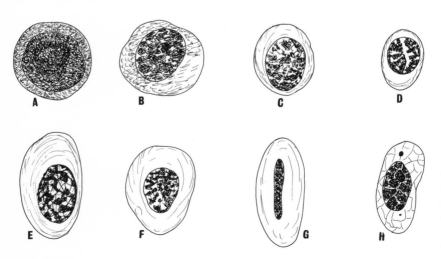

A   B   C   D

E   F   G   H

THE CIRCULATORY OR CARDIOVASCULAR SYSTEM

The Blood and Circulation

Blood is a mixture of living and non-living substances in the form of solids and liquids. It consists of proteins, fats, oils, carbohydrates, vitamins, minerals and water. It transports everything the animal needs, the raw material, manufactured substances, and the waste products.

Characteristic features of blood are the red and white blood cells—erythrocytes (RBCs) and leucocytes (WBCs), respectively, (Figs. 15 and 16). Erythrocytes contain haemoglobin, a red pigment including iron which is capable of absorbing and releasing oxygen and carbon dioxide; oxygen is taken up in the lungs and released to the tissues, whilst carbon dioxide is absorbed and released in the lungs.

The erythrocytes of birds are much larger than those of mammals. They are oval and range in size from 10-14 by 5-8 microns (thousandths of a millimeter) and contain a nucleus. This nucleus is evidence of the close relationship of birds to reptiles. Avian RBCs are complete cells, whereas mammalian RBCs are not, having no nucleus.

The WBCs are of various shapes and sizes, some of the so-called granulocyte series being highly plastic and adaptable to any shape which suits their environment. Like the amoeba, leucocytes ingest simple particles of food or bacteria by pushing out mobile projections known as pseudopodia, literally "false feet". This process of swallowing is called phagocytosis, signifying "cell-eating". The WBCs can pass through tissues, even the walls of capillary blood vessels, without leaving an opening. In this way they can reach all parts of the body.

Another group of WBCs called lymphocytes is concerned with fighting disease. The main function of these round cells appears to be the production of antibodies, they therefore play a rôle in maintaining immunity to disease. Other types of WBCs, such as the larger lymphocyte-like cells known as monocytes, are almost non-existent during health. These multiply at the height of disease and during the early stages of recovery and have an incompletely understood purpose. Another important and large group of cells, those lining blood and lymph vessels, the Kupffer cells of the liver and cells of the spleen and the bone marrow, make up the so-called reticulo-endothelial system; this is largely concerned with blood cell production and the disposal of old blood cells.

Erythrocytes are produced mainly in the bone marrow and a proportion is stored in the spleen. When they have been in circulation for several days they are removed from it by the reticulo-endothelial cells and carried to the liver. Here the valuable iron and other useful chemicals in the haemoglobin are stored in a compact form for future use. The bone marrow also produces white cells known as granulocytes which are destroyed in the liver after their work is done. Lymphocytes, as well as being produced by the bone marrow, are also produced by the spleen, the thymus gland, the Bursa of Fabricius and small areas of lymphoid tissue scattered throughout the body tissues, including the wall of the gut. As lymphocytes become worn out, they are disposed of by the various patches of lymphoid tissue, being replaced as they are withdrawn.

One function of blood which deserves special mention is its clotting mechanism. This process is often taken for granted and yet is vital for existence. If, however, clotting occurred readily in circulating blood, life would constantly be in jeopardy. In certain diseases, such abnormal internal clotting or thrombosis, can occur. The clotting process depends upon the production of a protein called fibrinogen which produces cobweb-like tangles of a solid protein known as fibrin. This process is brought about by the interaction of calcium, iron, enzymes, and other chemicals, some of which are produced by the liver and some by platelets, tiny particles produced in the bone marrow. The ultimate trigger is the release of chemicals by damaged tissues and the exposure of surfaces to the air. That the balance is delicate between liquid or colloidal fibrinogen and the precipitation of fibrin, can be seen by the speed and ease with which normal blood clots outside the blood vessels. Platelets (or thrombocytes) and blood cells are collected in the meshwork of fibrin making the blackish-red jelly which forms a clot. Soon the fibrin contracts, squeezes out serum and becomes firmer. Gradually, living cells, fine blood vessels called capillaries, and then fibre-forming cells invade the clot or thrombus, and eventually form a scar in the affected tissue. On the surface of damaged skin, a scab of dried lymph is formed which sometimes also contains dried and clotted blood.

The blood circulatory system consists of elastic tubes, the smallest branches of which are so minute that a red blood cell can only just pass through them. At this size they are called capillaries. Some of the best examples of a large capillary bed are the combs of domestic poultry and the cere of budgerigars. After the blood is pumped by the heart through the arteries and the arterial capillaries, it then starts its journey back to the heart by entering the venous capillaries which form the finest branches of the venous or return system. Any backflow of blood in the low-pressure venous system is prevented by valves situated at intervals along the larger veins.

The Heart

The cone-shaped heart is the centre of the circulatory system. The avian heart has four chambers, like that of mammals. It is enclosed in a translucent sac called the pericardium which keeps it moist and prevents friction and also acts as protection. If it fails to beat even for a few minutes, irreversible damage is done to the brain. Oxygen is carried by the blood and is required almost continuously to avoid permanent damage to or the death of brain cells.

The heart consists of two pumps each of which comprises a muscular, high-pressure output chamber known as a ventricle and a much thinner-walled, input chamber or auricle. The chambers are separated by valves to prevent backflow of blood when the heart chambers contract. Contraction of the right ventricle forces blood into the lungs; here carbon dioxide and other waste gases are removed and oxygen is absorbed. Blood pumped from the left ventricle supplies all other parts of the body with oxygen, including the internal organs, head and limbs. Blood returning from the lungs passes into a thin, muscular-walled left auricle and that from the rest of the bird into the right auricle. A plan of the blood vessels and heart is given in Fig. 17, which shows the general design of the circulation. Some of the blood from the left ventricle is diverted by branches from the aorta to the head and anterior parts of the body, whilst the remainder travels posteriorly to abdominal organs, and finally to the legs and tail. The return flow by the veins is very similar.

The heart-rate of birds varies considerably—see Table.

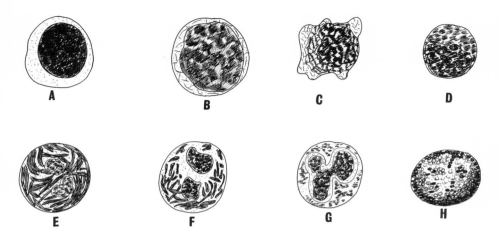

Figure 16 Greatly magnified types of white blood cells or leucocytes (A-H) of a gallinaceous bird such as the domestic fowl. A and B = common types of lymphocytes. C and D = types of monocytes, these vary in size and are often larger than lymphocytes. E and F = heterophils. G = eosinophil. H = basophil, a rare but distinct type of white cell. (Janet Keymer)

The Hepatic Portal System

The intestines and liver have a special venous supply of blood called the hepatic portal system. This enables blood which carries nutrients absorbed from the stomach and intestine to go directly to the liver for use and storage without having to travel round the body and thus lose nourishment. The nutrient-rich blood from the gut, which is also depleted of oxygen, passes from the capillaries of the gut situated in the absorptive folds of the intestinal lining and is drained into larger vessels and then into the great portal vein. This vein runs into the liver and branches out to supply capillaries to each liver unit. The blood filters through the columns of cells in each unit or lobule, becomes laden with blood-sugar and other cell nutrients and waste material, and is then collected into the capillaries of the hepatic vein. This vein then passes blood directly into the right auricle of the heart via the large vein called the posterior vena cava. Elimination of those wastes capable of becoming gaseous, occurs partly in the lungs, otherwise most excretion is by filtration through the kidneys. The liver prepares substances suitable for nourishment by cells and for elimination by the lungs and kidneys. A similar portal system, the renal portal system, by-passes blood from the intestine and rear parts of the body directly through the kidneys.

The Renal Blood Supply

Birds' kidneys have an interesting and complex circulation very different from the mammalian type. Instead of an arterial supply to each filtration unit and a similar system of collecting veins, the avian kidney has three main parts. Figure 17 shows the working of this unusual layout. The principle of such a renal circulation is that the kidney receives blood from the renal portal veins, and a large volume of slow-moving blood from the intestine augmented by venous blood draining away from the legs, and a relatively small arterial supply from the abdominal aorta. Two main vessels, each of which distribute this very mixed blood to the kidneys, finally drain into the renal vein and pass the blood back to the heart again.

The precise purpose of such a complex mechanism is not known, and experiments have shown that if this "portal system" is cut out by tying off blood vessels, birds can still thrive quite well. However, it can be seen from the diagram that the system of flow enables some of the waste matter in the kidneys to be removed without it first travelling around the entire circulation. The fact that nature no longer uses this system in mammals probably indicates that it is not as efficient as its mechanics would suggest.

THE LYMPHATIC SYSTEM

The lymphatic system consists of capillaries which unite into larger vessles. On their path, these lymphatic vessels—which have valves to ensure that the lymph flows in only one direction—pass through minute knots of lymph-rejuvenating tissue called follicles or plexuses which produce new lymphocytes; other sources of these cells are the spleen, the bursa of Fabricius in the cloaca and the thymus gland. It is important to realise that the lymphatic and blood systems meet. The blood passes on its out-going journey from the heart, to the smaller branches of the arterial system, its rate of flow becoming progressively slower. By the time it reaches the capillary network its move-ment is sluggish and largely governed by the activity of the organ or tissue in which the capillaries lie. At this point, some of the watery part of the blood leaks out as tissue fluid into the intercellular spaces, where it bathes the surrounding cells. Lymphocytes and some granulocytes actively force their way out as well. Having discarded its load of chemical raw materials (the anabolites), the tissue fluid absorbs waste products (katabolites), and drains slowly into other capillaries of the lymphatic system as lymph. Some less-burdened tissue fluid returns to the venous end of the blood capillaries. In addition to returning lymph or tissue fluid to the venous system the lymphatic vessels also carry absorbed fat.

Two relatively large lymph vessels known as the thoracic ducts empty into the right and left jugular veins at several places. Lymphoid tissue in mammals is aggregated into large masses called lymph nodes. In birds, however, such nodes are rare, although ducks and geese are stated to have cervical and lumbar, lymph nodes. In the embryos of all birds and also adults of some species like the ostrich, there are sacral or pelvic lymph vesicles known as "lymph hearts", which are muscular and pulsate.

The unusual nature of the avian, lymphoid system may account for the comparative rarity of recognizable abscesses in birds. General proliferation of diseased lymphoid tissue is best seen in lymphoid leucosis ("lymph cancer"), or "big-liver disease" of poultry, which occasionally occurs in budgerigars and other species.

When the lymphatic vessels are blocked due to inflammation or by tumours, lymph cannot drain adequately from the tissue and they become waterlogged or dropsical. If the abdominal organs only are affected, fluid accumulates in the body cavity as ascitic fluid. If the

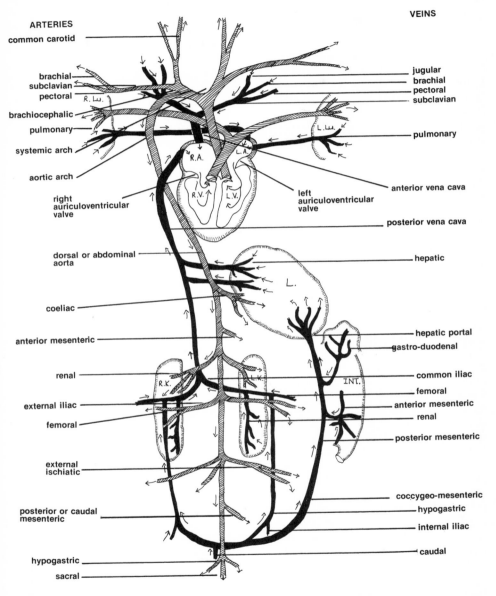

ARTERIES

VEINS

common carotid

brachial
subclavian
pectoral

brachiocephalic
pulmonary

systemic arch

aortic arch

right
auriculoventricular
valve

dorsal or abdominal
aorta

coeliac

anterior mesenteric

renal

external iliac

femoral

external
ischiatic

posterior or caudal
mesenteric

hypogastric
sacral

R. Lu.

R.A.

R.V.

L.V.

L.A.

L. Lu.

L. K.

R. K.

INT.

L.

jugular
brachial
pectoral
subclavian

pulmonary

anterior vena cava

posterior vena cava

hepatic

hepatic portal
gastro-duodenal

common iliac
femoral
anterior mesenteric
renal

posterior mesenteric

coccygeo-mesenteric
hypogastric
internal iliac

caudal

left
auriculoventricular
valve

Figure 17 Cardiovascular system of a bird. R.Lu. = Right lung; L.Lu. = Left lung; R.A. = Right auricle; L.A. = Left auricle; R.V. = Right ventricle; L.V. = Left ventricle; H = Heart; L = Liver; R.K. = Right kidney; L.K. = Left kidney; INT. = Intestine. Arrows show direction of blood flow. (Janet Keymer)

fluid is in the limbs or generalized throughout the body, it tends to gravitate and produces a puffiness of the tissue which dents under pressure, the presence of this fluid being called oedema.

THE NERVOUS SYSTEM

The avian nervous system is similar to that of mammals and consists of central, peripheral and autonomic systems. Its functions include the transmitting of stimuli from sense organs by nerves to the brain and spinal cord, the storage and analysis of this information, and the transmission of motor stimuli to the limbs and viscera.

The central nervous system comprises the brain and spinal cord (Fig. 18) protected respectively by the cranium of the skull and the chain of ring-like vertebrae which form the backbone. Twelve pairs of cranial nerves pass from the brain to supply movement or sensation to the eyes and eyelids, the organs of smell, ears, jaws, tongue, pharynx, larynx and a few muscles of the upper neck. Behind the brain, the spinal cord has a pair of spinal nerves between each vertebra to supply the remainder of the body with sensation and movement. These paired nerves, their branches distributed throughout the entire body, make up the peripheral nervous system. This pairing is a relic of the early days of evolution, and indeed of the embryonic development of the bird itself, when the head and body were clearly divided into segments somewhat like the Michelin tyre man of the advertisements. A typical avian nervous system is illustrated in Fig. 18.

The brains of birds show several areas, which are grouped for convenience into three continuous sections, the fore, mid and hind brain.

The cerebrum forms the bulk of the forebrain and is concerned with interpreting sensations and acting on them, giving conscious orders to make the bird run or fly, for example. The mid and hind brain areas tend to overlap. The mid brain contains a small part of the cerebellum and also the optic lobes. The hind brain includes the bulk of the cerebellum and the medulla oblongata. The cerebellum is a large cauliflower-like mass placed above the hind brain and is highly developed in birds; it has a co-ordinating action on the various movements of the body, organizing the muscles to act effectively upon an order from the cerebrum. The lower part of the hind brain, known as the medulla oblongata, carries several masses of nerve cells, as opposed to mere nerve fibres; it is really a primitive brain.

When the cerebrum cannot function due to injury a bird can still eat and drink when food is put in the mouth and it can also move its legs and wings in a reasonably organized manner. If the cerebellum is extensively damaged, some form of consciousness and movement is possible but co-ordination and purposeful movement are not. When the hind brain alone is undamaged a bird can live for a short time as a limp vegetable-like creature, the heart and lungs continuing to function. Some of the more basic instincts, such as hunger, thirst, fighting, or fright, are governed by hind brain activity.

Through the brain stem, bundles of nerves pass to the cerebrum and cerebellum from the body. Some of these carry back sensations to the brain: these are called afferent or sensory nerves. Others are known as efferent or motor nerves and send out instructions to a similar range of organs and tissues. Examples of the sensory kind are the optic (visual), olfactory (smell) and auditory (hearing) nerves. Motor nerves include those which control the eye and tongue movements.

Nerve impulses pass between the various parts of the body and the special areas of the brain via the spinal cord. They travel through a series of nerve cells and the tendril-like fibres projecting from them, the individual nerve unit or neurone acting as a miniature control panel, condenser and alarm.

The nerves which can be seen easily when dissecting a carcase, are bundles of tendrils emanating from nerve cells in the spinal cord, which in turn make contact with cells in the brain. The nerves, as they emerge in pairs from the spinal cord, carry both motor and sensory fibres. Branches of these nerves, when they split up to serve the various organs and tissues, may be purely motor, purely sensory, or mixed. A nerve severed by a wound may therefore deprive of sensation, mobility, or both, that part of the body which it serves.

The autonomic nervous system is a delicate and scattered web of nerve fibres diversifying throughout the body. It is concerned with that part of the nervous function which is beyond the conscious control of the bird. It regulates such processes as the secretion of digestive juices and the workings of the endocrine glands, gut movement, the volume of blood flowing in and out of the organs, variations in the heart-rate, kidney and liver function. Where several fibres join together they form a "nerve knot" or ganglion. A familiar ganglion is the solar plexus, found just below the spine near the kidneys. The system is connected to the central nervous system and functions in harmony with it by a series of fine nerve branches through its entire length from brain to tail. In this way all the numerous functions of a bird are co-ordinated. Some effects on distant organs, however, are brought about chemically by the ductless glands without the intervention of nerve fibres: this control is called a humoral mechanism. Sometimes a tissue or organ can be affected by both humoral and nervous stimuli.

THE ENDOCRINE SYSTEM

Endocrine, tubeless or ductless glands manufacture fluid and pass it into the surrounding tissue or directly into the blood stream. The secretions, which are known as hormones, influence almost instantaneously, on their release from the gland, all those tissues of the body sensitive to their presence, no matter how distant. The endocrine glands are some of the most important but least understood organs of the body.

The Pituitary Gland is situated in a small, bony cavity in the floor of the cranium and is surrounded by a cushion of small blood vessels. The secretions of this gland have a marked effect on all the other ductless glands, stimulating or inhibiting their action. The pituitary gland has been referred to as the conductor of the glandular orchestra. It is ideally placed, being attached to the base of the brain where it can be influenced by stimuli from the eyes, ears, the bloodstream and the masses of nerve cells or centres in the brain which deal with such vital matters as body temperature and heat regulation, heart and respiratory rates and the blood requirements of various organs. The numerous functions of the gland are performed by only two types of pituitary tissue, which are in its anterior and posterior parts. The pituitary hormones take their names from the ductless gland which they control: for example, the thyrotrophic, adrenocorticotrophic or gonadotrophic hormones. The anterior pituitary gland stimulates the sex glands seasonally and this appears to depend on the effect of light; progressive lengthening of the daylight period by artificial light can often induce egg production out of season and even mating. The lactogenic hormone or prolactin influences the production of "crop milk" in pigeons and probably proventricular "milk" in budgerigars. It also leads to broodiness and sometimes to the production of brood patches. The anterior pituitary gland may produce in birds the hormones concerned with growth of all parts of the body, but this is not yet known for certain. The posterior lobe of the gland is in direct nervous communication with the brain and it probably controls movement of the oviduct.

The Thyroid Gland consists of two roughly oval structures lying in the chest near the syrinx and the jugular or main neck veins. They are usually red or damson colour and vary in size according to species, age, the individual, and seasonal changes. The thyroid is mainly concerned with maintaining and altering the metabolic rate so the glands increase in size when greater demands are made on the metabolism of the body, in cold climates for instance and during egg laying, (see Chapter 19). Thyroxine, the thyroid hormone, can be produced only when sufficient iodine and tyrosine (an amino acid) are available in the body. If thyroxine production fails or the gland is surgically removed, the mental and physical development of young birds is stunted, whilst adults become sluggish as body processes slow down and the condition of their plumage deteriorates. In an effort to increase hormone production, the gland enlarges. Enlargement is quite common in budgerigars and frequently caused by deficiency of iodine. In some species, however, enlargement does not necessarily imply deficiency in thyroxine production: in many, enlargement of the gland is accompanied by over-secretion of thyroxine, which leads to hyper-excitability or nervousness, excessive moulting and incomplete growth of feathers. In young birds, sexual precocity may also be seen. Both these types of enlargement are called "goitre", (see also Chapter 19).

The Parathyroid Glands are very small structures situated close to the thyroids. The parathyroid hormone controls the calcium and phosphate levels in the blood as well as deposition in bones and liberation from them; it also regulates their absorption from the gut and utilization for the production of egg-shells. It is believed that the parathyroid is not under the control of any other endocrine organ, but is stimulated by the level of calcium in the blood. The level of minerals in the blood of healthy birds is very constant, but in certain diseases it may fall markedly and result in softening of the bones.

The Adrenal or Suprarenal Glands lie near the kidneys as their name indicates, being situated at their anterior ends. They are just visible to the naked eye in the smaller passerine birds, as pink or creamy-grey specks. Each gland is composed of two main parts, as in mammals, but the tissues are not demarcated into an outer cortex and inner medulla, the two types being mixed.

The "medullary" type of tissue is under sympathetic nervous control and produces adrenalin. This hormone immediately increases the heart rate, raises the blood sugar level and prepares the body in a variety of ways for sudden emergencies, for fighting or fleeing. The "cortical" tissue is equally important, but its action is less conspicuous and lasts longer. It secretes the adrenocortical hormones, (cortisone for example), which are concerned with assisting the body to combat stresses of heat, cold, disease or starvation by influencing the carbohydrate and protein metabolism. It may be described as a "fortitude" hormone, whereas adrenalin is reserved mainly for emergencies. Other cortical hormones are concerned with salt and water metabolism. A third group in conjunction with the pituitary gland affects development of the gonads and therefore the special modifications of the body associated with sexual display, such as plumage. Sometimes the hormones of the pituitary gland may be attempting to stimulate the gonads, while the adrenal cortical hormones may be striving for the opposite effect because of other more pressing commitments. The converse may be equally true.

Damage to the cortical areas as the result of infection, tumours or other destructive influences may make the bird susceptible to quite slight environmental changes. It is then possible that a 5°C. drop in aviary temperature, the presence of a marauding cat, a fight, rough handling or even a change of diet, can produce sudden death, which is probably due to stress.

The Islets of Langerhans (Pancreas) are tiny groups of endocrine cells known as beta cells which are scattered throughout the pancreas. The Islet tissue produces insulin; this hormone determines blood-sugar levels and takes sugars out of the circulating blood to store them in the liver in the form of glycogen, or to distribute them to the skeletal muscles and other organs where they are temporarily stored for emergencies. Other endocrine cells—alpha cells, mainly in the splenic lobe of the pancreas—produce a hormone called glucagon, which mobilises blood glucose. At rest, blood sugar in mammals is fairly contant at 80-130 mg. per each 100 ml. of blood, but in birds it is as high as 150-250 mg.

In mammals, challenges are met by the liberation of such hormones as adrenalin, which can almost instantly mobilise liver glycogen to form glucose and then encourage the muscles to take up this fuel for their activity. Adrenalin raises the level of glucose in the blood and if it exceeds a certain amount, the glucose is excreted by the kidneys. This process has not been well studied in birds, but in *diabetes mellitus* —the well known disease of mammals, including humans—the "sugar-squandering" propensities of the adrenal are not counteracted by the thrifty effects of insulin because the Islet cells have been destroyed. The liver's glycogen stores are therefore depleted and loss of weight results, with excessive thirst, hunger and debility. This disease, however, has not been reported in birds, and the effect of insulin on the level of the blood sugar is much less marked than in mammals—except apparently in carnivorous birds. It seems that adrenocorticotrophic hormones have a much greater effect than insulin on the level of blood sugar. Excessive insulin, which can only result from Islet tumours or the injection of insulin, causes lowered blood sugar in mammals, and if the level falls too low, convulsions, coma and death result. The danger point in birds has not yet been determined accurately, but is probably about half the normal level.

The endocrine activities of the gonads are described at the beginning of this chapter and in chapter 19.

Although this account of the endocrine system is necessarily brief, it is hoped that it gives a general idea of how the functions of the various parts of the body are integrated and controlled; it should be read in conjunction with the section on the nervous system.

The Thymus Gland
The function of this gland is poorly

understood in man and other mammals; even less is known about its activities in birds. It appears to be involved in lymphocyte and antibody production.

The gland is most highly developed in the young and gradually gets smaller as the animal develops. It is composed of a chain of small fat-coloured lobes closely related to the jugular veins in the base of the neck. In some species such as the budgerigar the gland may extend into the submandibular region. In a few birds it increases in size temporarily during the breeding season, but the reason for this is not clear.

SPECIAL SENSES: SIGHT, HEARING, TASTE AND SMELL

The Eye. The eyeball has a tough, outer fibrous layer called the sclera. The small, exposed surface is transparent and called the cornea. The middle layer of the eye is the pigmented, vascular choroid, whilst the inside of the eye is lined with the light-sensitive tissue known as the retina. The contents of the eye form two unequal parts. The front or superficial portion immediately behind the cornea contains a watery liquid, and is separated from the posterior and larger part by the iris diaphragm, the crystalline lens and the ciliary body. The back of the eye contains the pecten and a jelly-like substance called the vitreous body. The iris diaphragm in front of the lens has a pupil or opening which is controlled by constrictor and dilator muscle fibres. The organ is pigmented and is responsible for the eye colour of birds. The pecten is peculiar to the avian eye; it is smallest in nocturnal birds and largest in diurnal birds of prey. Although its true function is unknown, it is believed that it provides oxygen and nutrition to the retina, since it is a highly vascular organ. The impulses generated by light fall on the retina through the cornea, pupil, lens and the ocular fluids, and are carried to the brain via the optic nerve. This is a stalk of nerve tissue which is associated with the blood vessels which run from the eyeball beneath the pecten to the brain. The muscles of the ciliary body move the lens; by pulling at its periphery and flattening the curvature, they alter the optical power of the cornea, and thus allow focusing on objects at varying distances.

In spite of its vulnerable position and its relatively large size, the eye usually suffers little damage. The finer particles of dust and other minor irritants are swept away by the translucent third eyelid or nictitating membrane which comes across the eye from its nasal corner. Nearby objects or the threat of injury cause the two vertically moving eyelids to close rapidly, at the same time washing the eye with the constantly secreted tears; these are produced by the lachrymal gland in the roof of the bony orbit. The tears drain away into the nasal cavity through the lachrymal duct. A large gland known as the Harderian gland also produces a lachrymal secretion.

The layout of the muscles which move the eye is not important in birds, because in most this movement is negligible. The muscles are concerned with pulling the eye into the orbit (thus avoiding stretching the optic nerve) with turning, and with rotating the eyes. Special cranial nerves control these extrinsic muscles and are distinct from the optic nerve which connects to the retina.

The avian eye varies considerably in different species (Fig. 19). Those with poorer vision tend to have a bulb-shaped eyeball, while those with more acute vision have a conical or almost cylindrical eye. In many birds, the eye is surrounded by a cylinder or collar of bone which is separate from the skull.

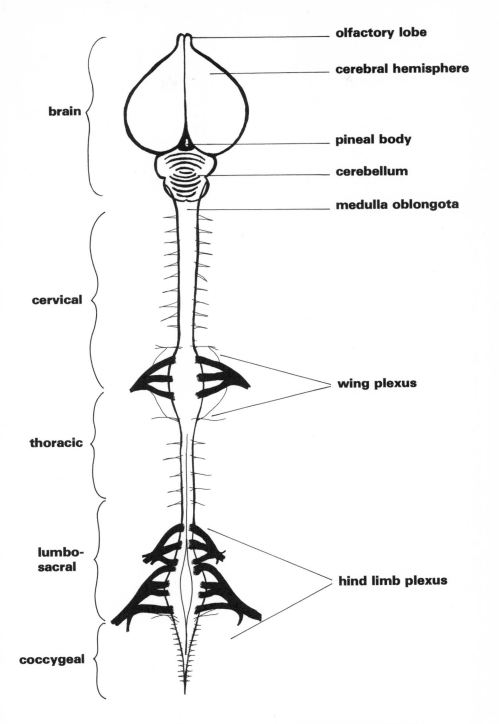

Figure 18 Central nervous system of a bird. (Janet Keymer)

olfactory lobe

cerebral hemisphere

pineal body

cerebellum

medulla oblongota

brain

cervical

thoracic

lumbo-
sacral

coccygeal

wing plexus

hind limb plexus

The owl is a typical example. Birds possess proportionally much larger eyes than mammals. Some have eyes adapted to night vision, while most can see well only in daylight. Probably all diurnal birds have colour vision.

The position of the eye varies according to the feeding habits, and the angles through which vision is possible, vary tremendously. Species which have their eyes on the side of the head cannot see directly in front without moving it, when they see with one eye at a time. In owls and to a lesser extent in many other birds of prey, vision is binocular: they see objects with both eyes at once and can more quickly judge distances. Such predatory birds have excellent vision, enabling them to hunt for prey from several hundred feet in the air.

Birds have varying powers of focussing or accommodation. This implies that they can move the lens or greatly alter the shape of the cornea in order to focus on objects over a wide range of distances. In the great majority of birds with monocular vision, the power of judging distances and size of objects would be poor were it not for the fact that a bird's head is in almost constant movement, thus enabling it to look at an object from several slightly different viewpoints almost at the same time. It should be noted too that movement of the head is necessary since the eye is almost immobile in its socket. From these glimpses, the brain can interpret size and distance. Exceptions are some diving birds like penguins, which have more eye movement because of better developed eye muscles.

The Ear

The ear of birds (Fig. 20) is much simpler than that in man and most mammals. The external ear comprising an ear flap or pinna, is absent in birds. The outer ear is a short, simple, feather-lined tube or canal leading to the tympanum. It is placed a little behind the eye and can be readily seen by gently parting the feathers in this region, although in vultures and the ostrich it is unfeathered and exposed. The tympanum is a delicate sheet covered on both sides with bone and a vascular skin, which extends across the base of each ear canal like a drum skin.

The tympanic membrane or drum forms the outer wall of the middle ear. This is an air-filled cavity transversed by a minute bone called the columella, which transmits vibrations produced by sounds from the tympanum across the chamber to the "oval window" or *fenestra ovalis* of the inner ear. From the middle ear a fine tube, the eustachian tube, passes down to the pharynx. This serves as another passage to the exterior and thus equalises the pressure in the ear. When the ears "pop" it is due to a small amount of air suddenly bursting out into the pharynx via the eustachian tube as the result of changing atmospheric pressure.

The inner ear houses the cochlea or hearing organ, and the vestibule. The cochlea in birds is only slightly twisted, whereas in man and the higher mammals it is a tightly-spiralled tapering tube. In birds some variation exists and this is related to the complexity of the song which the bird sings. The words cochlea and vestibule simply mean "snail" and "little room" by a fanciful resemblance of the organs to these objects. The vestibule is the organ of balance. It contains three arched tubes lined by hairs and contains fluid. Because of their arrangement in three planes, tiny particles of solid material floating in the fluid come to lie on different hairs in each tube. When the hairs are thus stimulated, information is carried to the brain, which then interprets the bird's position relative to its environment. When these structures are damaged a bird is unable to walk, fly or

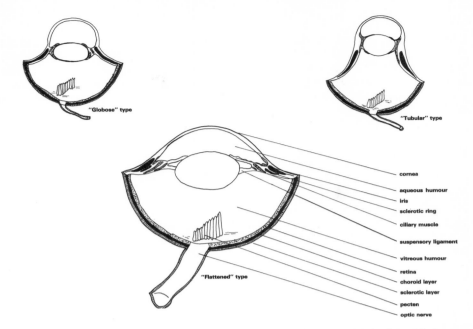

Figure 19 Three types of birds' eyes. The Globose type which gives high resolution at considerable distances. It has a rather flattened lens and a highly curved cornea. This type occurs in predators such as diurnal birds of prey (Falconiformes). Tubular type seen in owls (Strigiformes) is developed for nocturnal vision. The eye is elongated so that more light enters the eye and produces a brighter image on the retina. The flattened type is the commonest form and represents the least specialized "all-purpose" eye, as seen in the ducks, geese and swans (Anseriformes). (Janet Keymer)

even stand properly and may experience dizziness.

Taste and Smell

It is believed that most birds possess a poor sense of taste compared with mammals. Certainly the shape of food plays a great part in its selection, and in species with mobile tongues such as the parrot family, "tasting" movements and sampling an object prior to swallowing, probably constitute recognition by the sense of touch. Colour appears to be a more important factor than taste in the selection of food.

Birds have taste buds similar to mammals in structure, but confined to the soft area at the base of the tongue. They are, however, considerably fewer in birds, but some birds are believed to be able to detect such simple tastes as salt, sweet, acid and bitter. The ninth or glossopharyngeal nerve transmits the stimuli to the brain. Heat and cold are sensed by the mucous membrane of the mouth.

The olfactory lobes in the forepart of the brain are the centres for interpreting smells. Their restricted size in most birds is probably related to their poorly developed sense of smell. The tiny olfactory lobe and the absence of any sniffing behaviour, strongly support the contention that smell and taste perception is at a primitive level in birds.

67

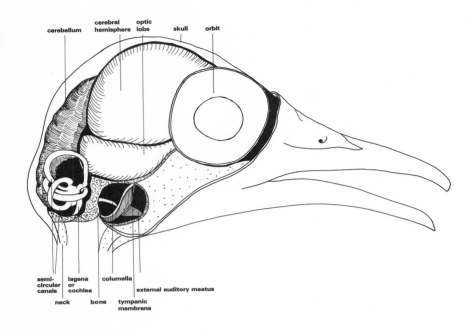

cerebellum · cerebral hemisphere · optic lobe · skull · orbit

semi-circular canals · lagena or cochlea · columella · external auditory meatus

neck · bone · tympanic membrane

Figure 20   Side view of head of pigeon showing structure of ear. (Janet Keymer)

THE EXOCRINE GLANDS

The exocrine glands are the glands of external secretion.

A gland is a group of cells which produces chemicals which start chemical or physical actions in various parts of the body. The active part of the secretion is often an enzyme or organic catalyst. Secretions may simply diffuse through the wall of the gland cells, or by budding-off cells liberate batches of secretion from the parent cell. Sometimes even the whole cell may burst, shedding its contents. Some gland cells produce only mucus and act as lubricators and protectors of the various hollow organs. The mouth, crop, proventriculus, pancreas, intestines, respiratory tract, oviduct, ureters, cloaca and preen gland abound for example, in gland cells.

Exocrine glands are to be found everywhere in the body and supply various organs by means of ducts. The gland cells are grouped into the linings of clefts beneath the surface of the skin or mucous membranes, while some actually form solid masses. Examples of their secretions are bile, saliva and other digestive juices, and preen gland oil.

68

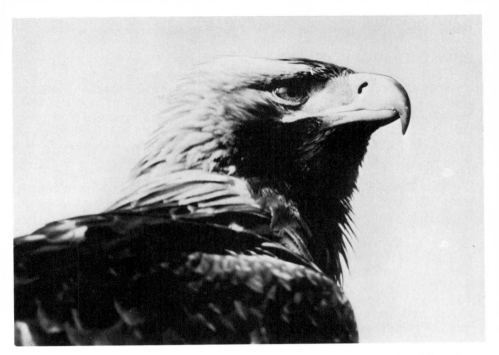

The eagle is a diurnal bird of prey with keen eyesight. The eye is of the globose type and contains a pecten. See Figure 19   The geese, in the photograph below, have flattened type eyes, set in the sides of the head, providing them with monocular vision. The eagles, above, have binocular vision.

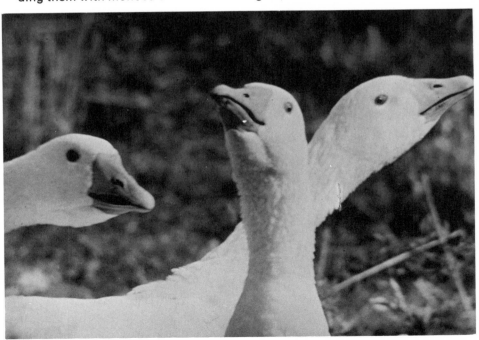

SELECTED BIBLIOGRAPHY

AREY, L. B. (1965). *Developmental Anatomy.* 7th Ed. London. W. B. Saunders. 695pp.

BRADLEY, O. C. (1960). *The Structure of the Fowl.* 4th Ed., revised by T. Grahame, Edinburgh, Oliver & Boyd, 143pp.

CHAMBERLAIN, F. W. (1943). *Atlas of Avian Anatomy,* Osteology—Arthrology—Myology. East Lansing, Michigan State College, 45pp.

DARLING, L. & DARLING, L. (1962). *Bird.* Boston, Houghton Mifflin Company, 261pp.

EVANS, H. E. (1969). *Anatomy of the Budgerigar. In* Diseases of Cage and Aviary Birds, p.45–106. Ed. Petrak, M. L., Philadelphia. Lea & Febiger.

FARNER, D. S. & KING, J. R. (1971). *Avian Biology.* New York and London. Academic Press. Vol. I, 586pp. Vol. II, 612pp. Vol. III, 573pp.

GRASSÉ, P-P. (1950). *Traité de Zoologie,* Vol. 15. Oiseaux. Paris, Masson et Cie., 1164pp.

LUCAS, A. M. & JAMROZ, C. (1961). *Atlas of Avian Hematology.* Agriculture Monograph 25, Washington D.C., United States Department of Agriculture, 271pp.

LUCAS, A. M. & STETTENHEIM, P. R. (1965). *Avian Anatomy. In* Diseases of Poultry, p.1–59. Eds. Biester, H. E. and Schwarte, L. H. 5th Ed. Ames. Iowa. State University Press.

McLEOD, W. M., TROTTER, D. M. & LUMB, J. W. (1964). *Avian Anatomy.* Minneapolis, Burgess Press, 143pp.

MARSHALL, A. J. (1960 and 1961). *Biology and Comparative Physiology of Birds.* New York, Academic Press, Vol. I, 518pp. Vol. II, 468pp. '

OLSON, C. (1965). *Avian Hematology. In* Diseases of Poultry, p.100–119. Eds. Biester, H. E. and Schwarte, L. H. 5th Ed. Ames, Iowa. State University Press.

ROMANOFF, A. L. (1960). *The Avian Embryo, Structural and Functional Development.* New York, The Macmillan Company, 1305pp.

ROMANOFF, A. L. & ROMANOFF, A. J. (1949). *The Avian Egg.* London, Chapman and Hall, 918pp.

STRESEMANN, E. (1934). *Aves. In* Handbuch der Zoologie. Kükrenthal W. and Krumback, I. eds. Berlin, Walter de Gruyter & Co. Vol. 7. 899pp.

STURKIE, P. D. (1965.) *Avian Physiology.* 2nd Ed. Ithaca. New York, Comstock Publishing Associates, 766pp.

THOMSON, Sir A. Landsborough, (1964). *A New Dictionary of Birds.* London and Edinburgh. Thomas Nelson Ltd., 927pp.

WORDEN, A. N. (1956). *Functional Anatomy of Birds.* London. Poultry World, 136pp.

NUTRITION AND METABOLISM

Metabolism may be described simply as the utilization of food and its effects within the body. These include the building up (anabolism) and breaking down (katabolism) of the chemical substances from which the body is made. The processes vary from species to species depending upon inherited biochemical characteristics and also upon individual variations, which include age and activity as well as environmental factors such as diet and exposure to heat or cold.

Carbohydrates

Carbohydrates are the main and most readily available form of energy. They are the so-called storage foods or starches, which form a large part of the normal diet and are found in high proportions in such foods as cereals, grains and fruit. Meat also has quite a high carbohydrate content. All carbohydrates contain atoms of carbon, hydrogen, and oxygen, combined together in chains or rings with various side branches. The structural units from which carbohydrates are formed are known as sugars. The simple 6-carbon sugars are called monosaccharides; the more complex ones such as lactose and sucrose are known as disaccharides, while the starches and cellulose with numerous molecules are termed polysaccharides.

Glycogen is manufactured by the liver, other active organs and muscles, from simple carbohydrates or sugars.

The glycogen is stored and can be mobilised by various nervous and chemical mechanisms at extremely short notice when a sudden flood of energy is needed.

Fats

Fats and oils (unstable fats) consist of organic acids called fatty acids. They are also mainly composed of carbon, hydrogen, and oxygen. Fats are long-term reserves of concentrated stored energy which also furnish heat insulation and some protection against injury. In addition, they help to maintain the health of skin and plumage and aid in the absorption of fat-soluble vitamins. When food is short, fats are utilized by the body. Fat is also a source of certain unsaturated fatty acids which are essential ingredients of the diet.

An excessively high level of fat in the diet slows the emptying of the stomach and consequently the digestion of all food in the digestive tract. It is therefore wasteful and interferes with the utilization of other vital nourishment.

Proteins

Proteins are long chains of smaller compounds, called amino-acids which contain carbon, hydrogen and oxygen plus nitrogen and occasionally sulphur. They are used in the formation of body tissue needed for growth, to replace proteins broken down in bodily functions, and to furnish the proteins required in making eggs. Proteins are also present in high proportion in most

71

organs and tissues of the body, particularly feathers, skin and appendages, the heart, liver, kidney and eggs.

Protein is the third and last storehouse of energy. In starvation or prolonged disease, after most of the fat storage depots have been depleted, the body starts to use this only remaining material. Muscle wastage then becomes noticeable, particularly over the breast and limbs in birds. The protein breaks up by discarding its nitrogen-containing element and becomes a carbohydrate-like substance which can be readily utilized. Much of the nitrogen is excreted in urine. The resultant loss of weight in birds is spoken of as "going light".

In certain circumstances, for example when there is an imbalance of protein in the diet (especially of such psittacine birds as budgerigars and parrots), the metabolism becomes deranged and waste by-products accumulate in the body, producing gouty deposits near the joints of the limbs and in the internal organs.

There are about twenty different types of amino-acids. Some of these can be manufactured by the bird, and therefore are called non-essential amino-acids. The other group, the essential amino-acids, cannot be manufactured by the bird and must be supplied in the food. Plant proteins tend to be deficient in certain essential amino-acids and therefore it is often desirable to add special protein supplements to the diet of seed-eating birds kept in captivity. In the wild state, such birds would eat a wide variety of invertebrates and also feed them to their young, thereby obtaining animal protein and the essential amino-acids.

The precise requirements of the different amino-acids for birds are unknown, even for poultry, and differ according to species. Tyrosine and lysine appear necessary for feather pigmentation, while the former is also used in the formation of the thyroid hormone, thyroxine.

VITAMINS

The term vitamin is applied to widely differing groups of chemical compounds which are essential to nutrition but do not necessarily bear any structural or functional relationship to each other. It is important to remember that nature provides an adequate amount of all vitamins—provided that a wide variety of fresh foods is eaten. When foods are stored for long periods, especially in damp containers, and are fed day after day with no variety, relative deficiencies of one or other vitamins can and do occur. Diets which are low in vitamins are often low in some of the essential amino-acids which make up good quality protein, and such complicating factors make the diagnosis of vitamin deficiencies difficult. Disease also increases the demand for vitamins and may interfere with their absorption or utilization. Freshly gathered natural foods such as leaves, fruit, or seeding grasses are a better and more balanced vitamin and mineral tonic than many commercial products. Proprietary vitamin supplements should normally be necessary only for sick birds and those unable or unwilling to eat normal food. Single vitamin deficiencies rarely occur naturally and are the province of the experimental worker in avian diets who may create them to order, for research purposes.

Unlike carbohydrates, fats, and proteins, vitamins are catalysts and are able to aid chemical processes and remain unchanged at their completion. In cage birds, vitamin requirements vary with species, and owing to their differing natural diets some birds are more likely to be affected than others.

Vitamin C, also known as ascorbic acid, is the only well-known vitamin which most birds are unlikely to need in their diet since, as in many mammals, it can be manufactured by the body. There is evidence, however, that vitamin C is required in the diets of certain fruit- and nectar-eating birds, because in at least one species of bulbul the enzyme which converts glucose to vitamin C in the liver, appears to be absent.

The vitamin is involved in the formation of certain types of connective tissue. It is also believed that vitamin C and E are mutually protective regarding their storage in the liver.

Vitamin A is essential for growth, maintenance of a healthy skin and mucous membranes, and for good vision. A deficiency of the vitamin has an adverse effect on the epithelial lining membranes of the respiratory, alimentary and reproductive tracts and allows infections to gain ready entry to the body. It has sometimes been called the "anti-infective vitamin". It does not really protect or combat organisms trying to invade, but does assist the membranes to function normally, that is to act as a barrier to disease. Vitamin A is stored in the liver and is found only in animal tissue. Its precursor carotene is found in all green plants and yellow seeds and is converted by the body into vitamin A.

Vitamin D is required for the normal production and maintenance of bone, the absorption of calcium and phosphorus for making egg shells and also for maintaining the quality of beak and claws. The amount needed varies. Vitamin D promotes the retention of minerals by increasing absorption or decreasing their excretion. Sun-ripened seeds and leaves, eggs and fish liver oils are rich sources of vitamin D_2. Vitamin D_3 is the form available for birds, being found mainly in eggs and fish liver oils. Vitamin D is synthesized in the skin, especially the unfeathered parts, by the action of direct sunlight. It is also believed that the secretion of the preen gland is converted into the vitamin by the action of sunlight when it is spread on the feathers.

Vitamin E consists of a group of fat-soluble, unstable, organic compounds known as tocopherols, and is believed to have several far-reaching effects in the body, although even in man, domestic animals, and poultry, its functions are not clearly understood. In most birds it is probably needed for normal development of skeletal muscle, nerve cells of the brain, maintenance of protein levels in the blood, the health of male germ cell-producing tissue of the testes, and especially for the development and growth of embryos. The tocopherols are found in the germ oils of many seeds and in fresh green foods. The effects of the vitamin, however, are very easily negated through oxidation by unsaturated fatty acids in rancid oils and minerals. If cod liver oil is mixed with seed and stored this may happen. Administration of liquid paraffin or other oil prevents the absorption of vitamin E.

Vitamin K is necessary for clotting of the blood. It is present in most green leaves and grass. Bacteria of the lower intestine synthesize some vitamin K, but this is probably significant only in species where considerable fermentation occurs, e.g., in those seed-eaters which have well-developed caeca and colorecta. Deficiency rarely occurs but could result from indiscriminate use of antibiotics, especially if mixed in the food or water, when they are more likely to cause changes in the intestinal, bacterial flora and thus affect the synthesis of the vitamin.

73

The **Vitamin B Complex** is a large group which contains several important and separate vitamins. Most play an important rôle in metabolism.

VITAMIN B1, THIAMINE OR ANEURINE, is a water-soluble compound, unstable in heat. It is important to all cells of the body, including nerve cells, since it is involved in the metabolism of carbohydrates; without it death soon occurs, preceded by severe nervous disorders. Cereal grains and their by-products usually contain a sufficiency of this vitamin, but certain seeds such as mustard, hot rape, and fresh fish, contain substances which destroy the vitamin.

VITAMIN B2, OR RIBOFLAVIN, is a heat-stable and water-soluble compound. It takes part in several chemical processes in the tissues involving the building up, normal function, and breakdown of cells, and the metabolism of oxygen and other gases carried by the blood. It is contained in most green foods, yeast, liver and milk.

VITAMIN B6, OR PYRIDOXINE, is a stable member of the vitamin B complex and is necessary in various chemical reactions concerned with the metabolism of proteins and fat. Requirements vary greatly between species, and even breeds, of birds. Since the vitamin is widespread in avian foodstuffs, it is unlikely that deficiencies of pyridoxine will occur.

VITAMIN B12, OR CYANOCO-BALAMIN, OR COBALAMIN, is water soluble. It has numerous functions in the metabolism of many food substances and chemicals of the body and is not produced by plants or animals above the most primitive forms of life, e.g., single-celled organisms and bacteria. Having the metal cobalt in its make up, it can be compared with the pigment chlorophyll of plants, which contains magnesium, and with the haemoglobin of vertebrates, which contains iron. The vitamin is absent from green plants and seeds but is found in meat, milk products and yeast. Although it is synthesized by intestinal micro-organisms a dietary source is also necessary. Deficiency is particularly likely to arise when the bulk of gut bacteria are killed by excessive administration of sulphonamides, antibiotics, or other antibacterial drugs.

Deficiency has deleterious effects on skin, feather and horn, and also retards growth, causes poor appetite, and reduces hatchability of eggs.

The vitamin is often used as a tonic, to stimulate numerous body processes. Its part in feathering is related to the intake of methionine, choline, and folic acid, since methionine, for example, is an important sulphur-containing amino-acid essential for the production of several tissue proteins including those of feathers.

Pantothenic acid, which is easily destroyed by heat, plays an important part in the metabolism of the three main food constituents, carbohydrates, fats and proteins. Other functions include the production of acetyl choline, vitally important in the conduction of nerve impulses and in their translation into muscle movements and other functions under nervous control. There is evidence that in some birds the requirements for this vitamin depend to a large extent on the amount of vitamin B12 in the diet. Although seeds such as wheat and oats provide an adequate supply of pantothenic acid, the richest natural sources are yeast and liver.

Nicotinic acid and niacin are closely related compounds which are involved in the metabolism of the three main food constituents, but at a different stage from pantothenic acid. Some seeds such as maize (known in the U.S.A. as corn) and oats are relatively poor sources of these substances. Tryptophane is usually adequate in the diet.

Folic acid, which is fairly stable, plays a restricted but important part in the synthesis of certain body proteins and is also stated to be an anti-anaemia factor. Seeds and grains are not generally rich in the vitamin, but yeast and liver will supply any deficiency in the normal diet.

Choline, like pantothenic acid, is essential for the formation of acetyl choline and is also involved in fat metabolism. The richest sources are yeast, liver, fish meal and fish solubles. The amount required in the diet is dependent on the vitamin B12 intake.

Biotin or vitamin H is stated to prevent perosis and poor hatchability, although no definite metabolic rôle has yet been established for the compound in birds. It is a complex sulphur-containing substance and occurs in many foodstuffs including yeast and milk by-products. Unheated egg white contains a protein which can react with biotin in the intestinal tract and thereby render it unavailable to the bird, thus producing a deficiency of the vitamin.

MINERALS

The bodies of all warm-blooded animals include metallic elements in addition to the organic chemicals, which always contain carbon, hydrogen, oxygen, nitrogen and water. These elements, in combination with their salts, are referred to as "ash" in analyses and represent the unburnable parts of the body. This ash consists of a high proportion of dehydrated tissues and contains calcium (as the phosphate and carbonate), sodium (as the chloride), magnesium, potassium, and much smaller amounts of iron, copper, sulphur, iodine, manganese, fluorine, zinc, cobalt, molybdenum, and selenium. Such minerals are called trace elements, and although minute and measured in parts per million as opposed to percentages of the total body weight, are nevertheless essential to normal development and health. Minerals enter into the composition of bone and give the skeleton rigidity and strength to support the soft tissues. They also combine with protein and other substances and help to form the body tissues. Other tasks include a rôle in the functioning of protoplasm, the transport of oxygen and the maintenance of degrees of acidity and alkalinity.

Calcium is a major constituent of bone, egg-shell and muscle. It is necessary for the conductivity of nerves, the function of the heart and other muscles, blood-clotting and many metabolic processes. Most seeds are deficient in calcium, and therefore in captivity it is essential to provide a calcium supplement which is provided traditionally in the form of cuttle fish bone or crushed oyster shell grit. Calcium is required in larger amounts than any other mineral and its metabolism is linked with that of phosphorus and vitamin D, adequate amounts of these nutrients being necessary for its proper utilization. The normal calcium/phosphorus ratio required for the growing domestic fowl is between approximately 1.5 : 1 and 2.0 : 1. It is probably similar for most species of birds. In growing birds, most of the calcium is used for bone formation; later in life it is used by hens for egg production. The requirements of calcium and also phosphorus (see below) are dependent to some extent upon the level of vitamin D in the diet. When large amounts of vitamin D are fed the amount of the minerals can be reduced. A deficiency of vitamin D on the other hand can be counteracted to a large extent by increasing the quantities of calcium and phosphorus in a suitable ratio.

Phosphorus is important in the metabolism of fats and carbohydrates. It is combined mainly with calcium in bone and egg-shell, as well as being an important constituent of all living cells, especially muscle. In severe kidney disease, the calcium stores of the body are squandered while phosphorus is retained. The rôle of vitamin D_3 in calcium and phosphorus metabolism has been discussed above and is also referred to under skeletal disorders. Phosphorus is widely distributed, occurring in plants, milk and fish.

Magnesium, although found in the body in much smaller quantities than calcium and phosphorus, is also an essential constituent of bone. Most of the mineral is present as a carbonate. Egg-shells also contain an appreciable quantity of the mineral and it is necessary for carbohydrate metabolism. Most diets contain magnesium and it should not be necessary to provide supplements.

Potassium is found primarily in the cells of the body, including bone. It plays a rôle in metabolism which is not clearly understood and is necessary for the oxygen-carbon dioxide exchange in red blood cells and for normal activity of the heart, having a relaxing effect by reducing contractibility, the opposite effect to that of calcium. Potassium allows certain chemical exchanges through the cell membranes to occur more easily. The mineral is widely distributed in food of both plant and animal origin so that deficiencies are unlikely to occur.

Sodium is usually combined with chlorine to produce common salt or sodium chloride and is found mainly in the fluids of the body (blood and lymph) in contrast to potassium, which occurs inside cells. The sodium content helps to keep the body from becoming too acid, being involved in the acid-base equilibrium and regulation of the pH of the blood which prevents marked changes in acidity or alkalinity. Together with potassium and calcium in proper balance, it is essential for heart activity. Excess chloride is discarded in the urine, while some is retained for use in digestion as hydrochloric acid. As sodium occurs fairly widely in combination with chlorine or as the carbonate or phosphate of compounds, especially in foods of animal origin, it is seldom necessary to supplement the diet of cage or aviary birds. Should this seem necessary, it must be done with great care as an excess of salt is toxic to many birds.

Other elements and trace elements are required in much smaller amounts; yet their lack can lead to spectacular effects. IRON is well known as a constituent of the haemoglobin of the blood, but even smaller amounts of COPPER are necessary as well for the formation of this pigment. Iron and copper are also necessary for the function of various enzymes and, as with other essential chemicals, they are required in increased quantities during the period of egg-production. Stores of iron are present in the liver.

SULPHUR is a constituent of certain amino-acids, methionine and cystine, used in the formation of muscle protein, egg yolk, egg albumen and keratin in skin, horn and feathers. IODINE is used almost exclusively by the thyroid gland. Without it the hormone thyroxine, secreted by the gland, cannot be made. MANGANESE is only known to be essential for avian development by the bone and joint defects such as perosis which result from its deficiency, though it may play a part in egg production. FLUORINE may play a part in bone metabolism of birds, although this is doubtful. The main interest of this element is that toxic levels can occur in birds and poisoning result if large quantities of fluorine-containing minerals are fed. SELENIUM is another element of doubtful necessity in cage birds although it may help in the retention of vitamin E. In the domestic fowl it prevents encephalomalacia ("softening" of the brain) and muscular dystrophy. ZINC seems to be necessary in minute quantities for all warm-blooded creatures being essential for growth. In poultry, high intakes of dietary calcium increase the requirements of zinc. MOLYBDENUM is also necessary for normal growth. COBALT, the metallic atom in vitamin B12, does not appear to be necessary alone for birds, providing that vitamin B12 is supplied in sufficient quantities in the diet or is synthesized by gut bacteria.

FIBRE OR ROUGHAGE

Mammals and birds have evolved to occupy a special place in nature. Each has become adapted to its changing environment and the availability of its food and, as Darwin discovered, only the fittest and most adaptable survive to thrive in this niche.

Apart from most plants and some primitive and parasitic forms of life, animals depend on food manufactured from the bodies or remains of other living creatures. Their food is thus a mixture of the digestible, absorbable, and indigestible. In times of food shortage, the readily digestible and absorbable ingredients are scarce while the intrinsically valueless ones are available. Individuals with digestive processes most efficient at dealing with poorer quality food are therefore more likely to survive and breed.

Birds and mammals have an efficient digestion, each species with its own modifications enabling it to deal with a wide range of plant or animal food material. Part of that efficiency depends on the maintenance of tone or muscle power in the complicated tube comprising the alimentary canal or gut. The muscular tone of the gut depends on work, like its counterpart in the skeletal musculature. Dealing with roughage ensures that the muscles of the gut and also the secretory activity of its glands are exercised and maintained. A sick bird can be kept for a short period on readily absorbable liquid foods. If on recovery, however, it is suddenly provided with normal food only, a digestive upset is likely.

Dietary requirements vary considerably in birds—from the predominantly nectar, fruit and flower-eating species, through the insectivorous, flesh and carrion eaters, to the grain, grass, and bark feeders. Fruit and flowers, although very high in water content, are also quite rich in fibre. No flying bird can afford to carry much surplus weight and the quantity of food carried in the gut of most species at any one time tends to be smaller than with purely terrestrial animals. Nevertheless, some roughage is needed by almost all birds. It is also needed to give a favourable environment for multiplication of the micro-organisms which aid digestion and produce such vital substances as vitamin B12. If the percentage of roughage is greatly increased, there is a tendency for impactions of the crop, gizzard, or sometimes the intestine to occur, these being most frequently seen in badly nourished and debilitated birds.

WATER

About 70 per cent of the tissues of most

higher animals consists of water. Birds cannot, as flying creatures, carry excess water. The amount consumed differs considerably between individuals as well as between species. In cases of poisoning by common salt, for example, there is a great increase in thirst.

Fruit-eating birds such as mynahs and lorikeets, seldom need to drink. Their problem is to eliminate the excess water. This results in extremely sloppy, watery droppings in which both the urine and faeces fractions are highly diluted. The appearance of the excreta should not be mistaken for diarrhoea or kidney disease.

Water is needed for every chemical process of the body and since the amount of "spare" water lying in the various parts of the alimentary tract at any one time is small, it must be available at all times. Withdrawal of water can rapidly produce distress in many species, especially in a high environmental temperature. It leads to panting, gaping, collapse, convulsions, and death. Much water is lost via the lining membranes of the respiratory system. Respiratory water loss cannot be easily controlled and in fact increases when the bird becomes distressed. A small amount of water is lost in urine and faeces but it is regulated largely by the reabsorption of water in the large intestine.

It will be appreciated that because of the great variation of water intake in the diet, and the relative humidity of the environment, the use of medicated drinking water for treatment is a relatively inaccurate method of dosing.

GRIT

Insoluble grit is essential in the diet for seed-eating birds which have a well developed muscular gizzard. The grit aids in the grinding of the seeds and other hard particles of food, and should therefore be hard with sharp edges, for example, quartz. If the grit is too fine it will fail in its function and may cause impaction of the gizzard. It is equally important that the particles are not too large for the size of the bird. Special grit for cage birds can be purchased, but where birds are kept in aviaries with a soil base this is not so important as the birds may find suitably sized particles for themselves.

Insoluble grit should not be considered as a source of minerals. These may be provided in the form of such substances as broken-up oyster shells and cuttlefish bone.

DIETS FOR DIFFERENT TYPES OF BIRDS

Small psittacine birds, (non-breeding), e.g. Budgerigars, Lovebirds, Cockatiels and Parrotlets.

Canary seed	3 parts
White or yellow millet	1 part
"Panicum" or spray millet	1 part
High protein seed	1 part
(Equal parts Rape, Teazle, Hemp, Flax (Linseed), Gold of Pleasure, Niger and crumb or dry mash supplement)	1 part
	7 parts

The "crumb" or mash is composed of as many of the following items as possible: dried egg yolk, alfalfa leafmeal, dried skimmed milk, iodised salt, wheat germ, yeast, dried parsley flakes, vitamins A, D_3 and B_{12}.

Breeding Budgerigars
The crumb or mash supplement mentioned, should be mixed with a little millet and canary seed and fed in a

separate container in increasing amounts according to the requirements of breeding birds during egg-laying, growing, feeding chicks, etc.

Large Psittacine Birds, e.g. Parrots, Cockatoos and Macaws. Most, except those of the subfamily Loriinae, will thrive on the following:

Canary seed	2 parts
White millet	1 part
Panicum or spray millet	1 part
Turkish hemp	1 part
Sunflower seed	1 part
Peanuts	1 part
	7 parts

Small quantities of green food, fruit (apple, grape) and other nuts may be added.

Larger parrots, such as Amazons and Macaws, appreciate chillies and maple peas. All psittacines should be encouraged to eat a little meat or mealworms.

Canaries: Adult, non-breeding and youngsters over 6-8 weeks:

Canary seed	5 parts
Rape seed	3 parts
White and yellow millet	1 part
Panicum or spray millet	1 part
	10 parts

A further soft food supplement suitable for breeding canaries is as follows:

Dried breadcrumbs	14 parts
Dried skimmed milk	2 parts
Bran	1 part
Wheat germ (Bemax)	1 part
Peanut oil	1 part
Cod liver oil or Shark's liver oil	1 part
	20 parts

Breeding Canaries and Young Birds
A mash similar to that for breeding budgerigars may be fed *ad lib*. Niger, crushed oats, rape, sesame, flax and poppy seed may be offered in place of, or up to half of the basic canary diet.

Other Small Hardbills, *e.g.* other seed-eating finches:
The seed mix can be of the basic budgerigar type, although rape seed can be omitted if not taken readily or it can be replaced by crushed oats or coarse oatmeal.

Supplements which are accepted readily, regularly or occasionally according to species, time of year and whether or not breeding, include:

(a) Various commercial "condition" foods
(b) Green food
(c) Fruit—particularly small berries.
(d) Live food—small flies, gentles (*i.e.* blowfly maggots), mealworms, spiders.

The commercial soft foods should be available at all times, whereas live food is essential only during breeding and perhaps moulting periods. In planted aviaries shrubs and other plants attract insects, but plants (or their fruits) which are poisonous to birds, should of course be avoided, (see Chapter 22).

Softbills, *i.e.* predominantly insect-eaters.
This group includes birds which also eat fruit and seeds. All take some of the following as food—flies, spiders, worms, maggots, other larvae, moths, butterflies, slugs, snails, beetles, woodlice and cockroaches.

It is possible, however, to breed or culture houseflies, blowflies, locusts, fruitflies, mosquitos, midges, maggots, wax moths, mealworms, bee larvae and certain beetles.

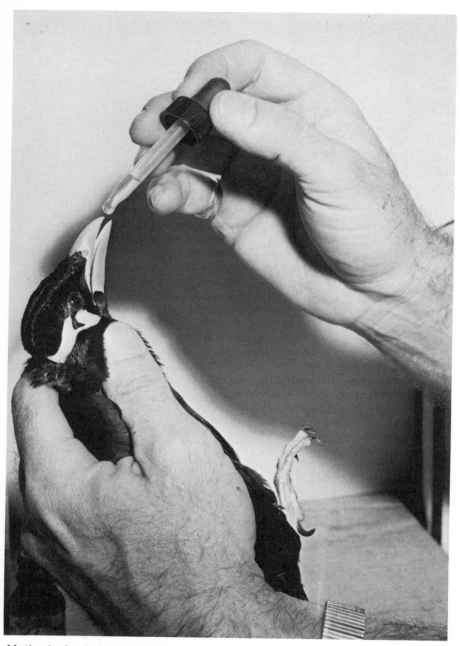

Method of administering fluid vitamin solutions to birds such as mynah, using a dropper or pipette.

As a substitute for live or insectile foods various mixes may be given, e.g.:

(a) Fine biscuit meal .... 7 parts
    Dried whole milk .... 1 part
    Wheat germ (Bemax) ...... 1 part
    White fish meal .... 1 part
                                   ──────
                                   10 parts
                                   ──────

To a kilogram of the above add 50 g. of dried yeast, 50 g. Arachis oil and 10 ml. cod liver oil.

(b) Fine biscuit meal or baby
    rusk .... 2 parts
    Dried flies or shrimp
    meal .... 1 part
    Animal fat (oily)............... 1 part
    Ants' "eggs", i.e. pupae 1 part
    Hen's egg (dried) .... 1 part
    Honey .... 1 part
    Wheat germ....................... 1 part
                                   ──────
                                   8 parts
                                   ──────

To 1 kg. is mixed 10 ml. of fresh cod liver oil. Raw, minced, lean meats, grated carrot, turkey starter mash, and peanut butter have been recommended as substitutes for part of the above.

Fruit and Nectar Eaters
This group includes lories, toucans, hummingbirds, sunbirds, honey-eaters, white-eyes, honeycreepers and flowerpeckers.

A nectar substitute called "Mellins Food" (a mixture of maltose, dextrin plus thiamine mono-nitrate, ferric glycero-phosphate and potassium bicarbonate) is available. Evaporated milk and honey, at the rate of one teaspoonful of each per cup of water is an alternative. Fresh, sweet, ripe fruit should also be provided for fruit eaters.

For larger members of this group, e.g., lories and lorikeets, whole rice boiled in milk, plus brown sugar or honey; fruit, mashed potatoes; coarse ground, brown bread; plain and fruit cake with beef extract (e.g., "Bovril") or vegetable extract ("Marmite") may be added. Baby foods, canned, fruit cocktails and mealworms may be added or substituted.

Other Groups
The reader is advised to seek information on special diets for waterfowl, gamebirds and the larger gallinaceous species in the textbooks devoted to these species. Some zoological societies will supply information on special diets for birds not specifically included here, such as cranes, flamingoes, bustards, emus, rheas, ostriches, etc., etc. Many are mostly grain eaters, although some are omnivorous and carnivorous to a certain extent.

Scientific names of seeds and plants mentioned above:
CANARY SEED (*Phalaris canariensis*)
MILLET (*Panicum* **spp.**)
RAPE (*Brassica* **spp.**)
TEAZLE (*Dipsacus* **spp.**)
HEMP (*Cannabis sativa*)
FLAX (*Linum* **spp.**)
ANISEED (*Pimpinella anisum*)
GOLD OF PLEASURE (*Camelina sativa*)
NIGER (*Guizotia abyssinica*)
SUNFLOWER (*Helianthus annus*)
SESAME (*Sesamum indicum*)
POPPY (*Papaver* **spp.**).

SELECTED BIBLIOGRAPHY

DAVIDSON, S. & PASSMORE, R. (1969). *Human Nutrition and Dietetics,* 4th Ed. Edinburgh and London. E. & S. Livingstone Ltd. 899pp.

HUNGERFORD, T. G. (1969). *Feeding of Poultry. In* Diseases of Poultry including Cage Birds and Pigeons, p.28–97. 4th Ed. Sydney, London, Melbourne. Angus and Robertson.

MASSEY, D. M., SELLWOOD, E. H. B. & WATERHOUSE, C. E. (1960). *The amino-acid composition of budgerigar diet, tissues and carcase.* Vet. Rec. 72, 283–286.

NORRIS, L. C. & SCOTT, M. L. (1965). *Proteins, Carbohydrates, Fats, Fiber, Minerals and Water in Poultry Feeding. In* Diseases of Poultry, p.144–180. Eds. Biester, H. E. and Schwarte, L. H. 5th Ed. Ames, Iowa. State University Press.

SCOTT, M. L. & NORRIS, L. C. (1965). *Vitamins and Vitamin Deficiencies. In* Diseases of Poultry, p.181–219. Eds. Biester, H. E. and Schwarte, L. H. 5th Ed. Ames, Iowa. State University Press.

TAYLOR, T. G. (1958). *Feeding Exhibition Budgerigars.* 2nd Ed. London. Illiffe Press, 52pp.

TAYLOR, T. G. (1965). *Nutrient requirements of budgerigars.* Mod. vet. Pract. *46* (9), 60–66.

TOLLEFSON, C. I. (1969). *Nutrition. In* Diseases of Cage and Aviary Birds, p.143–167. Ed. Petrak, M. L., Philadelphia. Lea and Febiger.

WATERHOUSE, C. E., HUTCHESON, L. M. & BOOKER, K. M. (1961). *Food consumption and palatability studies in budgerigars.* J. Small Anim. Pract. *2,* 175–188.

WINTON, A. L. & WINTON, K. B. *The Structure and Composition of Foods.* Vol. 1, (1932), Cereals, Nuts, Oil Seeds. Vol. 2, (1935), Vegetables, Legumes, Fruits. Vol. 4, (1939), Sugar, Cocoa, Coffee, Tea, Spice Leaves. New York, John Wiley & Sons.

HYGIENE

Prevention of many diseases can be achieved through forethought, common sense and reasonable cleanliness.

Sanitary premises do not necessarily mean those which have undergone meticulous removal of every particle of debris, nor saturating the environment with disinfectants, or burning with blowlamp or flame gun. In fact, as has been shown with some protozoan diseases, the disturbance of a dry litter can stir up latent organisms and cause a veritable epidemic; here balance is required. Sterilization of premises may sometimes be necessary, but it is a heart-rending process when stock has to be destroyed in order to make it effective.

Most organisms, be they bacteria, viruses, fungi, protozoa, helminths or arthropods, are susceptible to certain factors in their environment. These include drying, excessive cold or heat, sunlight, or lack of suitable hosts. Most of these organisms thrive in the presence of moisture, warmth, decaying organic matter, overcrowded and weakened hosts, undisturbed nooks and crannies, and darkness. There are certain exceptions in all groups; but for each the remedy is usually self-evident.

If adult birds are known to harbour pathogenic organisms, it is foolish to allow them contact with young nestlings and fledglings if this can be avoided. Nevertheless, since the normal environment is far from germ-free, it is equally foolish (and usually impossible) to avoid entirely infection or infestation. Birds reared in a near-sterile environment develop no immunity when suddenly confronted by hordes of pathogenic organisms. It must be stressed, however, that certain highly dangerous organisms which are also pathogenic to poultry and sometimes to mammals, including man, should be avoided if at all possible. Pasteurellae, salmonellae, Newcastle disease and avian pox viruses, trichomonads, the ornithosis agent, or others capable of causing disease, must be rigorously controlled. Some ectoparasites and intestinal worms can be safely tolerated in most temperate countries providing they are kept to an absolute minimum by a high level of management. Details of control are to be found in chapters on specific infectious diseases.

ISOLATION AND QUARANTINE

Any newly purchased bird, one borrowed for breeding or recently returned from a show, is a potential source of micro-organisms to all birds with which it comes into contact. In some countries, quarantine laws necessitate such birds being isolated at the port of entry in special quarantine premises. The name quarantine comes from the old French official method, *Quarente* representing 40 days isolation, but nowadays it tends to be applied also to private isolation. Quarantine is a valuable tool in preventing entry of epidemic disease foreign to the receiving country, or preventing

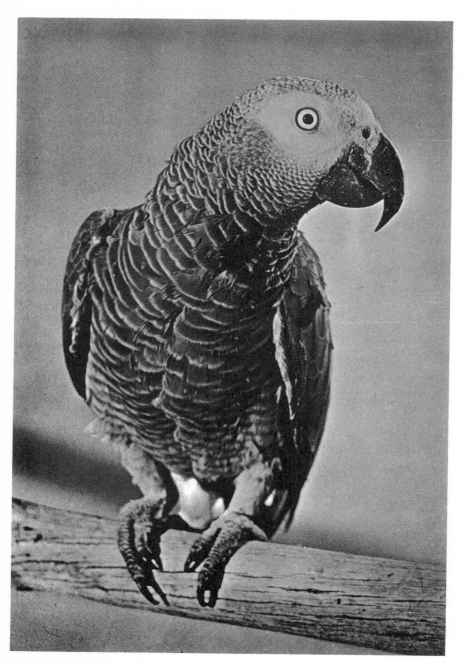

The African grey parrot (*Psittacus erithacus*) is the most popular of all parrots. It usually adapts well to cage life and household conditions and if acquired when young readily learns to mimic the human voice.

re-entry of those which have been eradicated. The suppression of livestock diseases such as tuberculosis, brucellosis glanders, rinderpest, and rabies in some countries has been made possible only by quarantine laws. On a smaller scale, isolation or quarantine can prevent entry of disease from another breeder or dealer, if the same principles are applied to all recently acquired stock.

HUSBANDRY

Any keen bird keeper knows the importance of good quality food, regular cleaning of premises, protection from marauding cats, dogs, rodents, and (where possible) wild birds. Soundly built and easily cleaned structures cut maintenance to a minimum. A little thought and money spent on good design and materials amply repays the outlay. Lighting, water, litter disposal, and other facilities should be adequate, whilst tidy habits reduce the opportunities for filth and pathogens to accumulate. The temptation to try the cure-all mixtures advocated for "loss of appetite, voice, feathers, etc." must be resisted. The first thing to do with any form of illness is to determine the source of the trouble by checking all points of husbandry, sources of possible contamination of foodstuffs, age groups and species affected, contacts, direction of spread if any, and recent additions to stock or other factors. By the time the illness is found to be more than a temporary malaise, much of the information which is necessary for diagnosis,

treatment and the prevention of further spread of the disease will have been acquired.

Good husbandry does not mean cossetting your stock. One reason why the most prized birds seem to be the ones which die first in an epidemic is that they are frequently exhausted by excessive warmth. A newly imported bird from a warmer climate may require extra heat, but it must be remembered that reducing ventilation to contain heat favours concentration of airborne infected water droplets and the multiplication of micro-organisms and parasites in the litter and environment. Excess local heat may lead to heatstroke. A fan heater introducing warm air from outside the building is a useful means of ventilation and heating in humid climates and for birds is preferable to air-conditioning which humidifies as well. A low-powered ultraviolet lamp is useful for air sterilization but should not be directed upon the birds themselves, or skin burns and conjunctivitis may result. Cold, dampness, draughts and enforced inactivity in cramped quarters combine to lower a bird's resistance to disease. The obvious good state of health seen in subtropical birds, however, in North America or European winters when they are provided with open wire netting flights in addition to sheltered perching and nesting quarters, illustrates how easily these birds can adapt to more severe conditions. Such birds happily spend most of their time in active pursuits in open windswept flights and are much healthier than those which are pampered.

SELECTED BIBLIOGRAPHY

HINSHAW, W. R. (1965). *Principles of Disease Prevention. In* Diseases of Poultry, p.120–143. Eds Biester, H. E. and Schwarte, L. H. 5th Ed. Ames, Iowa. State University Press.

HUNGERFORD, T. G. (1969). *Disinfection, p.18–22, and Fumigation, p.22–25. In* Diseases of Poultry including Cage Birds and Pigeons, 4th Ed. Sydney, London, Melbourne. Angus and Robertson.

CLINICAL EXAMINATION

A person who lives closely with animals acquires a "oneness" with them. The old groom who used to sleep next to the stables, and the shepherd living alone on the moor would quickly notice restlessness, changed breathing, and other slightly abnormal signs even without seeing the affected animal. Close association with all animals, especially when one spends hours merely watching them and when they have long since lost interest in and accepted one's presence, is not only a valuable way of learning to understand them but is also intensely absorbing and rewarding. The behaviour of living creatures undisturbed by human intrusion is a fascinating study; and in fact knowledge of normal behaviour is essential in order to recognise signs of ill health.

Preliminary Examinations

Patience and careful observation are frequently required in order to detect early signs of illness; they depend upon the full utilization of the senses of sight, hearing and touch. A fourth, the sense of smell, may sometimes be of help.

Visual Observations
A common error is to approach the subject much too quickly. The bird should first be viewed from a distance, preferably in its normal surroundings and long enough for it to lose any apprehension produced by one's sudden appearance. Features that can be seen in this way are the following:

The posture—huddled, tail up or down; position of wings, drooped or elevated; position of feet and toes; the attitude of the head, thrown back or drooping forward; eyes and beak, open or closed.

The respiratory rate and nature of breathing.

The degree of steadiness on the perch, teetering or slipping of the feet, rocking or loss of balance due to bodily weakness or affections of the nervous system.

The state and colour of the plumage, ruffled or tattered, moulting or faded. The appearance of the skin where it is visible.

Any variation in the contour of the body, such as swellings or other deformities.

Signs of asymmetry, one wing drooped, a hanging leg, a patch of matted feathers suggestive of local injury.

A closer look is then desirable. This may reveal less obvious abnormalities. The bird can now be disturbed from its perch and encouraged to move in order to see if there is any unsteadiness of the legs, lameness, impaired or weakened flight, partial paralysis or incoordination. In this way it is also possible to detect blindness (as shown by bumping into objects), limb damage, brain and spinal cord dysfunction, gout, arthritis and numerous other signs, as well as detecting respiratory distress and the degree of listlessness and ill health.

Birds show signs of pain and discomfort to a much lesser extent than mammals. In this fact lies much of the difficulty in making a diagnosis. Early signs of illness are often very slight and the majority of diseased birds, other than those with external injuries, may be seriously ill before the owner has become aware of the situation. By then, appetite or digestion may be badly impaired and signs of illness follow rapidly upon the self-imposed starvation. The smaller the bird, the more severe the diseased condition can become before it is recognized.

Observations are also made of the bird's environment; the food and fluid intake, the output of waste material. A search of the cage may reveal clusters of feathers or smears of blood and indicate that some predator has attacked the bird. Scattered food or water containers may suggest the presence of an unwanted visitor and account for head or other self-inflicted wounds or sudden death. Patches of nibbled paint may account for illness due to poisoning, especially if the paint contained lead. Evidence of vomit may be an indication of regurgitation in the courtship display of budgerigars or it may be due to ingestion of mouldy food or the result of some other digestive upset. The appearance of the droppings should be noted. They may be small and hard or copious and soft, contain watery or creamy white (urinary) fraction, or watery or semi-solid mucoid, grey, green or yellow (intestinal) fraction. The significance of these findings is discussed later.

Aural Examination or Auscultation
Although special instruments have been or could be devised, the unaided ear is quite adequate for detecting normal and abnormal sounds. Some clinicians, however, prefer a lightweight stethoscope with a small but sensitive chest-piece for heart, lung and air sac examination.

The ear should be placed systematically over various areas of the body, and care should be taken to avoid being pecked or scratched by the claws.

First the ear is held close to the nostrils. Clicking sounds may indicate partial blockage of the upper respiratory passages in the head and neck. This may be due to the movement of exudate, worms, foreign bodies or swollen folds of mucous membrane in the pharyngeal region. Some species can produce voluntary clicking sounds apparently by means of the tongue, glottis and associated throat muscles. Involuntary "sneezing" may indicate gapeworms, mobile masses of solid exudate or pressure of growths on the syrinx.

By applying the ear over the frontal bones of the head, hissing or whistling sounds may indicate partial blockage of the external or internal nares by exudate. This may occur in deficiency of vitamin A, or with infections of the nasal sinuses by organisms such as *Mycoplasma* (see Chapter 7), or as the result of beak injuries. Changes in the voice are audible from a distance but are clearer on direct auscultation.

Other areas which should be auscultated are the lower surface of the neck and the sides of the thorax and the back, especially the anterior half. Occasionally, listening to the abdomen may yield sounds of gut movement but generally only when large amounts of gas are present. This can be regarded as abnormal, except perhaps in those birds with large caeca. Back or thoracic auscultations reveal information about the state of the respiratory tract and the heart and great vessels of the circulatory system.

The squeezing or tapping of a suspected diseased area with simultaneous auscultation assists the detection of gas under the skin or gas or fluid in the abdomen. Much practice is necessary to identify sounds of oedema and congestion of the lungs, and of fluid or thick exudate in the trachea, bronchi or airsacs, as well as the normal sound of inflation and collapse of the airsacs. Pressure on the syrinx by the thyroids or as the result of crop enlargement may also affect these sounds and interpretation is best left to a veterinarian. In most of the species with which we have to deal, the heart sounds are so rapid as to be uncountable, except perhaps in very large birds. The quality of the heart beat is shown by the pitch and clarity of the sounds. The use of a much slowed-down tape recorder would be necessary for a specialist to interpret abnormalities. In a bird which has fits it is sometimes possible to detect irregularity or cessation of heart beats for a fraction of a second when circulatory failure is the cause. Valvular murmurs are generally undetectable.

The heart rate and respiratory rates (see Table), of birds even at rest vary considerably and are of only limited practical value.

Digital Examination: Palpation and Manipulation

The tips of the fingers have more sensory nerve endings to the square inch than almost any other part of the surface of our bodies. They are therefore invaluable when examining a bird in order to detect movements, approximate temperature, shape and size as well as the consistency of the areas palpated.

Owing to wide variations in the size of birds kept in captivity, there are certain limitations regarding the extent to which an examination can be carried out. Dangers may exist both to the bird and to the examiner. With tiny varieties, it can be difficult to hold the patient without interfering with breathing or causing injury and yet permit enough of the bird to be seen for examination purposes. The stronger parrots can be very difficult to restrain sufficiently with one hand while adequately investigating the various areas of the body, without a vice-like claw or beak grasping the examiner. A heavily gloved hand affords some protection but impedes examination. It is advisable therefore for an experienced assistant to hold the patient whilst the bird is clinically examined by another person.

When a bird is handled, it is easier to estimate its weight, muscular development, bodily condition, the distribution of fat and any abnormal body contours due to such factors as growths, ruptures or fractures. In fact palpation will often reveal more than close observation.

Next, a combination of manipulation with visual and aural faculties can be brought into play. The beak is opened and the lining membranes of the tongue, palate, internal nares, pharynx and glottis are examined for discolourations, exudate, ulcers, wounds, gapeworms and other obstructions. It is also worth smelling the odour of the mouth. When examining the body, plucking a few feathers, parting them by blowing or with the fingers, enables the skin colour or any superficial abnormality to be examined. Any stiffness, swelling or other deformity of joints may be auscultated while the diseased region is gently pressed, twisted or angulated. Clicking, crunching or grinding noises, known as crepitations, are associated with fractures, cancer of the bone and arthritis. Soft, fluctuating swellings over the neck and body, which on manipulation produce clear crackling sounds (also called crepitation) signify the presence of air or other gases trapped under the skin, a condition called subcutaneous emphysema. Shivering can be both felt and heard as a coarse humming sound due to rapid muscular movements.

A difficulty inherent in the structure of the avian skeleton and muscular system, especially of strong fliers with well developed pectoral muscles, is the almost total enclosure of the thorax and much of the abdomen by the sternum, associated musculature and ribs. Species vary in the proportion of the soft, ventral, abdominal area which can be palpated. The heart and lungs can never be reached in palpation. The thyroid, tracheo-bronchial region and crop can sometimes be felt in the V formed by the clavicle, except when the crop is absent or empty. Sometimes the pulse may be detectable here in the great blood vessels if the finger can be inserted a little way into the V cleft.

If the pubes of the pelvic girdle are sufficiently separated, various abdominal organs can be palpated through the abdominal wall. The gizzard is the most obvious structure in grain-eating birds and can be easily mistaken for a growth or egg unless the grating of its gritty contents is detected. Loops of small intestine, the U-shaped duodenum and caeca if present, can sometimes be felt. During the breeding season when the oviduct contains an egg or is enlarged due to a pathological condition, it may be easily palpated, but at other times it is too small or flaccid to be readily identified. The gonads are too deeply placed for palpation unless grossly enlarged through disease. The kidneys too, lying in the hollow below the lumbar spine and pelvis, are impalpable unless grossly enlarged due, for example, to tumour formation which sometimes occurs in budgerigars. The liver varies slightly in size according to the species, but when normal, not more than the sharp edge of one of its lobes can be palpated. In some diseases such as leukosis an enlarged liver may fill much of the abdomen and the bulk of this organ may then be felt. The spleen, unless markedly enlarged, is rarely palpated, since it has limited movement in mid-abdomen.

A further difficulty in diagnosis is the remarkable tolerance which birds show to painful stimuli. Mammals will often wince and cry out when a painful area is touched, but in birds it is seldom possible to get even a "cheep" when a diseased organ or limb is handled. Sometimes an injured limb may be withdrawn when handled or a spasm of fluttering may occur. Handling the head may produce momentary closing of the eyes, especially when pain is present. The pain threshold appears to be very high except in certain specialised areas: the angles of the beak, the cere, nostrils, around the eyes and the feet. Elsewhere cutting the skin or stitching a wound produces little evidence of pain although stretching or undermining of the skin may provoke some fluttering or struggling. Visible response to pain is suppressed by fear especially in the less domesticated species. Abdominal pain, accentuated by finger pressure is demonstrated by respiratory sounds, although this may only indicate respiratory embarrassment.

It is common for bird keepers to misinterpret clinical signs shown by birds. They frequently state that a patient has a "gastric stomach", or "asthma", or is "egg-bound", or "lazy", when what is really meant is that food is being regurgitated; the breathing is rapid, laboured, or noisy; the abdomen is enlarged, or the bird is in a very weak state.

It is essential to be conversant with the normal activity, appearance, or habits of the particular species examined, because without this knowledge an accurate diagnosis cannot be made.

Measurement of body temperature

Instruments generally available are mainly those designed for examining humans or domestic mammals: they are large, clumsy, and generally unsuitable for all but the bigger birds.

The clinical thermometer, the primary tool of the doctor and veterinarian, is a glass-sheathed instrument containing mercury, which can be used to advantage in birds the size of a pigeon or larger. It is inserted in the vent and can be pushed very gently into the rectum by slight deviation of the point to the bird's right while it is in the cloaca. Directing it to the left in the female may force it into the oviduct where infection from the excreta can all too easily be carried high up the reproductive tract with dire results. It is impossible to make glass thermometers small enough for finch-sized birds, but electrical thermometers (pyrometers) have been made with probes as small as 3 mm. × 0.5 mm. These, however, are very expensive and designed for experimental studies in mice, or other small creatures, when large numbers are being examined simultaneously. They are impracticable for lay use because of expense and the great care needed in their use in order to avoid rupturing the cloaca when the bird moves. See Table in Appendix for the ranges of body temperature for several types of birds. A rise of much more than 1°C (2°F) above these figures suggests the possibility of an acute infection or heat-stroke, whilst lower figures denote excessive loss of body heat due to severe chilling, shock, or imminent death. Struggling during handling can also significantly raise the body temperature.

It has been found that the body temperature of adult birds may vary from 40°C (104°F) for some larger birds, to at least 44°C (112°F) for small species such as some humming birds. The temperature, as well as the general body processes or metabolism, varies considerably with muscular activity and the time of day. Often a seasonal variation occurs, all within a range which can be regarded as normal.

When the temperature of the surroundings is altered greatly from that to which the bird is accustomed, body temperature control is severely affected. This is especially the case when the surroundings are draughty, when the plumage is in poor condition, or when birds are tightly packed in crates during transport. If control of the body temperature fails, the bird becomes chilled or dies of heat stroke, depending upon the circumstances. When a bird is too cold it shivers and fluffs up its feathers to form a more efficient and insulated covering by trapping air in the plumage. A weak, shocked or exhausted bird will do the same. When it is too hot, it cannot sweat so it stretches its neck, gapes and pants, whilst holding the wings away from its body. In extreme cases it may elevate the feathers fully to expose the skin in a desperate effort to lose heat.

Under certain conditions these mechanisms fail. A time when this may happen is when the humidity of the air is very high. This lessens the effectiveness of the panting type of breathing, especially when the temperature is also raised. In cold, moist conditions the efficiency of the feathered overcoat is impaired. Similar types of atmosphere are found in some badly designed nest boxes. Here, although the outside air may be warm and dry, the nest may be hot and steamy when the parent is sitting, but cool off by evaporation when the parent leaves the nest. Such a condition of "sweating" occurs with bad ventilation in leaky buildings, when birds have diarrhoea, broken or addled eggs, all or any of which may cause dirty nests.

Healthy adult mammals and birds can in normal circumstances control their body temperature to about 0.25°C (0.5°F) above or below their normal, and are known as homeothermic animals.

In new-born animals, including birds, which during development show characteristics of their more primitive ancestors, this maintenance of body temperature is not present. This applies even to the human being, and like the fish and reptile, a new-born baby is for a time, poikilothermic or "cold blooded", the body temperature varying with that of the environment. In some species of birds the young are four or five days old before any degree of temperature stabilization is achieved and it may take a similar period before full control is attained.

Sampling

Common specimens examined by veterinary and medical laboratories include excreta, saliva, swabs from the mouth, cloaca or rectum; scrapings of skin, scaled areas of the beak, the cere, and eyelids; feathers; blood; swabs from wounds and infected tissue; snippets of tissue (biopsy specimens) such as abnormal skin, ulcers, horn, and tumours; fluid from cysts or from other soft swellings and of course intact carcases or organs from dead birds. The tests that may be carried out on these samples are too numerous and technical to be included here. Many are complicated and expensive and are used when there is a danger of a flock epidemic, recurrent losses, or cross infection to other birds, animals or man; or when a bird is of special individual value or interest.

Samples can be examined under the microscope (after suitable preparation) for types and numbers of bacteria, fungi, and parasites or their eggs. The organisms may be tested for drug susceptibility to avoid using drugs which are not effective against the particular infection. Droppings and various body fluids can be tested chemically to determine their nature or origin, if in abnormal sites. Blood cells can be examined also for abnormal shape, size, or numbers. Tissues suspected of abnormality can be cut into sections which are only a few thousandths of a millimetre thick, stained, and then examined microscopically for evidence of inflammation or for the presence of tumour-cells. In this way it is often possible to determine the growth rate of a tumour, its potentiality for invading other tissues, and the prospect of its recurrence if an attempt is made to remove it surgically. Very exacting work is required to identify some bacteria and viruses. To ascertain the importance and dangers of some organisms it is necessary to inoculate them into experimental animals or birds. Within the *Salmonella* group alone, the list of bacterial species runs into hundreds. Bacteria can be identified by complicated tests which involve growing them in cultures containing sugars and other substances. Tests using sera are also used to classify and help in the identification of bacteria and viruses.

X-ray Examination or Radiography

Radiography, or x-raying, of parts of the body, head, or limbs is an additional aid to diagnosis that can be used occasionally. Again, it is the tool of the specialist and most people are aware of the dangers to the operator. It is not possible to position a conscious bird or animal for x-ray and expect it to stay still while the radiologist retires behind a protective screen. Protective gloves tend to obscure the patient and are not 100 per cent safe, therefore a general anaesthetic or strong sedative is usually necessary. An x-ray assists in deciding whether a swelling on a limb is a fracture, a soft, harmless tumour or a bone-destroying cancerous growth. They may also be used to show the position of a piece of metal or other inedible material which has been swallowed.

Occasionally depressed fractures of the skull and internal growths may be detected.

Laboratory tests, x-ray, and other advanced techniques are seldom a short cut to diagnosis. They are primarily a means of confirming a suspicion or tentative diagnosis. They are aids to clinical examination, or extensions of it, not alternatives. In some circumstances, especially epidemic disease or prolonged illness, they may help to pinpoint diagnosis and suggest specific treatment.

SELECTED BIBLIOGRAPHY

STONE, R. M. (1969). *Clinical Examination and Methods of Treatment. In* Diseases of Cage and Aviary Birds, p.177–187. Ed. Petrak, M. L. Philadelphia. Lea & Febiger.

INTRODUCTION

"Infection" implies a disease which may be caught, (usually from another living creature), by entrance into the body of some agent or organism capable of causing illness. Infectious organisms include not only the ultramicroscopic viruses, the microscopic rickettsiae, bacteria and protozoa, which are non- or one-celled, but also fungi which consist of groups of cells and the larger many-celled creatures, such as fleas, lice, bugs, ticks, mites, roundworms, tapeworms and flukes. All these organisms are living with the possible exception of viruses, there being some doubt as to whether a virus protein is a living creature or merely an inert chemical which develops in a similar fashion to a crystal of sugar growing in a pot of homemade jam.

Although members of all these groups live in or on the bodies of birds, and at the expense of their hosts, and are called "parasites", this term is usually confined to the protozoa and large multicellular creatures such as helminths (worms) and the arthropods (joint-legged creatures). Some authorities also include fungi as parasites. Instead of "infection" the term "infestation" is used for multicellular organisms such as helminths and arthropods.

Most of the lower forms of life clearly belong to the animal or plant kingdom. The multicellular worms and arthropods are obviously animals, while bacteria and fungi are considered to be plants although they lack the green pigment chlorophyll, of the higher forms of plant life. Protozoa, however, are animals, in spite of having no chlorophyll. The place of viruses and rickettsiae is indeterminate.

Infectious diseases were first studied in man, then the domesticated animals and birds. Because the study of cage bird diseases is a recent one, well-recognized poultry and mammalian infections were discovered and studied first. Epidemic diseases with high mortality rates were next studied scientifically, having been recognized earlier as distinct entities by observant aviculturalists. The number of people engaged in the study of cage bird pathology, either full-time or part-time, is still small, but it is already clear that cage birds are capable of contracting a wide range of infections.

93

When numerous birds are kept closely together, there is a corresponding concentration of their infections and infestations. As a result, unless vigilance is maintained, sooner or later outbreaks of disease are bound to occur. Even under conditions of apparently ideal management, infections can gain a permanent hold or become endemic. This is due partly to limitations of our knowledge and partly to the fact that an environment which is unfavourable to one organism may be a haven for others. Dry, dusty litter may, for example, encourage transmission of fungus spores. A cool environment may make birds huddle and favour transference of external parasites; moist warm air aids survival of airborne infection such as virus particles in water droplets and speeds up the rate of reproduction of certain disease-carrying flies and their larvae. Some creatures prefer darkness for their activity, others daylight. Few of the organisms capable of causing disease flourish or even survive in strong direct sunlight.

VIRAL AND RICKETTSIAL INFECTIONS

Viruses and rickettsiae are particles or chains of protein material which have the power to multiply. Most can only survive inside living animal or plant cells. They vary from 10-500 millionths of a millimeter in size (10-500 millimicrons), and unlike bacteria can pass through the pores of special unglazed, porcelain filters as used by virologists.

New viruses are continually being discovered and there is little doubt that many more have yet to be classified. Of the dozen or so viral and related diseases of poultry, only four appear to be sufficiently common in other species of birds to warrant a full description here, namely, pox, ornithosis, Newcastle disease and Herpes virus infection of pigeons. The remaining diseases mentioned are either uncommon, found mainly in free-living birds, or are of doubtful identity or occurrence.

Pox or avian diphtheria

Avian pox has been recognized as a distinct disease for centuries and has been a scourge wherever birds have been kept closely together.

Avian pox viruses are akin to the pox diseases of man and other mammals. They produce the same type of lesion, although avian pox viruses do not generally affect mammals and vice versa. There appear to be several strains, the best known being those viruses infecting poultry, turkeys, pigeons, and passerines such as canaries. In the latter, pox is sometimes referred to as Kikuth's Disease. Most strains do not keep strictly to the species giving them their name and their virulence or disease-producing ability varies. Some strains are capable of becoming more virulent in an unusual host and less so in their normal host. This adaptability, however, is variable, and some strains may be completely unable to cause disease in an unnatural host species.

The ability of pox viruses to stimulate the production of antibodies differs in the various species. In any bird where clinical illness is produced, infection is always followed by strong immunity or protection from further attacks in those which recover. Some strains, while causing little obvious disease, also produce immunity to one or more avian pox

95

viruses. Most pigeon pox strains protect pigeons against both the pigeon and canary-type virus. Some strains capable of causing a high death rate in canaries will produce little evidence of disease and a high level of immunity in pigeons and poultry.

CLINICAL SIGNS Pox primarily affects the skin and lining membranes of the head and its cavities. The virus grows in cells of the skin to such an extent that it destroys and bursts the cell, stimulating the production of lymph. The skin lesions start as vesicles or blisters of various sizes which separate the surface layers into pockets of watery fluid rich in multiplying virus. These swellings burst to the surface and the skin over them becomes yellow and necrotic, whilst the fluid or lymph congeals to form scabs. The scabs fuse together and may form a continuous crust or wart-like growths (Plate 1/6 and 2/6). Bacteria can now gain access and produce purulent discharges and further necrosis (Plate 3/6). These are particularly noticeable around the eyes where the exudate may cause the eyelids to adhere, producing blindness.

Conjunctivitis often occurs; it is manifested by a clear watery discharge from the eyes accompanied by congestion and oedema of the eyelids, giving them a puffy, half-closed appearance. The third eyelid is usually partly drawn across the eye. The face feathers become soiled. Sometimes a slight loss of activity or appetite occurs in the most seriously affected birds. In other respects the birds are normal. Within a few days several or all the birds may be affected. By then the earliest affected often have thickened, ocular discharge which may be sticky and mucoid or contain pus. The clear discharges are at first usually bacteriologically sterile but later become infected with bacteria such as *Staphylococci* or *Escherichia coli*. Lesions also occur near the nostrils, the angles of the beak and on any special structures, such as the cere, wattles and other fleshy parts. When the scabs fall off they may leave a scar. Canaries, pigeons and other affected birds also often show scabby lesions on the legs, feet and various parts of the body. In the mouth, throat and on other moist mucous surfaces, the lesions consist of white, moderately raised areas of sloughing, dead sheets of cells. This lifting up of the dead epithelium produces a so-called diphtheritic membrane, and the false membrane formed by coalescence of several such areas leaves a raw, red and eroded surface when the dead tissue is removed. Breathing may become difficult when throat lesions are present. In addition to these typical pox lesions, a generalized illness occurs caused by the presence of virus in the blood (*i.e.*, a viraemia). The viraemia occurs early in the disease and can cause death.

With certain strains of virus in some species, the viraemia has little or no effect on the bird. In severe cases of canary pox, however, the virus may multiply within the internal tissues, as well as the skin and mucosae. Clear exudates (plate 4/6) and sometimes haemorrhages are then seen at necropsy on the serous membranes lining the body cavity and the pericardium. Oedema of the lungs may also occur.

DIAGNOSIS Although not the only disease in birds capable of causing extensive scab formation on the skin, false membranes in the mouth, illness and death, these signs are sufficient to warrant a suspicion of avian pox. The disease can only be accurately diagnosed using special laboratory tests. These involve the inoculation of virus-rich discharge into experimental birds or embryonated eggs, and successfully transmitting the disease. Microscopic and other examinations may also be necessary. When strongly suspected by your veterinarian, a programme of vaccination (in those countries where suitable vaccines are available), isolation or culling can be undertaken on his advice. It is important to realise that the disease is contagious and also highly infectious and can exist in dried scabs for long periods.

DIFFERENTIAL DIAGNOSIS Other diseases which can give rise to one or more of the signs of pox include:
1. Trichomoniasis (canker) of the mouth and throat.
2. Herpesvirus infection of pigeons.
3. Candidiasis (thrush, oidiomycosis, moniliasis).
4. Hypovitaminosis A (nutritional roup).
5. Ornithosis (ocular forms of the disease).
6. Knemidocoptic mange (scaly face).
7. Mosquito and other insect bites.
8. Favus (ringworm).
9. Some skin tumours.
10. Some local bacterial infections.
11. Some allergic reactions.

TREATMENT AND PREVENTION As with most viral infections, no drug has any direct effect on the virus, and prevention in the form of vaccination is probably the best means of control. There are breeders who claim successful treatment using flowers of sulphur, applied to skin lesions or given orally. Removal of skin lesions with sodium bicarbonate washes, careful removal of diphtheritic membranes in the mouth to prevent choking, and the raising of the environmental temperature to about 15–20°F (8–11°C) below blood heat will probably be equally effective. The main danger, however, with these manipulations is that they may spread the infection to other parts of the skin via the hands and utensils.

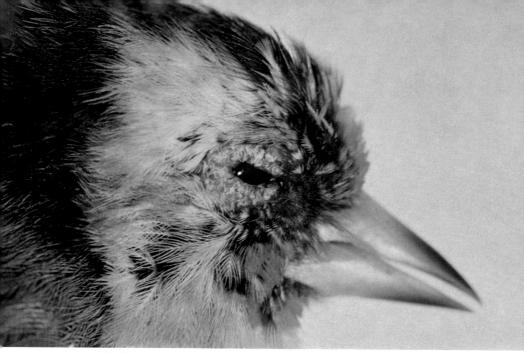

Plate 1/6. Head of a goldfinch showing raised wart-like lesions of the eye-lids probably caused by passerine pox virus. (I.F. Keymer)

Plate 2/6. Head of a racing pigeon showing typical wart-like lesions due to a chronic, severe infection with pigeon pox virus. (I.F. Keymer and T.C. Dennett, Zoological Society of London — Z.S.L.)

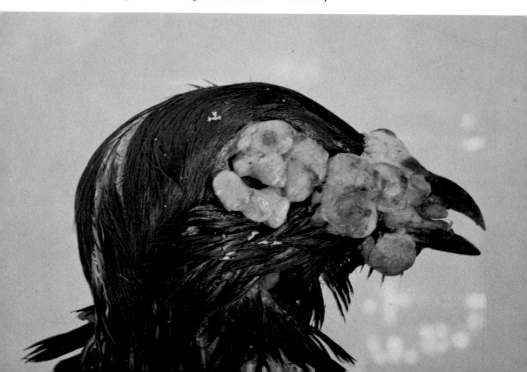

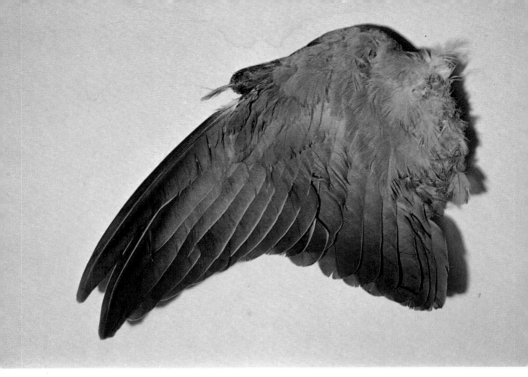

Plate 3/6. Wing removed from an immature woodpigeon showing chronic, necrotic lesion of pigeon pox affecting the terminal digits. (I.F. Keymer)

Plate 4/6. Exudate covering most of the internal viscera in a canary infected with pox. (D.K. Blackmore)

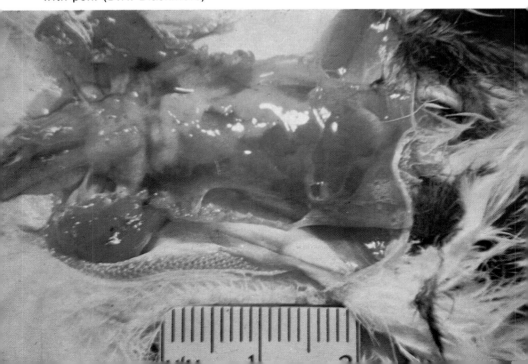

Bathing the eyes with 1-2 per cent saline solution followed by the application of a broad spectrum, antibiotic ointment containing chlortetracycline or oxytetracycline helps to combat conjunctivitis by eliminating bacteria. The infection, however, will run its course and usually clears up spontaneously, Nevertheless. bathing the eyes with a saline solution aids recovery, which may take at least a week.

A crude method of vaccination, which may protect healthy birds which cannot be isolated from those infected, is to dip the tip of a sterile scalpel into a freshly ruptured and discharging sore of an affected bird, and with it scratch a small area of skin on the wing, back or legs of each healthy bird. The slow dispersal of the virus from the scarified area allows antibodies to develop without a general infection arising and before most of the birds have time to become naturally infected. If the disease is already incubating, this procedure will not give protection and may even actively aid the invasiveness of the disease. The decision whether or not to practice this method of vaccination should be left to the veterinarian, who may be able to suggest a commercial vaccine rather than the use of the homegrown virulent virus.

Avian pox is most common in the temperate parts of the world and occurs mainly in the summer. Insects are probably responsible for some of the transmission from one premises to another, while wild birds can account for outbreaks spread over wider areas. Although primarily a contagious disease spread by direct contact, the survival of virus in scab particles, in feather debris and other substances, may result in infection via the mouth by contamination of food.

Ornithosis, Psittacosis or "Parrot Fever"

Probably more has been written about ornithosis than any other avian disease. It was first recognized and named in 1879. Because the disease is infectious and sometimes even fatal to human beings, the importation of psittacine species or parrot-like birds has been controlled in several countries as these species are especially susceptible to the infection. It was originally thought that a virus caused the infection, but it has now been established that the agent is a rickettsia-like organism, which is usually referred to as *Bedsonia* and more recently called *Chlamydia*.

Ornithosis, which literally means "bird disease" started its recognized life with the names psittacosis and parrot fever, because it was originally believed that only parrots were affected. When the seriousness of human infection was realised and cases arose in people not in contact with parrots or budgerigars, investigations were carried out on numerous other species. It is now known that many species in a variety of families of birds and small mammals also carry the disease, often with little or no clinical signs in the creatures themselves. Although psittacine birds still appear to account for the greatest number of cases, ornithosis also occurs occasionally in domestic poulty, (especially in turkeys, ducks and pigeons), certain seabirds and some other species. In Britain ornithosis is now common in parrots and also in budgerigars.

The virulence of the disease varies from species to species and from outbreak to outbreak. Investigations in England, have shown that a high percentage of pigeons develop an immunity to the disease, while a smaller number harbour the ornithosis agent with little clinical effect. Human infections derived from pigeons appear to be less serious and less common than those contracted from parrots. It is possible that birds in the parrot family have the power of increasing the disease's virulence for man. Alternatively, more virulent strains may survive best in psittacines.

The ornithosis agent is susceptible to some antibiotics, especially tetracyclines. It is of worldwide occurrence and is endemic in the bird population of many countries, as is shown by the detection of antibodies in the sera of many species. Only quite brief contact may be necessary for one bird to infect another or a human being. Transmission is by inspiration of the organism in water droplets or dust. A less common method of infection is via the mouth.

Although showing no clinical signs of disease, many birds excrete the organism in the droppings or nasal discharges, while the feather dust and debris may also be contaminated. Repeated passages through a succession of individuals occasionally results in an intensification of the virulence for that species, until some birds show obvious signs of the disease and even die. The most commonly infected cage, aviary and ornamental birds are the psittacines, including the entire range of parrots, parrotlets, parakeets, budgerigars, macaws, cockatoos, cockatiels, lories, lorikeets and lovebirds, as well as all types of pigeons and doves. Gamebirds, including pheasants, partridges, certain ducks and also species of hummingbirds, magpies, tits, thrushes, various finches including the Java sparrow, canaries and cardinals, and some members of the troupial family are occasionally infected. No list can be complete because new host species are frequently being found.

CLINICAL SIGNS Clinical signs of the disease include green or grey diarrhoea, listlessness, huddling, closing of the eyes and conjunctivitis, droopiness, occasionally a watery or pus-like discharge from the nostrils and/or beak, rattling respiratory sounds, rapid laboured breathing, lack of appetite, loss of weight, prostration and death. Flight is inhibited in older birds due to weakness and listlessness. Young stock are

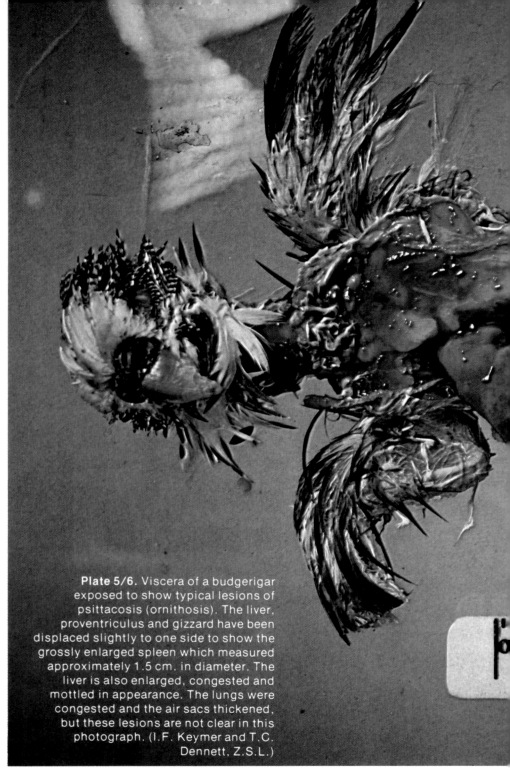

Plate 5/6. Viscera of a budgerigar exposed to show typical lesions of psittacosis (ornithosis). The liver, proventriculus and gizzard have been displaced slightly to one side to show the grossly enlarged spleen which measured approximately 1.5 cm. in diameter. The liver is also enlarged, congested and mottled in appearance. The lungs were congested and the air sacs thickened, but these lesions are not clear in this photograph. (I.F. Keymer and T.C. Dennett, Z.S.L.)

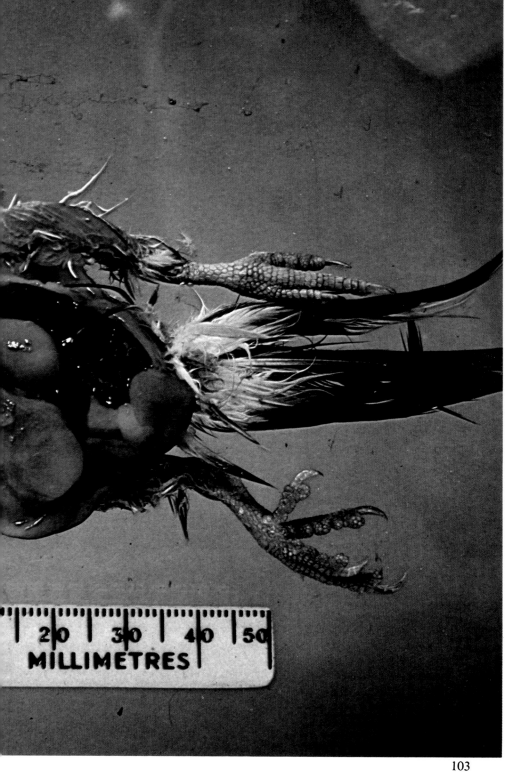

particularly susceptible. Intensively kept birds, such as those kept in large numbers in an aviary and bred collectively are most vulnerable to serious outbreaks. As with all diseases, the infection is less likely to occur in collections of birds where the hygiene is good and a balanced diet is fed.

It is important to realize that birds which survive the disease may carry the causal organism for long periods, excreting it continuously or intermittently. These dangerous birds are called carriers, and may never show signs of illness. Although it is still not certain, it appears possible that some species can transmit the infection to the embryo by laying infected eggs. The shell may also become contaminated and infect the chick on hatching if the parent does its own brooding, or alternatively the adult may directly infect the nestlings.

When transported long distances, birds are often subjected to stresses such as change of diet, fluctuating temperatures and restricted activity caused by overcrowding in cramped containers. Adverse conditions of this nature frequently lower the birds' resistance to disease and especially to ornithosis. The survivors, however, reach the dealers and pet shops, where, when weak and therefore tame, they may be sold by unscrupulous people to unsuspecting members of the public. Under such circumstances the disease often becomes virulent for man and other avian species. The isolated parrot imported by a seaman for his family and kept under good conditions usually becomes acclimatized by the time he gets it home, and if by then it is still healthy, it is likely to remain so. It may still, however, be a carrier and a potential source of infection to its owner or any other birds with which it comes into contact.

DIAGNOSIS It will be appreciated from what has been said that clinical signs are far from specific or diagnostic, although in typical cases the *post-mortem* lesions are fairly characteristic (Plate 5/6). The disease may be suspected from the pattern of infection in an area or premises. Confirmation, however, requires highly specialized laboratory techniques. One method is serological testing for antibodies of the disease. This is the usual method when human beings are involved. It is merely a method of measuring the amount of resistance the man or bird has developed in response to meeting the disease. If this happened a long time ago, the antibody level will be low. When the disease is being actively fought, however, the level rises rapidly. A fairly recent infection produces a high level of antibodies which only falls slowly over months or years.

Other stages such as complete recovery, the carrier state, or lack of adequate antibody response to infection all give inconclusive results. The presence of the infection in a bird can only be demonstrated with certainty after death by infecting a susceptible host, such as a mouse. This involves inoculating an extract of a piece of diseased liver, spleen or other internal organ into the brain or peritoneal cavity. Death of a proportion of inoculated mice showing certain characteristic lesions confirms the diagnosis. The disease can also be diagnosed by inoculation of the extracts into the yolk sacs of living embryonated eggs.

TREATMENT Infected birds should be destroyed. It is unwise to attempt treatment unless the dangers of the situation are appreciated and the premises and stock are self-contained. Treatment should be carried out only under the strict supervision of a veterinarian. The owner should not underestimate the considerable danger to himself, his family and others who may come into close contact with his birds or himself. The tetracyclines are the best drugs where treatment is thought prudent. They check, but do not necessarily kill the causal organism. Symptomatic treatment and careful nursing should accompany the specific antibiotic therapy.

Newcastle Disease (Fowl Pest)
This is a highly infectious and serious disease of poultry, being virtually world-wide in distribution. It is commonly called "fowl pest" in Great Britain, although this term also includes a similar viral infection of poultry more correctly known as "fowl plague". In some countries the disease in poultry is notifiable and if suspected it must be reported, so that the official veterinary officers can take steps to control the spread of infection. Many species are susceptible to the disease, but it occurs mainly in gallinaceous birds such as pheasants, partridges and quail, and birds of prey including owls, pigeons and psittacines. Except for recently imported parrots and other psittacines, which have undergone various stresses, most species usually become infected from poultry, particularly chickens. In the majority of species young birds are probably more susceptible than adults.

CLINICAL SIGNS Signs shown by pheasants, partridges and other game birds are similar to those seen in the domestic fowl. They vary according to the virulence of the virus but include difficulty in breathing with discharge from the nostrils, greenish or yellowish diarrhoea, tremors and paralysis of the legs and wings. Sometimes there is loss of balance and usually depression and ruffled feathers. Birds of prey may exhibit head shaking and sneezing, whilst pigeons show nervous rather than respiratory signs. In some species or when relatively mild strains of virus are involved, the signs

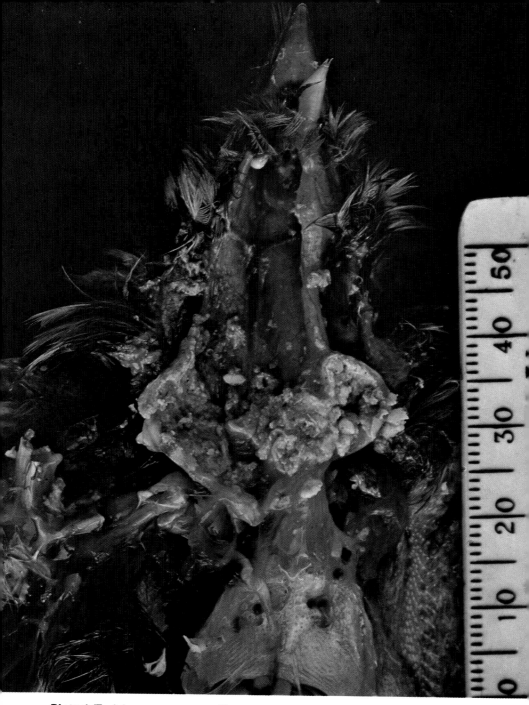

Plate 1/7. A house sparrow affected with *Salmonella typhimurium* infection of the crop. The ventral surface of the neck and thorax have been opened to show the soft, yellowish necrotic lesions affecting the crop epithelium. (I.F. Keymer and T.C. Dennett, Z.S.L.)

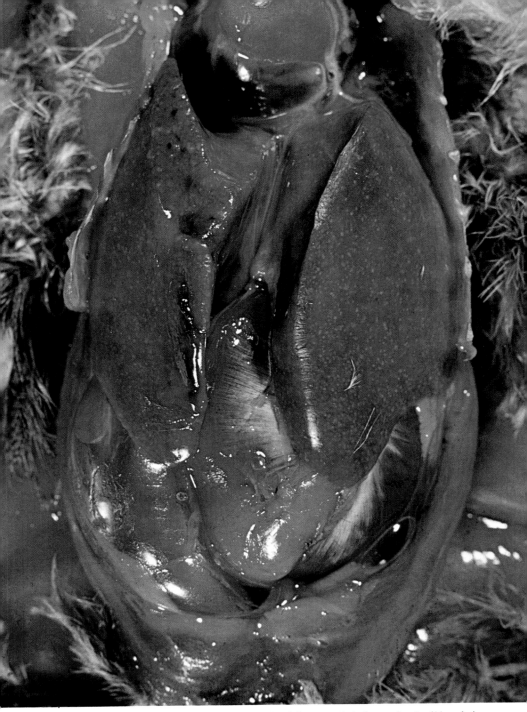

Plate 2/7. A common partridge infected with pseudotuberculosis (*Yersinia pseudotuberculosis* infection) showing minute, yellowish, necrotic foci evenly distributed throughout the liver. (I.F. Keymer)

may be vague, birds showing little more than depression and ruffled feathers.

In most species the infection is likely to be acute, birds dying within a few days of showing signs of illness.

DIAGNOSIS Whenever deaths occur in birds which are in close proximity to confirmed outbreaks of the infection in poultry, the disease should be suspected immediately. Although in some species the clinical signs may denote the possibility of the infection, it is not possible to confirm the disease without a proper *post-mortem* examination, including isolation and identification of the virus. The demonstration of antibodies to the disease in blood samples taken from live birds is also an important aid to diagnosis.

TREATMENT AND PREVENTION There is no treatment available. Prevention of the disease is important. Birds should be kept well away from domestic poultry, especially as the virus is capable of surviving for long periods under favourable conditions of temperature and humidity. All recently acquired birds, especially recently imported psittacines, should be kept in strict isolation for about a month, before being introduced to a collection. Ideally this means that they should be kept on different premises and cared for by a person who has no contact with other birds. Day-old chicks, raw poultry meat and feathers should never be used for feeding carnivorous species such as birds of prey, because they may be contaminated and are therefore a dangerous potential source of the virus. The infection is also easily transmitted to other birds via excreta and nasal exudates.

Vaccines are available for gallinaceous birds such as the domestic fowl. The vaccines may be either "live" or "dead", that is containing living or artificially inactivated virus. Both types of vaccine afford protection from the disease for only short periods of time. Although the "live" vaccines contain only mildly virulent strains of virus, their use should be confined to gallinaceous birds, because they may be fatal to many other species. Although there is little information available regarding the value of vaccination for birds other than poultry, there is some indication that it may help to protect birds of prey from the disease. The types of vaccines available vary in different countries and a veterinarian should always be consulted for advice regarding their use.

Herpesvirus Infection of Pigeons; Smadel's Viral Infection; One-eyed Roup or Ophthalmia

The clinical signs shown by racing pigeons infected with *Herpes* virus or ornithosis are similar and impossible to diagnose in these birds without laboratory examination. It follows therefore that the diseases, known by pigeon breeders as roup, ophthalmia or "eye-colds", may be either of these diseases or indeed *Mycoplasma* infections.

CLINICAL SIGNS Birds under a year old are mostly affected. Watery eye discharge indicating a conjunctivitis and nasal discharge due to rhinitis or inflammation of the nasal passages, are almost constant features of the disease, and some may also show respiratory distress caused by the mucous membrane of the larynx being coated by a diphtheritic membrane. Small ulcers and yellowish-brown cheesy material may be present in the pharynx, larynx and oesophagus, and tracheitis or inflammation of the trachea is sometimes present. Without microscopical and other laboratory diagnostic methods the mouth and oesophageal lesions are indistinguishable from trichomoniasis. Lesions in the internal organs include hepatitis and nephritis.

TREATMENT There is no specific treatment for the virus itself and in the absence of a confirmatory laboratory diagnosis, cases should be treated as recommended for ornithosis, *Mycoplasma* infection or trichomoniasis, depending upon the circumstances.

Other Viral Infections

It is not within the scope of this book to deal with all the other viral infections which may be met in birds. Textbooks on poultry diseases should be consulted for information on infectious laryngotracheitis, infectious bronchitis, encephalomyelitis (epidemic tremor), fowl plague, the lymphoid leukosis complex including Marek's disease, avian monocytosis and infectious synovitis. All of these are virtually confined to the domestic fowl, although infectious laryngotracheitis has been diagnosed in pheasants, and fowl plague in waterfowl. Books on poultry diseases should also be consulted for information on viral diseases of waterfowl: duck plague or duck virus enteritis and duck virus hepatitis.

Several species of seabirds become infected with a virus known as puffinosis or vesicular dermatitis. Quail bronchitis is mainly confined to game-bird farms in North America.

Lesser known viral infections of non-domesticated species of birds include rabies, viral hepatosplenitis of owls, Pacheco's parrot disease, avian influenza and a "virus hepatitis". Perhaps least is known about the last mentioned infection.

Aegyptianellosis, which is probably a rickettsial infection although previously believed to be due to protozoa, is mainly a disease of geese and the domestic fowl.

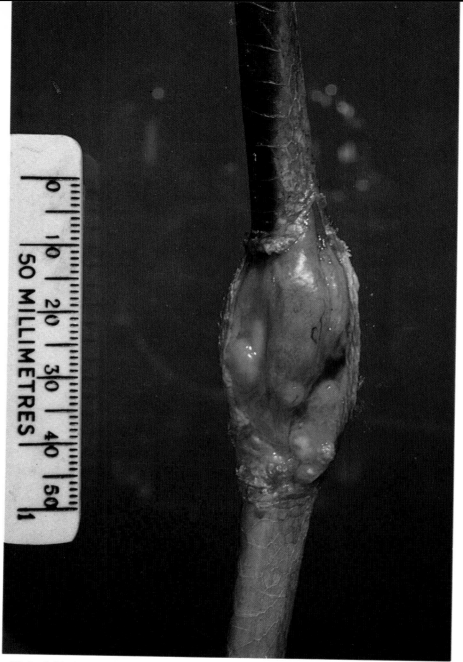

Plate 3/7. Anterior aspect of the exposed femero-tibiotarsal (hock) joint of an Eastern purple heron showing lesions of staphylococcal synovitis and arthritis. The joint is swollen, the tissues around the joint capsule are congested and small, yellowish-white lesions are present containing pus from which *Staphylococcus pyogenes* bacteria were isolated. (I.F. Keymer and T. C. Dennett, Z.S.L.)

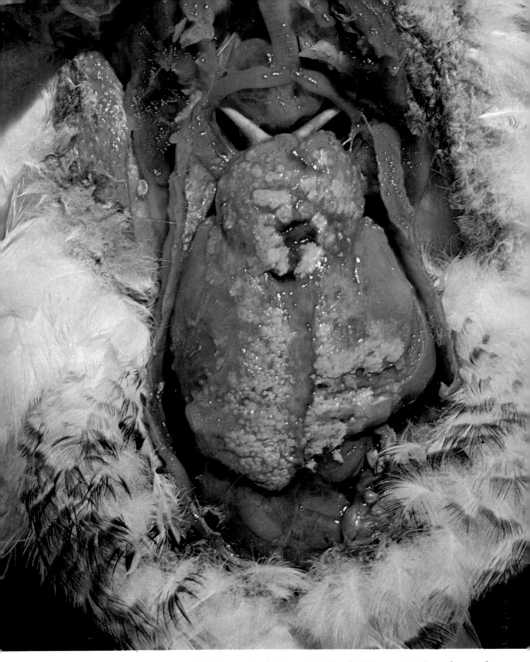

Plate 4/7. A severe case of tuberculosis in a shelduck. The ventral surface of the body has been opened to expose extensive, caseous, yellowish necrotic lesions covering the pericardial sac (enclosing the heart) and the liver (below). The liver is enlarged and is obscuring most of the intestinal tract. In addition to pericarditis, peritonitis was also present and the spleen was virtually replaced by necrotic tissue. Pneumonia of a relatively acute type was also present. (I.F. Keymer and T.C. Dennett, Z.S.L.)

Many species of free-flying birds carry viruses belonging to the arthropod-borne encephalitides. Some of these so-called arboviruses are important infections of man and domestic mammals, but they seldom seem to be responsible for clinical disease in birds.

It can be stated categorically that poliomyelitis virus is not a natural inhabitant of avian tissues. The observation which eventually reached the newspapers a few years ago concerning the isolation of the virus from a budgerigar and the presence of antibodies to poliomyelitis virus in serum from one of these birds merely indicated contamination with the virus from an infected human contact. No evidence could be found that this or other individuals of the species were truly susceptible to the disease.

SELECTED BIBLIOGRAPHY

ARNSTEIN, P. & MEYER, K. L. (1969). Psittacosis and Ornithosis. In *Diseases of Cage and Aviary Birds,* p.384–391. Ed. Petrak, M. L., Philadelphia, Lea and Febiger.

BIESTER, H. E. & SCHWARTE, L. H. (1965). *Diseases of Poultry,* p.512–843. 5th Ed. Ames, Iowa. State University Press.

BURKHART, R. L. & PAGE, L. A. (1971). Chalmydiosis (Ornithosis—Psittacosis). In *Infectious and Parasitic Diseases of Wild Birds,* p.118–140. Eds. Davis, J. W., Anderson, R. C., Karstad, L. and Trainer, D. O. Ames, Iowa. State University Press.

CAVILL, J. P. (1969). Viral Diseases. In *Diseases of Cage and Aviary Birds,* p.373–383. Ed. Petrak, M. L., Philadelphia. Lea and Febiger.

HUNGERFORD, T. G. (1969). *Diseases of Poultry including Cage Birds and Pigeons,* p.119–122. 4th Ed. Sydney, London, Melbourne. Angus and Robertson.

KARSTAD, L. (1971). Pox. In *Infectious and Parasitic Diseases of Wild Birds,* p. 34–41. Eds. Davis, J. W., Anderson, R. C., Karstad, L. and Trainer, D. O. Ames, Iowa. State University Press.

MEYER, K. F. (1965). Ornithosis. In *Diseases of Poultry,* p.675–770. Eds. Biester, H. E. and Schwarte, L. H. 5th Ed. Ames, Iowa. State University Press.

PALMER, S. F. & TRAINER, D. O. (1971). Newcastle Disease. In *Infectious and Parasitic Diseases of Wild Birds,* p.3–16. Eds. Davis, J. W., Anderson, R. C., Karstad, L. and Trainer, D. O. Ames, Iowa. State University Press.

BACTERIAL INFECTIONS

No method of naming diseases is completely satisfactory; for in only a small proportion of cases does a single known microbe cause a recognizable disease. Frequently, one infection can produce several merging or distinct manifestations in various groups of birds, it may also show different signs in different species. Alternatively, one well-recognized group of clinical signs may be caused by several bacteria or viruses as the result of a variety of different pathological changes. Organisms, while not in themselves capable of causing a recognizable disease, may often produce a weakened bird which is the prey to other more pathogenic bacteria capable of creating a clearer picture of disease.

In this section diseases will be described which are caused by specific bacteria or groups of bacteria. Clinical diseases in which the cause is multiple or unknown or which are of a local nature, will for the most part be found under the region or system concerned.

Salmonellosis, Paratyphoid or Infectious Enteritis

These names are given to the disease caused by any one of the numerous related but different species of bacteria called *Salmonellae*. They are closely related to *Escherichia coli* and paracolons mentioned later and belong to the family of gut organisms *Enterobacteriaceae*. Minor reclassification is constantly going on and new members are frequently being discovered. Although only a proportion of species or serotypes are of importance in birds, the disease they produce may under some circumstances be severe. Many of the avian species and strains of *Salmonellae* are also capable of infecting reptiles, mammals and man.

Paratyphoid infections are of special importance in many species of cage birds, especially in mixed aviaries, breeding establishments, pet shops, and indeed all places where a number of birds are kept closely together. Because of the relatively high incidence of the organisms in some wild birds, *e.g.* house sparrows (Plate 1/7), their presence in rodents and the almost inevitable presence of mice and rats near aviaries, attracted by spilt seed and other food, transmission

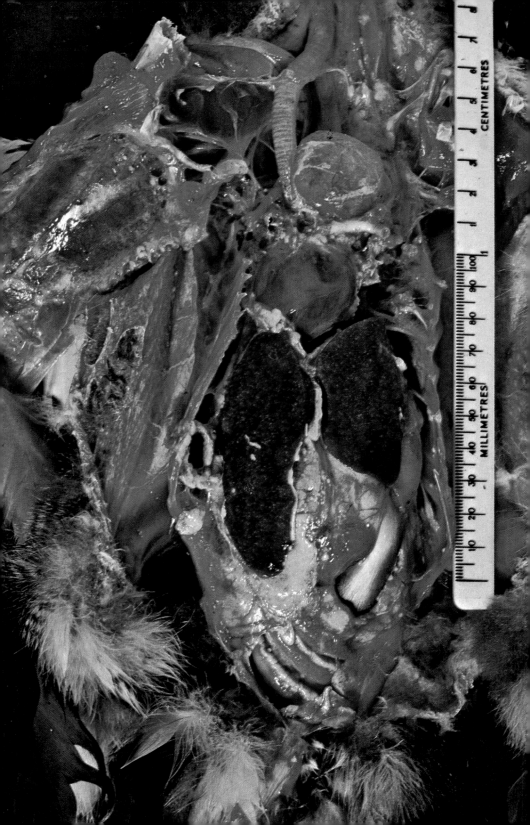

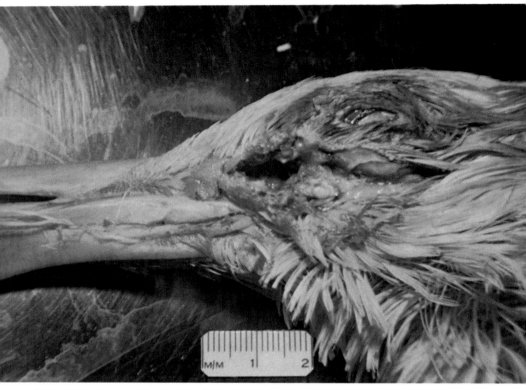

Plate 1/8. Aspergillosis infection of the infra-orbital sinus of a herring gull. Note the presence of whitish, caseous necrotic material in the opened sinus. (D.K. Blackmore)

Plate 5/7. Internal viscera of an ashy-headed goose exposed to show lesions caused by tuberculosis. The liver is the most conspicuous organ and shows multiple pale areas and minute, whitish foci of necrosis through-out. Below the liver lesions of peritonitis can be seen, characterized by yel-lowish-white, necrotic fat with adhesions to the gizzard and loops of the in-testine. (I.F. Keymer and T.C. Dennett, Z.S.L.)

of infection to captive birds is a constant danger. In indoor aviaries, with brick floors and very fine mesh netting, such unwelcome species can usually be excluded.

Salmonella typhimurium, S. enteritidis, S. oranienburg, S. anatum, S. thomson and *S. paratyphi* are examples of the many types which may be encountered in a wide variety of species which include among many others, doves, quail, pheasants, water birds of all kinds, canaries and other finches, sugar birds, parrots, budgerigars and robins. The majority of infections are caused by *S. typhimurium* and smaller numbers by other *Salmonellae*. In some birds, especially waterfowl and poultry, these infections can affect embryos in the egg by contamination of the shell with infected droppings. Less frequently, and notably in waterfowl, embryo infection may be derived from an infected ovary. Because cage-bird eggs are almost all hatched in the nest and seldom artificially incubated, most *Salmonella* transference to nestlings is probably from the parent birds soon after hatching. Incubator hatching, if perfected for cage birds, would in most species greatly limit spread in the young. The infection of adult or growing stock occurs in three main ways:

1. Contamination of food at source; proprietory egg food is a potential danger.
2. Contamination of food or water by rodents or wild birds in the aviary or store.
3. Contact with a newly-acquired infected bird.

Less commonly, infection is spread at shows or as the result of handling by visitors who have been in contact with the bacteria. Spread throughout an establishment is aided by overcrowding, allowing food to become stale, scattering seed and food where it can attract vermin, and other unhygienic practices. Flies and some parasites are also capable of transmitting the disease, while *S. typhimurium* is able to live for almost four months in stagnant water in temperate climates.

CLINICAL SIGNS In an outbreak, the initial picture may depend on the source of infection and the age groups first affected. The severity may also depend to some degree on the type of *Salmonella* responsible. The severest and most acute outbreaks are usually seen in young chicks, for example, when infected egg food is fed to parents and later to offspring. The parents at this stage may show little evidence of disease. However, low hatchability rates, dead-in-shell or weak newly-hatched chicks, and chicks "fading" during the first few days of life are strongly suggestive of the infection. The blood, other tissues and droppings of such chicks as well as the parents' excreta, are rich sources of the organisms. As little as 10 per cent of all eggs incubated may hatch, and all of these chicks may die before leaving the nest. The effect of a long-

116

established infection, however, may be much less spectacular. Newly-hatched chicks which are affected are likely to be small, weakly, bedraggled and produce loose droppings, giving rise to the condition called "sweating" by some breeders. It is sometimes thought that a single hen has merely been clumsy when the flattened dead chicks are later found in or thrown out of the nest, but poor hatchability in several nests should point to a more serious cause.

Losses usually start a few days to two weeks after eating contaminated seed or other food. According to the virulence of the organism and the susceptibility of the species concerned, clinical signs may last only a day or two with occasional losses over several weeks or, within 10 days of the first death, as much as 90 per cent of the growing and adult stock may be dead. Signs range from sudden death to gradual onset of depression over one to three days, accompanied by huddling of the birds, fluffed-up feathers, unsteadiness, shivering, loss of appetite, markedly increased or absence of thirst, rapid loss of weight, accelerated respiration, and watery yellow, green, fawn, or occasionally grey or blood-tinged droppings. The vent feathers become matted with excreta, the eyes begin to close, and immediately before death some birds show apparent blindness, inco-ordination, staggering, tremours, or other nervous signs including convulsions. In addition pigeons sometimes show arthritis, especially of the wings. A really sick bird seldom recovers even with appropriate treatment.

DIAGNOSIS Diagnosis cannot be made on the basis of clinical signs alone. Confirmation depends on isolating the bacteria from the heart blood or lesions of dead birds and the droppings of live, recovered carriers, but this can only be done in a properly equipped laboratory. In an establishment where occasional losses have been experienced in several age groups, examination of droppings from birds which have been in close contact with the dead birds should be made because salmonellosis can be well established before it is even suspected. When an infection is well distributed throughout the stock and established, but not causing heavy losses, it is said to be endemic or enzootic. When an infection suddenly wreaks havoc in an aviary, causing a high incidence of clinical disease and deaths, it is referred to as an epidemic or epizootic. Paratyphoid or salmonellosis can produce both situations.

The blood-testing methods for antibodies (agglutination tests) used in the related pullorum disease or bacillary white diarrhoea (B.W.D.) of poultry and caused by *S. pullorum*, and fowl typhoid (*S. gallinarum* infection) have not been used very much for cage birds, but represent a useful means of identifying carrier birds harbouring a particular strain of

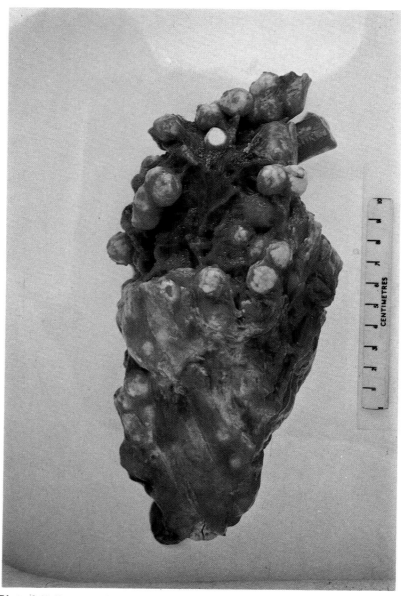

Plate 2/8 (Intact lung). Chronic, severe aspergillosis in the lung of a king penguin showing numerous granulomatous nodules. The photograph on page 119 shows a section of this same lung. (I.F. Keymer and T.C. Dennett, Z.S.L.)

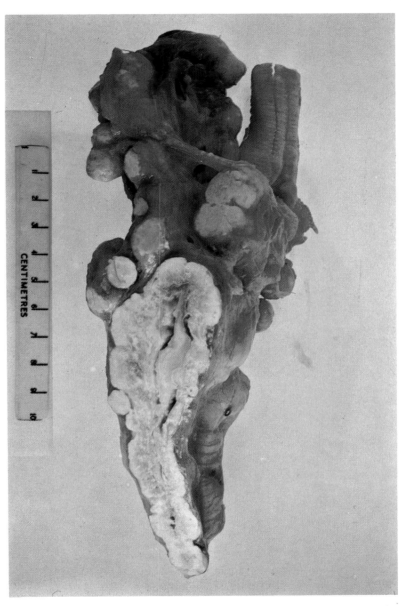

Plate 2/8 (Section of same lung). Aspergillosis in the lung of a king penguin. The section through the lung shows that many of the lesions have fused to form an elongated mass of necrotic material which towards the centre is deposited in layers. The air sacs were also affected. (I.F. Keymer and T.C. Dennett, Z.S.L.)

119

organism. Unfortunately, when small birds are infected, blood testing is impractical as sufficient blood cannot be obtained without seriously jeopardising the birds' lives. Negative results also sometimes occur in birds previously known to have been infected. However, in cage birds, recognition that a pathogenic strain of *Salmonella* is present in carcases or in droppings is sufficient warning to commence remedial measures.

Infectious diseases of cage birds, particularly those of an acute nature, often present similar features regardless of cause. Salmonellosis therefore, especially in adults, can be confused with such infections as pasteurellosis or pseudo-tuberculosis.

TREATMENT AND PREVENTION It must be stressed that, short of destroying all infected birds, carriers and those in contact, it is unlikely that an establishment can be entirely cleared of the infection. If rodents or wild birds can gain access, they will soon be acting as a reservoir of the organism. Because of the individual financial and sentimental value of cage birds, treatment is more generally attempted than in the case of poultry. This reduces mortality and greatly slows the onset of new cases of clinical illness but masks infected birds by turning them into symptomless carriers. Treatment must be prolonged, and repeated at intervals in all valuable birds. Breeding should also be discontinued for the current year. Some would say that once birds are infected they should never be used for breeding again. Minor or major fresh outbreaks are to be expected in following seasons, especially if sudden change of food occurs, also during a cold spell or breeding, or indeed during any conditions of stress. The greatest success in treatment has occurred with the drugs furazolidone and spectinomycin. Sulphonamides, particularly sulphadimidine and sulphadiazine are also quite effective in reducing losses and checking clinical signs. The tetracyclines, chloramphenicol and neomycin generally appear to be less effective, although some strains respond reasonably well. It is advisable therefore to combine or alternate two or more of these drugs. Where drug-sensitivity tests are available, which indicate the particular efficiency of either one or more drugs, these drugs should of course be used.

No commercial vaccines and sera are available, but some success has been reported with vaccines made from *Salmonella* isolated from birds on the affected premises. These "autogenous vaccines" are said by their advocates to be helpful in controlling outbreaks where the infection is established.

The most important factors for prevention are cleanliness, care in the choice and origin of foodstuffs, vermin-proof premises, isolation of new stock and all stock after visits to shows, and the avoidance of buying any but healthy birds, no matter how much of an asset their possession might appear to be.

Other *Salmonellae* and Related Bacteria of the Gut. *Salmonella pullorum* and *S. gallinarum*

These are both pathogens of poultry and only affect a relatively small proportion of the birds with which we are mainly concerned. Most species appear to be resistant to pullorum disease and fowl typhoid (*S. gallinarum* infection), but canaries, parrots and some finches in particular can become infected occasionally. Reports are few and signs differ so much between outbreaks that no purpose would be served by listing them. The symptoms are very similar to those described for paratyphoid above, and bacteriological examinations are essential for an accurate diagnosis.

Paracolon infections are even less common, the bacteria being distinguished by their biochemical properties rather than from the disease which they produce.

Escherichia coli

Coliform organisms, of great importance in calves, pigs and several other domestic mammals, are closely related to *Salmonella*. They are mostly normal inhabitants of the guts of healthy animals. A few strains are capable of causing disease in cage birds, especially when introduced into a different part of the body, for example, the oviduct, or abdominal cavity. It is possible that some underlying illness—such as chilling or a viral infection—enables *Escherichia coli* to gain access to these sites. In cage birds *E. coli* may give rise to a septicaemia; an inflamed oviduct associated with egg-binding or retained egg material; peritonitis; pneumonia in association with a failing circulation or aspergillosis; septic arthritis such as "bumble foot", and chronic air sacculitis. The organism is seldom discovered until necropsy is performed and bacteriological examination carried out. Diarrhoea or sudden death are often the only signs with septicaemic and peritoneal infections; young, previously weakened birds are most likely to succumb. Canaries, pigeons, quail and budgerigars are among species liable to be infected. *E. coli* is not a normal inhabitant of budgerigars' intestines and the finding of this organism, even in the droppings from apparently normal birds, should be looked upon with suspicion.

TREATMENT When there are surviving, ailing, birds, the tetracyclines, furazolidone, or sulphonamides are most likely to be effective.

121

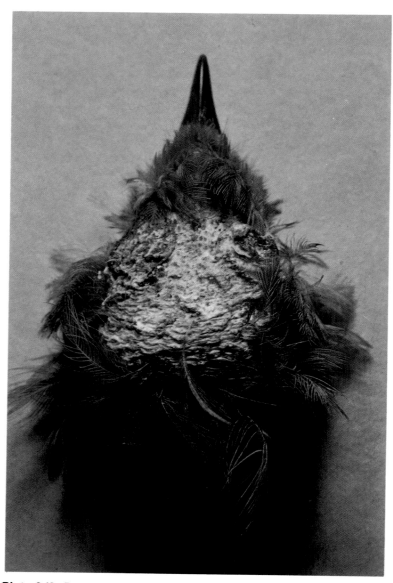

Plate 3/8. Dorsal aspect of the head of a European robin showing skin lesions probably caused by a *Trichophyton* sp. of fungus. There is complete loss of feathers in the affected area and the skin is thrown up into dry, thickened and whitish encrustations. (I.F. Keymer)

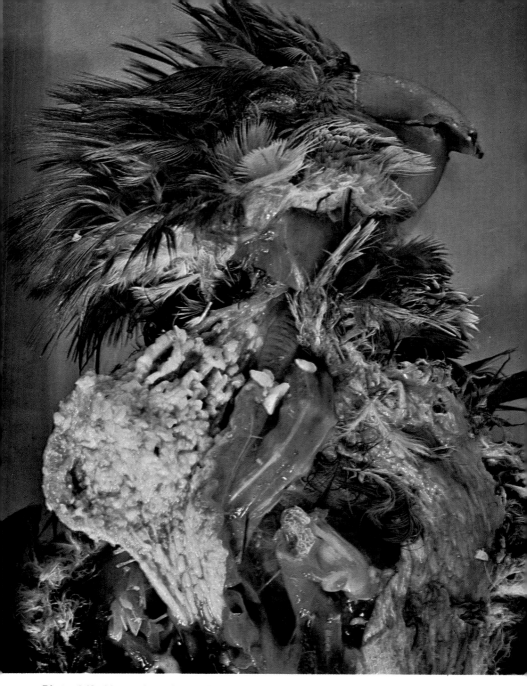

Plate 4/8. Ventral surface of the neck and thorax of a quaker parakeet exposed to show lesions of candidiasis caused by *Candida albicans* involving the epithelium of the crop and parts of the oesophagus. The lesions are present in the form of a thick, soft, whitish deposit which is mainly loosely attached to the underlying epithelium. (I.F. Keymer and T.C. Dennett, Z.S.L.)

Infections with *Pasteurella septica* occasionally occur in cage and aviary birds. The disease may occur either in epidemic form or sporadically. Some birds may remain carriers, shedding a few bacteria in nasal discharges or droppings for at least a year. As with other infections, external parasites and flies are of importance in infecting a hitherto clean establishment. Vermin, including wild birds contaminating the aviary with droppings, are probably a more dangerous source.

Transmission occurs by inhalation of infected material in the form of water droplets or dust and by eating infected food.

Probably all avian species, including poultry, gamebirds, waterfowl, some birds of prey, pigeons, and numerous species kept as cage birds or in zoological gardens are susceptible to some degree.

Pasteurellosis, Avian Cholera, or Haemorrhagic Septicaemia (*Pasteurella septica; P. avium* or *P. multocida* infection)

CLINICAL SIGNS The pattern of disease varies. Multiple rapid deaths with few warning signs may occur three to ten days after introduction of the infection. Sometimes the illness may last a few days and show a wide range of clinical signs, while a residual group of birds which are sickly may survive and become carriers. When a bird actively shedding bacteria is introduced into a "clean" aviary the mortality is likely to be high and can approach 100 per cent. A previously fit bird may suddenly become quiet and depressed and sit motionless on the perch or floor. Within a few hours the depression deepens, the eyes close, feathers become fluffed up, the bird becomes unsteady on its feet and collapses. Before death, fluttering or convulsions may be noted, or the bird may stiffen, throw back its head, or possibly utter a squeaking sound and become limp. Rapid breathing is frequently seen in the early stages. Death can occur during flight, or while eating or scratching, without being preceded by any signs of malaise.

When birds become infected later in an outbreak, and in more resistant individuals or species, the symptoms are clearer. Again, there is a degree of listlessness, shivering, and huddling. There may be pasty, fawn, or yellow droppings and sometimes rattling respiratory sounds, sneezing and sticky nasal discharges. The feathers around the vent, eyes, and beak may become matted. Appetite may persist, at least until late in the disease, and the thirst is also often unaffected. The droppings may become blood-stained due to ulceration of the intestines. Death in this type of the disease is not inevitable and survivors tend to show signs of the chronic type of the infection. The chronic disease is characterized by marked loss of weight, moderate loss of bodily activity and appetite, swelling of the abdomen, lameness and swelling of the joints, and in some cases scaly or crusty lesions on the unfeathered parts of the head.

124

Diagnosis depends on isolating the causal bacteria from blood or other tissues of a dead or sick bird. Blood-testing for *Pasteurella* antibodies is not yet reliable.

TREATMENT AND PREVENTION Vaccines have not yet proved effective or safe. Dead, chemically treated *Pasteurellae* as used in vaccines are poor stimulators of antibody production.

When an infectious disease such as pasteurellosis is suspected, remedial measures should be applied at once. Sulphonamides are the most effective drugs, particularly sulphadimidine. The antibiotics, except streptomycin which is too toxic for most species, are generally much less effective than sulphonamides both in lowering mortality and in checking the occurrence of the more chronic stages. Treatment must be continued during alternate weeks for at least six weeks to enable a reasonable check to be made on the disease. Severely ill birds, those with chronic nasal discharges, intermittent diarrhoea, and birds showing any signs of malaise should be treated in isolation if very valuable, but preferably killed and burnt.

If the general principles of good husbandry are observed, in particular strict hygiene, the risk of introducing this disease into a collection will be minimized.

Pseudotuberculosis (*Yersinia pseudotuberculosis* or *Pasteurella pseudotuberculosis* infection)

Pseudotuberculosis, so named because it produces yellowish or whitish, tuberculosis-like lesions in various tissues during the later stages of the disease (Plate 2/7), is primarily a disease of birds, rabbits and rodents. It is not uncommon in monkeys and may be more common in man than generally realized, because it produces symptoms resembling appendicitis. Numerous species of mammals and birds are susceptible. The disease tends to arise sporadically, infecting one or two individuals, rather than whole aviaries of birds. The disease was first reported in the canary and this together with turkey, is the species most commonly and severely affected. The infection also occurs in pigeons, sparrows, finches, toucans, members of the Corvidae (crow family) and gamebirds. The organisms are usually introduced into the body via the alimentary tract, or occasionally through skin wounds.

The disease begins as a septicemia which is very short lived and need not be apparent clinically. During this brief period the organisms can be isolated from the blood. In a few cases, especially with canaries, death may occur during this phase. More often, the infected bird survives a little longer and many of the bacteria are killed in the circulation, whilst others thrive and become localized in the liver, spleen, kidney, lungs, gut wall or under the skin, producing the characteristic cheesy masses or nodules.

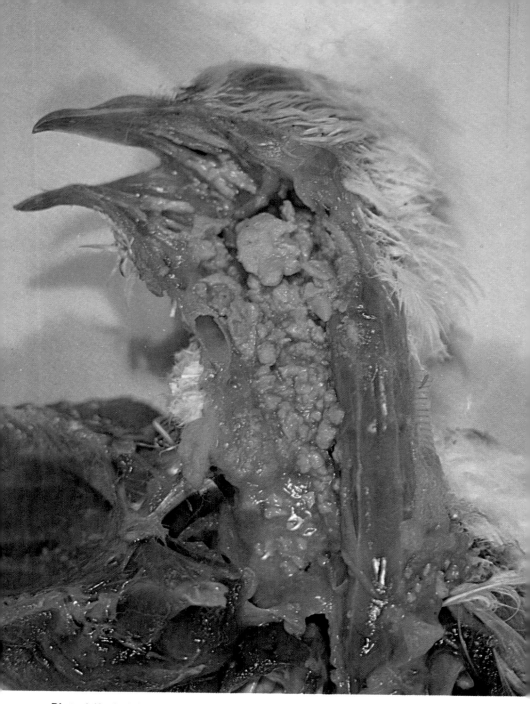

Plate 1/9. A domestic pigeon with severe, chronic trichomoniasis or canker involving the epithelium of the mouth, oesophagus and crop. The mouth and ventral surface of the neck have been opened to show the extensive necrotic lesions covering the epithelial surfaces. (I.F. Keymer)

126

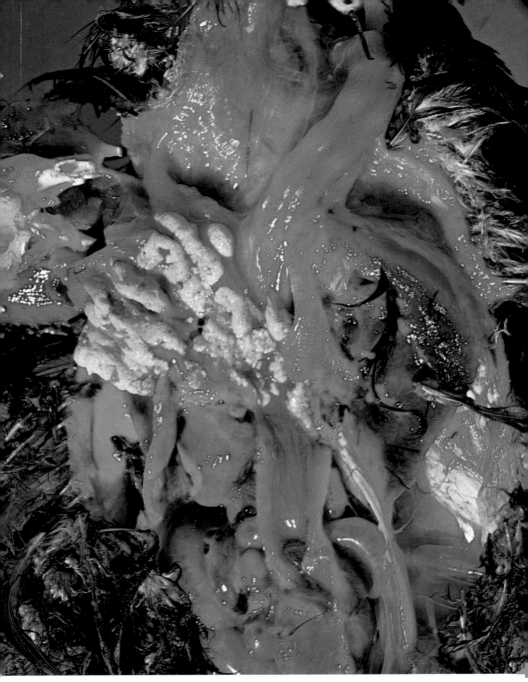

Plate 2/9. Lesions of trichomoniasis affecting the crop epithelium of a domestic pigeon. The ventral surface of the body has been opened, the liver removed and the crop lining exposed. Note the white lesions which are soft in consistency and cover the underlying reddened (congested) epithelium. Compare with Plates 1/7 and 4/8. (I.F. Keymer and T.C. Dennett, Z.S.L.)

CLINICAL SIGNS The incubation period between infection and development of clinical signs, varies from two days to two weeks. Short of unheralded death, the earliest signs are not distinct, being similar to any septicaemia with depression, fluffing of feathers, panting and diarrhoea including watery urate excretion. Those birds with a more chronic form of the disease show dullness, loss of weight, ruffled plumage, intermittent diarrhoea or occasionally abnormally hard droppings. The breathing may at times also be laboured. Loss of weight may extend to emaciation, this being one of the "going light" diseases of cage birds. As depression deepens, appetite falls sharply. The chronically affected bird is reluctant to move and, if hustled, may show a lameness or unsteady gait, marked weakness, or even appear paralyzed, according to the tissues mainly involved.

TREATMENT AND PREVENTION Broad spectrum antibiotics as indicated by sensitivity tests and given by injection, may help to reduce losses. No really satisfactory treatment is available, however, and no reliable vaccine has been produced. The disease is extremely difficult to prevent because it is carried by many species of free-living birds and rodents, which may contaminate both the quarters and the food.

Streptococcal Infections

These small, round bacteria, which tend to form chains, are capable of causing abscesses, infecting wounds and producing valvular disease of the heart. They are less important in birds than in mammals. Birds which may become infected occasionally, include canaries, various finches, sparrows, and parrots. The infection enters via wounds and probably the respiratory or alimentary tracts.

CLINICAL SIGNS The diseases caused by *Streptococci* in birds may be localized infections of repeatedly injured or pecked wounds, septic arthritis known as "bumble foot" or egg peritonitis. Generalized systemic or septicaemic illness may also occur. Septicaemia is the spread of infection throughout the body by the blood stream when the *Streptococci* are liable to cause death within 24 hours. The body temperature rises 2-4°F., and panting, fluffing of feathers, huddling, gaping, and depression may be observed 6 to 12 hours before death. At necropsy all the internal organs are congested, being a dark, purplish red in colour. They are also swollen, and samples of blood are found to be rich in *Streptococci*. The losses in an outbreak may sometimes be high, especially in canaries. In some birds the depression is replaced by nervous stimulation, the birds becoming excitable, jumping at a sharp sound, flash of light, or quick movement, and flying or blundering wildly against the bars of the cage or the aviary. Convulsive fits, with complete inco-ordination and nervous derangement may lead to self-inflicted damage, particularly to the head. For this reason haemorrhages over and within the cranium may be seen in this form of the disease. These haemorrhages, which are also found elsewhere in the body, are more likely to be the result rather than the cause of the inco-ordinated activity.

In cases of rapid death, there is the possibility that it is due to streptococcal waste products or toxins which are produced outside the body in stale food (especially egg food) and then eaten. The bacteria may also be eaten and digested, and the toxins absorbed.

Sometimes a more prolonged, chronic or gastrointestinal illness is seen. This takes the form of loose droppings of various colouration, occasional regurgitation, progressive and extreme loss of weight and dull plumage. During the course of one or two weeks canaries may develop a greenish diarrhoea. The bird loses weight and develops a preference for soft food. The body temperature slowly falls and is markedly subnormal shortly before death. Affected birds often continue eating until death is imminent, which may be preceded by twitching or other nervous signs. Although muscle wastage is severe, the abdomen is usually enlarged. The congested intestines and other organs give rise to a purplish colouration which is visible through the abdominal wall.

Differential diagnosis includes other bacterial and viral infections and poisoning by organo-phosphorus and other compounds. The disease therefore is virtually impossible to diagnose without recourse to bacteriological examination.

TREATMENT In an isolated case, it is unlikely that the cause will be recognized at least until necropsy and laboratory examinations have been carried out. It is inevitable therefore, for treatment to be empirical, as is so frequently the case when treating single sick birds. When a series of losses occur, it is essential to submit carcases for necropsy and bacteriological examination irrespective of which disease is suspected, so that treatment can be placed on a more secure, scientific footing.

Theoreticaliy, streptococcosis should respond well to antibiotics, because the bacteria are sensitive to most antibiotics when grown in the laboratory. Subject to laboratory recommendations, penicillin and the tetracyclines are most likely to be effective. The best route of administration depends on the drug to be used, the species and other factors. Good nursing, moderate warmth, a preliminary gentle laxative and an easily digested diet are essential.

For information on localized streptococcal infections, see "arthritis" and "bumble foot", (Chapter 21, Abscesses and Granulomas).

CLINICAL SIGNS *Staphylococci*, like the *Streptococci*, do not often produce purulent lesions in birds. Wounds most usually infected are those which are repeatedly pecked or knocked by the bird, especially on the breast, cere, bastard wing and eyelids. Foot lesions are commonly infected ("bumble foot") and also the most likely to develop pus formation.

Staphylococcal Infections

Joints are the characteristic sites for staphylococcal infections (see Plate 3/7), although the route by which they become infected is not always apparent. When one or both hock joints are involved, it is probable that infection arose through the skin in the region, but when several joints are affected it implies that the organisms were previously circulating in the blood and later became localized in the joints. Such a form of arthritis usually weakens the bird, causing loss of weight and eventually death.

Staphylococcal arthritis of the feet or legs causes lameness and usually swollen joints. Eventually the bird can only shuffle on its hocks and beak. The hocks and plantar surfaces or undersides of the toes are the most common sites, but any joint of the legs, wings, and even the spinal column can be involved. Swollen joints are painful when squeezed or manipulated. The "joint oil" or synovial fluid instead of being small in quantity and a clear, straw-coloured, slimy fluid, increases in amount and becomes opaque, filled with pus and later cheese-like in consistency. The circumstances in which staphylococcal arthritis can occur are partly managemental such as the use of coarse sand paper for cage floors, rough perches and hard, rough, concrete floor for aviaries. In outside aviaries frost bite may be a predisposing cause. Similarly birds with bone diseases and other affections causing partial paralysis of the feet or limbs are most likely to be affected, as well as those showing general weakness and debility. This is because such birds tend to spend a lot of time on the floor; minor abrasions and scratches easily occur and these are invaded by ever-present organisms. Eventually the affected joints fill with scar tissue, further restricting movement, and distortions of the limb due to tendon contraction result. It is usually adult and middle-aged birds which become affected and those with long toes and legs such as wading birds. These and various other semi-aquatic species when kept in captivity are particularly prone to arthritis. Indeed it is one of the hazards of rehabilitating previously oiled sea birds such as guillemots and razorbills.

Staphylococcal infection of the air sacs occasionally occurs if they have been directly exposed to the outside air by external injury, the organisms sometimes being associated with other bacteria and fungi such as *Aspergillus*.

TREATMENT AND PREVENTION Treatment with furazolidone or tetracyclines may limit the infection, especially by controlling infection of internal organs, but the arthritis is rarely cleared by such treatment. Incising the joint, scraping, and washing out the exudate with saline solution and packing it with an appropriate antibiotic and compound containing a digestive enzyme is more likely to succeed. Such treatment must of course be carried out by a veterinarian because it is very easy to cause permanent damage to joints.

Staphylococcal infections are nearly always sporadic and, although the organisms are ubiquitous, healthy, active stock is unlikely to be troubled. The infection can usually be avoided by good management and nutrition.

Erysipelas (*Erysipelothrix insidiosa* or *E. rhusiopathiae* Infection)

The bacteria which cause erysipelas are widespread and occur in soil. The disease occurs only occasionally in birds. The pig and turkey are its most usual hosts among domesticated animals and outbreaks in unvaccinated pigs are often severe. Rats and biting arthropods have been incriminated as sources of infection. In pigs, the bulk of outbreaks are at the height of summer, so it is believed that warmth encourages rapid multiplication of the organisms in the soil.

Many species of birds have been found to be susceptible to erysipelas, although susceptibility varies considerably. Most cases other than turkeys, have been described in gamebirds and pigeons, the latter being especially susceptible to this disease. It is probable that infection is through injuries to the skin or mucosal surfaces, particularly as the disease is commonest in male turkeys following fighting. Cage birds are not commonly affected, but should an outbreak occur, losses may be as great as 25 per cent.

CLINICAL SIGNS These include dullness, general weakness, lack of appetite and greenish-yellow, loose droppings. As depression deepens, affected birds huddle with "head-in-chest", eyes closed and tail down. There may be accentuated chest movements. In species with fleshy appendages of the head, these tend to fill with blood or oedematous fluid. Death occurs in 1 to 4 days according to species and individual susceptibility. Conjunctivitis has been observed as a symptom of erysipelas in budgerigars, the birds being reluctant to fly and preferring to move around the aviary by clinging to the wire netting and other obejcts by means of their beak and feet.

131

Diagnosis can only be made on *post-mortem* and bacteriological examinations. Recovered birds develop an immunity to further attacks and the antibodies representing this immunity can be measured by blood (agglutination) tests.

TREATMENT AND PREVENTION Erysipelas is fortunately quite responsive to treatment. Penicillin, either given twice daily as the soluble salt of calcium or in a longer acting form should rapidly cure most cases. All birds which have been in contact should also be treated. When response to this treatment is poor or doubt exists as to whether other infections are also present, then the tetracycline antibiotics can be used.

Erysipelas vaccines and serum are available. The vaccine has proved of practical value in preventing outbreaks in turkeys where annual occurrences are common. The serum, whilst not being particularly effective in the treatment of sick birds, is of value for the protection of other birds on affected premises.

Listeriosis or Listerellosis (*Listeria* or *Listerella monocytogenes* infection)

This organism only occasionally causes disease in cage birds, although it has been reported in other birds and mammals in widely separated countries. In canaries, outbreaks with quite high losses have been reported in both the Old and New Worlds.

CLINICAL SIGNS These range from sudden death in adults as the result of septicaemia, to a wasting disease in young birds. Occasional cases show central nervous system involvement. Diagnosis depends on bacteriological examination and isolation of the organism from various organs, especially the brain.

TREATMENT Broad spectrum antibiotics are likely to be the most effective drugs.

Tuberculosis (*Mycobacterium* infection)

There are three main types of tubercle bacillus (*Mycobacterium*) in warm-blooded animals: bovine, human and avian. Although the avian type occurs frequently in various species of mammals, the mammalian types are very rare in birds. However, parrots and other larger psittacines, such as macaws, are susceptible to both the human and bovine tubercle bacilli as well as the avian, whilst ornamental game birds are very susceptible to the latter. Budgerigars, canaries, and the hardier finches are fairly resistant, possibly due to their more complete adaptiveness to domestication.

Tuberculosis is a chronic disease with a slow, insidious stage of development during which the bird is apparently normal or only slightly off-colour. In a well nourished, active

132

bird this stage may pass with no further signs of illness. In such cases the tubercular lesions are walled off by scar tissue and become inactive. After many months, the organisms in the lesions die; but if another disease or stress challenges the bird in the meantime, the disease may again flare up. Birds which have been recently imported and which have undergone stresses on their voyage including change of diet are most likely to succumb to the disease.

Imported foreign birds are usually accustomed to very different climatic and other conditions from those they meet at their destination. Overcrowding, lack of sunlight, increased or decreased humidity or poor hygiene are all predisposing factors. Aviaries previously used for poultry, rearing pheasants, or waterfowl should never be used, as the disease is relatively common in these groups. Wild birds are often infected, especially woodpigeons in Europe and Great Britain. If possible therefore, aviaries should be protected from the droppings of wild birds.

CLINICAL SIGNS The main signs are pallor of mucous membranes, loss of weight, listlessness, usually diarrhoea, bedraggled, fluffed-up and dull plumage. Breathing often becomes rapid as the disease progresses, the eyes appear sunken, the bald parts of the head may be pale or greyish, and the sharp edge of the breast bone can be easily felt. In parrots, skin lesions appear as dry, flaking swellings, or raised ulcers mainly on the head. The picture is characteristically one of "going light" in bird keepers' terminology and is similar to any type of chronic, debilitating illness.

Although tuberculosis may probably attack birds of all species, especially adults, it must not be assumed that every bird "going light" over a period of weeks or months is tuberculous. Other chronic diseases, especially pseudotuberculosis and also pox, leukosis, heavy parasite burdens, aspergillosis, abdominal tumours, arthritis, gout and foreign bodies in the alimentary tract are all capable of causing slow debility with additional signs such as diarrhoea, skin lesions, lameness and anaemia. Although *post-mortem* findings may be highly suggestive of the disease, only microscopic identification of the characteristic organisms and other bacteriological examinations really confirm the diagnosis.

At necropsy, tuberculosis is easily suspected by the presence of whitish nodules or tubercles scattered throughout the internal organs, but more especially the liver and spleen (Plates 4/7 and 5/7). Without bacteriological examination it can be easily confused with pseudotuberculosis.

TREATMENT AND PREVENTION Treatment should not be attempted because the risk of fresh cases occurring is

133

too great and the response to drugs is too poor to warrant therapy. Added to this is the risk to other animals and sometimes to man.

The tubercle bacillus in addition to being relatively slow in producing disease is also a moderately resistant organism, capable of living for considerable periods in carcases and other infected material. All birds readily become infected by pecking at or eating contaminated matter and therefore diseased carcases, droppings, and other material should be incinerated. It is virtually impossible for practical reasons, to prevent the disease because infected birds or mammals are capable of shedding the organisms long before they become obviously ill. In one case infection and death of a parrot occurred long before the source of the disease was detected—the bird's owner. Tuberculin testing in order to detect the disease before clinical signs are apparent has not been developed for cage birds, but can be used for the domestic fowl. It may be tried, however, in larger species with fleshy head structures suitable for injection, such as ornamental gamebirds.

Spirochaetosis (*Spirochaete* infection)

This group of blood-borne organisms, which swim actively, is related to the causal organisms of syphilis and Weil's disease in man, and has occasionally been met with in birds other than the domestic fowl.

CLINICAL SIGNS The organisms are transmitted mainly by ticks from one bird to another, being introduced into the bloodstream by blood-sucking ticks. A spirochaete infection therefore usually indicates a tick infestation, and sometimes vice versa. Not all spirochaetes, however, are particularly pathogenic. In the more pathogenic species the incubation period is between three and seven days. In the early stages, during which period the organisms multiply in the bloodstream, signs· of fever, panting, thirst, fluffed-up feathers, depression and diarrhoea are seen. Later, coma and death may occur. Survivors thrive poorly. Isolated cases are liable to occur in birds recently imported by air from affected tropical or warm regions.

TREATMENT AND PREVENTION Penicillin has been found of some use in treatment of the disease in the fowl. It is also necessary to treat the affected bird for ticks and take steps to prevent further infestation (see Chapter 10).

Mycoplasmosis (*Mycoplasma* or P.P.L.O. infection)

Mycoplasma organisms have similarities both to bacteria and to the organisms known as rickettsiae. They are primarily

134

pathogens of cattle in which they produce a disease known as pleuropneumonia, hence the abbreviation P.P.L.O. which stands for pleuropneumonia-like organisms. Identical or very similar organisms affect poultry, turkeys, gamebirds, pigeons and various species of cage birds.

The organisms are sometimes associated with chronic disease of the respiratory tract. They occur in nasal and ocular discharges associated with infra-orbital sinusitis, and also in congested and oedematous lungs of pigeons, gamebirds and occasionally budgerigars, parrots and canaries. Both nestlings and older birds can become clinically affected, although youngsters are most susceptible. It is probable that transmission to young stock occurs from the parent through the egg; but opportunity for infection directly from parent to nestling is much more important, because the organisms can be transmitted by inhalation of infected water droplets in the air. Overcrowding encourages transmission.

CLINICAL SIGNS Infections are nearly always chronic and result in gradual debility and lowered susceptibility to other organisms, some of which may be present in normal healthy birds. Before clinical illness is apparent, stresses such as chills, exposure to draughts, or in the case of racing pigeons an exhausting flight, may result in the flare-up of an underlying infection and produce obvious illness. In racing pigeons this is reflected first in poor performance. Nasal and ocular discharges of various types, rattling respiratory sounds, partial closure of one or both eyes, depression, reduced appetite, progressive loss of weight, and "sneezing" are all signs which may be seen. In young birds and in some adult budgerigars, little is observed except for a day or two of slight dullness which may be followed by death. The infection can be endemic in an aviary with little evidence of its presence except for a few cases of vague respiratory signs, "one-eye colds", sinusitis or debility.

The disease is essentially an inflammation of mucous membranes resulting in congestion of blood vessels, swelling and discharges which may be watery at first and later become mucoid or cheesy. Mortality is usually low.

Diagnosis can only be made by identifying the causal organism in nasal or ocular discharges, nasal scrapings or air sac material in the case of dead birds. The main difficulty, however, is that the organism may be associated with bacteria or viruses and may not necessarily play the primary rôle in the production of disease.

TREATMENT Treatment is often unsatisfactory. In most cases the illness is mild or vague and laboratory confirmation is unlikely to be sought until a death occurs. Response to antibiotics is rather poor, but some success can be obtained by using tetracyclines given by subcutaneous injection or by nasal drops. Such treatment sometimes reduces the discharges and usually checks the loss of weight. In advanced cases, the thick exudate which accumulates in the airsacs, nasal chambers, sinuses and beneath the eyelids remains relatively unaffected. Eye and sinus lesions can, however, be treated by fomentation and by local applications of oily- or water-based antibiotic creams and curettage.

Only the most important infections have been dealt with above. But, as can be seen by reference to the Host List of Diseases (see Chapter 31) there are several others which have been reported in birds. Some of these are omitted because they are beyond the scope of this book, being mainly diseases of domestic poultry or intensively reared game birds, *e.g.*, infectious coryza caused by *Haemophilus gallinarum*, vibriosis due to *Vibrio metchnikovi* infection, vibrionic hepatitis, goose influenza and ulcerative enteritis of quail. Other diseases are rare and poorly documented in birds, such as anthrax, *Edwardsiella tarda* infection, *Corynebacterium ovis* infection and pseudomoniasis (*Pseudomonas aeruginosa* infection). These diseases can only be diagnosed after death with the aid of bacteriological and histological examinations.

Other Bacterial Infections

SELECTED BIBLIOGRAPHY

BIESTER, H. E. & SCHWARTE, L. H. (1965). *Diseases of Poultry,* p.220–493. 5th Ed. Ames, Iowa. State University Press.

FIENNES, R. N. T-W. (1969). Diseases of Bacterial Origin. In *Diseases of Cage and Aviary Birds,* p.357–372. Ed. Petrak, M. L., Philadelphia. Lea and Febiger.

HUNGERFORD, T. G. (1969). *Diseases of Poultry including Cage Birds and Pigeons,* p.223–332. 4th Ed. Sydney, London, Melbourne. Angus and Robertson.

KEYMER, I. F. (1961). *Post-mortem examinations of pet birds.* Mod. Vet. Pract. *42* (23), 35–38.

ROSEN, M. N. (1971). Avian Cholera. In *Infectious and Parasitic Diseases of Wild Birds,* p.59–74. Eds. Davis, J. W., Anderson, R. C., Karstad, L. and Trainer, D. O. Ames, Iowa. State University Press.

WETZLER, T. F. (1971). Pseudotuberculosis. In *Infectious and Parasitic Diseases of Wild Birds,* p.75–88. Eds. Davis, J. W., Anderson, R. C., Karstad, L. and Trainer, D. O. Ames, Iowa. State University Press.

FUNGAL INFECTIONS

Fungi belong to a group of primitive plants, The vast majority live independently but some are parasites on other plants, and relatively few mammals and birds. Most are in the form of filaments one cell thick, which grow into the material or tissue that nourishes and protects them. Because of their delicate structure, fungi are vulnerable to drying and most require moisture, warmth, and protection from light. These requirements are admirably provided for in the bodies of warm-blooded animals; oxygen and nutrients are also readily available. When the environment dries out, the filaments produce spores which are easily carried in air currents. Luckily only a few fungi have so far adapted themselves to become parasites of birds.

Aspergillosis, (*Aspergillus fumigatus* infection)

Aspergillus fumigatus is one of the common "green moulds" frequently seen in partly used jars of jam, on stale bread, decaying food and other organic matter. It is widely distributed throughout the world and together with related species is mainly found as a parasite of birds. In young chickens it causes "brooder pneumonia". It affects many species of birds as well as mammals and man, all becoming infected by inhaling or ingesting the fungus spores. The disease is particularly common in penguins, waterfowl and recently captured wild birds, especially if they have been subjected to adverse conditions of management and transport. Seeds, chaff, musty hay, straw and other dusty materials are rich sources. Small numbers of spores are tolerated by the body, but large numbers can cause disease. When established, the fungus can produce poisonous substances or toxins which damage various tissues in the same way as do some bacteria.

CLINICAL SIGNS Usually only debilitated birds suffer from the disease. Weak, overcrowded birds and those kept in unhygienic conditions are most prone, especially nestlings and old birds. The respiratory system is the favourite site for *Aspergillus*. The filaments multiply, branch, and mat with the tissue exudates. Then they tend to block the air passages and fill the airsacs. The internal nares or nostrils, sinuses, (Plate 1/8), and other cavities of the head, including those

137

under the eyelids become filled with cheesy, yellow masses. More frequently, the lungs (Plates 1/8 and 2/8) and air sacs, especially those in the thorax and abdomen are affected. Occasionally the fungus may resemble gouty deposits at *post-mortem* examination, unless microscopical examination is carried out.

The main signs in an affected bird are gasping, laboured and rapid breathing. Occasionally wheezing may be heard from a distance or when holding the chest to the ear. At times it is possible to hear clicking sounds indicating pieces of loose fungus or exudate flicking to and fro in the larger air passages. Although the disease can kill in a few days, in psittacines and some other species it tends to progress for weeks or even longer, especially in adults. Frequently death may occur with little previous outward sign except for loss of weight and progressive depression. In young stock, depression and sometimes convulsions are the main signs.

TREATMENT AND PREVENTION Prevention is almost entirely a matter of maintaining a high standard of nutrition, hygiene and housing, and having luck with weather conditions and in the purchase of clean seed. Dust is the main enemy, and birds living in a planted aviary free from loose litter are least likely to contract the disease. Untidy food stores with old grain sacks, bags, papers and other oddments strewn about, or dark, makeshift sheds are all ideal for the production of fungus spores, particularly when the weather is warm and humidity high.

Continuous use of antibiotics, for as little as two or three weeks, favours the establishment of fungal infections such as aspergillosis.

Treatment is unsatisfactory, especially as the disease is virtually impossible to diagnose during life. There appears to be no effective substance which can be used internally without eventually killing the bird. Some success has been claimed using potassium iodine in the drinking water as a preventive, but it is of doubtful value. Exposing birds to nystatin aerosol by the use of a nebulisor has also been suggested, but laboratory tests have shown that *Aspergillus* is resistant to this antibiotic. More recently, intra-venous amphotericin has been suggested, but it may well be toxic. The drug griseofulvin, which is effective in ringworm and other fungus infections of the skin has little effect on *Aspergillus*.

Favus is also known as the honeycomb fungus because of the rough, porous appearance of the scabs it produces on affected skin. It is an uncommon disease of birds but has been reported in wild European blackbirds and robins.

Favus or Ringworm (*Trichophyton* spp. infection)

138

CLINICAL SIGNS The fungus causes a chronic, skin lesion usually limited to the fleshy or thin-skinned areas of the head (Plate 3/8). It may also extend to the neighbouring feathered parts. Birds possessing combs, wattles and similar appendages are mainly affected. White spots develop which break off. Later a crusty layer appears which may be mistaken for knemidocoptic mange. However, on a closer examination characteristic mite tunnels are found to be absent. Scab samples or carcases should be sent to a laboratory equipped to deal with this type of investigation.

TREATMENT Spread from bird to bird is slow. Treatment of valuable specimens may be undertaken. Older remedies such as iodine, carbolic acid, mercuric chloride, formalin, phenyl mercuric nitrate or borate and the group of drugs known as quaternary ammonium compounds have been used in the form of tinctures. Ointments, oils, soaps and lotions have also been tried. The multitude of discarded remedies indicates the need for more effective and rapid treatment. Isolation of affected birds and oral administration of griseofulvin is suggested for the control of all types of dermatomycosis, as fungal infections of the skin are called. Killing and burning all affected birds, however, is safer and cheaper than treatment, especially when rare or otherwise valuable birds are not involved.

Candidiasis, Moniliasis, Oidiomycosis, Sour Crop or Thrush *(Candida albicans* infection) Turkeys, parrots, gamebirds and pigeons are mainly affected, and only occasionally other species. *Candida* are colonies of single, oval cells which bud and in some circumstances develop into chains or hyphae. They most frequently attack the epithelium of the crop. The infection can be induced by prolonged use of antibiotics, such as the tetracyclines, in the drinking water.

CLINICAL SIGNS The chief signs of infection of the alimentary tract are unthriftiness, listlessness and a bedraggled appearance, young birds being most prone to the disease. Patches of raised, whitish, dead epithelial material are occasionally seen in the mouth and these can easily be scraped off the mucous membrane. In this situation the lesions may affect the breathing. The crop and oesophagus are the main sites of the lesions (Plate 4/8). Less frequently, the epithelium of the proventriculus is affected and sometimes the yeasts are found in the intestinal tract. Occasionally regurgitation of food and loose droppings may occur.

Diarrhoea is more likely to result from some concurrent gut infection and vomiting is more likely to be associated with unsuitable food, gut obstruction or bacterial, parasitic

139

infestation of the alimentary tract. Pox infection may be confused with candidiasis in pigeons, but laboratory identification of the fungus will clinch the diagnosis.

TREATMENT AND PREVENTION   Prevention is largely a matter of good hygiene and management. Stale food, dirty premises, overcrowding and allowing water to slop over food or litter, all contribute to the build-up of an epidemic in young stock. In well-kept premises, however, the infection should never be a serious worry. Few treatments have appreciable effect, although powdered nystatin by mouth or copper sulphate in the drinking water have sometimes appeared to be effective. Dimetridazole also appears helpful especially in pigeons, probably because it prevents secondary infection by trichomonads (Chapter 9).

It is possible that certain nutritional deficiencies, especially of the vitamin B complex, may be predisposing causes of the disease. As young free-living partridges eat large numbers of ants, which contain formic acid, a deficiency of the acid has been suspected as a possible cause of the disease in these birds. Some success in reducing mortality has been claimed by spraying the food with 15 per cent formic acid at the rate of 20 ml./100 g. of food.

SELECTED BIBLIOGRAPHY

AINSWORTH, G. C. & AUSTWICK, P. K. C. (1959). Fungal Diseases of Animals. *Review Series No. 6 of the Commonwealth Bureau of Animal Health.* Farnham Royal, Bucks, Commonwealth Agricultural Bureau, 148pp.

BARDEN, E. S., CHUTE, H. L., O'MEARA, D. C. & WHEELWRIGHT, H. T. (1971). *A bibliography of avian mycosis.* 3rd Ed. College of Life Sciences and Agriculture, University of Maine, Orono. U.S.A.

CHUTE, H. L. (1965). Diseases Caused by Fungi. In *Diseases of Poultry,* p.494–511. Eds. Biester, H. E. and Schwarte, L. H. 5th Ed. Ames, Iowa. State University Press.

HUNGERFORD, T. G. (1969). Fungal Infections in Poultry, p.359–377. In *Diseases of Poultry including Cage Birds and Pigeons.* 4th Ed. Sydney, London, Melbourne, Angus and Robertson.

KEYMER, I. F. (1969). Mycoses. In *Diseases of Cage and Aviary Birds,* p.453–458. Ed. Petrak, M. L. Philadelphia. Lea and Febiger.

PROTOZOAN INFECTIONS

A parasite is an animal or plant organism which lives at the expense of another, the host. It derives food and protection from its host. An "obligatory" parasite is one which during the course of evolution has become entirely dependent on its host, while a facultative parasite is capable of living either free or as a parasite. Most successful parasites have learned to live in equilibrium with their host. Although they deprive them of food or body substances, they usually do not cause the host severe damage otherwise it would not be capable of maintaining the next generation of parasites. In a few cases, however, the parasites must kill the host in order to be released from the body and develop into another stage of the life cycle.

Coccidiosis (Coccidia infections) Coccidia of several different types occur in birds although the majority belong to two genera. These differ mainly in whether they produce oocysts or eggs containing four smaller cysts, or whether the oocysts contain two sporocysts: the former parasites belong to the genus *Eimeria* and the latter to *Isospora*. The two genera show a different distribution in their bird hosts. The genus *Eimeria* favours birds in the Orders Galliformes, Columbiformes, and Anseriformes, but also occurs in Gruiformes, Pelecaniiformes, Psittaciformes and Charadriiformes. The genus *Isospora* is more widespread, infecting birds mainly in the Order Passeriformes, but also the Struthioniformes, Falconiformes, Galliformes, Coraciiformes, Charadriiformes, Psittaciformes, Strigiformes and Piciformes. Unlike *Eimeria* spp. there is virtually no evidence that species of *Isospora* are pathogenic. Several species of *Eimeria*, however, produce disease in domestic poultry, various species of game birds such as pheasants and in peafowl.

Most species of coccidia occur in different areas of the intestines and penetrate the mucous lining. According to the species of bird and coccidia, the parasites occur at different sites, extending from the duodenum to the cloaca, including the caeca if present. Coccidia, including *Eimeria*, may infect the kidneys in some species of swans, geese, ducks and owls.

141

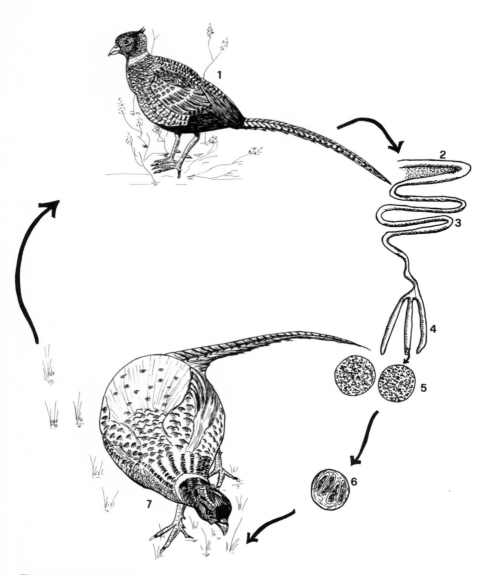

Figure 1/9. Not drawn to scale. Life cycle of coccidiosis (*Eimeria* spp.) in the pheasant (1). The parasites may live either in the duodenum (2), lower small intestine (3) or caeca (4) of infected birds depending upon the species of *Eimeria*. They undergo various stages in the gut epithelium and produce oocysts (5) which are passed out in the faeces. When conditions are satisfactory the oocysts develop into the infective stage (6). Pheasants become infected by eating (7) these oocysts and the life cycle is repeated.

Oocysts become mature and infective within one to three days after being passed in the droppings. If these oocysts are then swallowed by a susceptible bird, the stages known as sporoziotes are liberated in the gut by digestion of the oocyst wall. Here the parasites undergo rapid and complicated stages of asexual multiplication at various depths in the gut epithelium (see Figure 1/9).

Finally two dissimilar types of offspring unite to form an organism capable of producing further oocysts. The entire cycle takes from one to two weeks depending upon the species of coccidia.

CLINICAL SIGNS   During the life cycle the parasites may cause inflammation of varying severity in the gut wall according to species of bird and coccidia, the number of oocysts swallowed and the general health and age of the bird. The disease causes all stages of ill-health from mild diarrhoea to fatal dysentery. Signs include depression, anaemia, loss of weight, thirst, unthriftiness and watery, slimy greenish, or bloody diarrhea. The disease may be an acute or a lingering chronic process with or without fatalities. Rapid loss of weight leading to emaciation and dehydration precede death, particularly in young stock. Death is lingering in some birds with extreme depression and weakness. Tremors, convulsions or lamenesses are occasionally seen.

A mild or moderate infection in a fairly resistant bird results after a time, in immunity to further infection.

DIAGNOSIS   Diagnosis depends on microscopical examination and finding oocysts in the droppings. It is unlikely that epidemics of the magnitude seen in poultry will be encountered in cage or aviary birds. In most establishments a few birds harbour coccidia but show no signs of disease.

SPREAD AND CONTROL   The concentration of oocysts builds up most rapidly where birds are kept in overcrowded conditions, where food or water is readily contaminated with droppings and where litter is moist, warm, or not removed daily. Under these circumstances young stock which has not yet developed any immunity to the disease is particularly vulnerable. Attempts to rear birds in coccidia-free surroundings are almost bound to be followed by failure, but, if successful, leave the birds highly prone to the first oocysts which come their way. A light infection is probably preferable therefore, to a coccidia-free environment. Good hygiene therefore should prevent the disease causing any significant trouble. Removal of soiled food and wet litter will usually prevent serious outbreaks.

TREATMENT Numerous drugs have been used for the treatment of poultry. However, sulphonamides, especially sulphadimidine, sulphaquinoxaline, and also furazolidone are still among the most effective drugs. Certain other drugs are also used for poultry.

Trichomonas gallinae is a fragile protozoan which can swim actively by means of its five whip-like flagella and it possesses a wavy fin-like membrane down one side. It is the most important trichomonad of cage birds and it is especially pathogenic to pigeons.

Trichomoniasis, "Canker", "Frounce", or "Diphtheria" (*Trichomonas* spp. infection)

    Trichomonas gallinae affects various pigeons, doves, quail, falcons and hawks and occasionally other birds, including some of the smaller finches, Java sparrows and the canary. In the pigeon and dove family (Columbidae) it can cause severe epidemics. Wild species and feral pigeons frequently harbour the organisms and can be a source of infection.

CLINICAL SIGNS
In pigeons, the disease usually affects one to two week old squabs or sometimes older youngsters (squeakers), and less frequently adults. Characteristic lesions are sticky, creamy white or cheesy deposits in the mouth, pharynx, inner nares and oesophagus. As a general rule the wet, sticky type of exudate is seen mainly in the acute disease and the hard cheesy type in more chronic infections. The lesions sometimes extend to the crop, into the upper parts of the respiratory tract and even onto the outside of the beak (see Plates 1/9 and 2/9). As the result of such lesions, eating and drinking become difficult, food is refused or merely picked at, and respiration is often noisy. Lesions may occasionally extend down the alimentary tract, and cause cheesy, necrotic spots in the liver, spleen, lung or on the surface of the gut.

    Depression precedes early death in acute cases. In older or more resistant birds, great loss of weight occurs prior to death, and this may take up to three weeks or even longer. The disease is similar in diurnal birds of prey, such as falcons, hawks and eagles, and in these species it is often called "frounce". It is believed that birds of prey usually contract the infection by eating affected pigeons.

    The disease may be confused with candidiasis and vitamin A deficiency.

TREATMENT Treatment with dimetridazole is most effective against the organism provided the bird can swallow. The apparent success of tetracyclines and sulphadimidine is probably mainly due to the susceptibility of secondary bacterial invaders which flourish in the exudates.

144

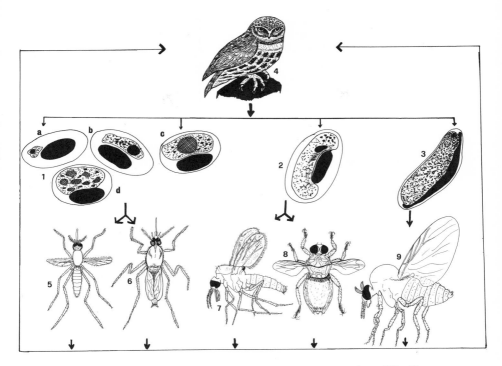

Figure 2/9. Not drawn to scale. Life cycle of *Plasmodium* (1), *Haemoproteus* or *Parahaemoproteus* (2) and *Leucocytozoon* (3). These blood parasites infect various internal organs of the host bird, *e.g.,* little owl (4) as well as the red blood corpuscles 1(a), (b), (c), (d) and 2. *Leucocytozoon* (3) usually infects the white blood cells and displaces the host cell nucleus (depicted in black in each blood cell). When a female blood sucking mosquito of the genus *Culex* (5) or *Aedes* (6) feeds on the blood of a bird infected with the *Plasmodium* (1) it takes up the parasites. These then undergo stages, firstly in the stomach and then in the salivary glands of the mosquito. When the mosquito feeds on a susceptible bird it becomes infected by stages of the parasite known as sporozoites which enter the subcutaneous tissues and blood. The life cycles of *Haemoproteus* (2) and *Parahaemoproteus* (2) (stages in blood identical) are very similar to *Plasmodium*, except that the vectors are not mosquitoes. *Culicoides* midges (7) transmit *Parahaemoproteus* and louse-flies or *Hippoboscids* (8) transmit *Haemoproteus*. The life cycle of *Leucocytozoon* (3) is also similar to that of the other parasites except that it is transmitted by black flies or simuliids (9). The blood stages also differ by containing no pigment derived from the host cell and stages known as schizonts are absent. Some species of *Leucocytozoon* infect red blood cells instead of white cells. (Janet Keymer)

Recovery from mild attacks produces an immunity to more virulent strains of *T. gallinae*. Severely infected birds should be destroyed, for even if they recover, they are likely to remain debilitated.

As trichomonads are susceptible to drying, heat and chemicals, it is perhaps surprising that they can be such a scourge. They are mainly spread by direct contact from beak to beak, especially when parent birds are feeding young. Indirect transmission, especially via the drinking water, also probably occurs. Direct spread is very difficult to control in a colony of birds. It must be remembered that trichomonads can be harboured in small numbers by certain birds without producing clinical signs.

Giardiasis (*Giardia* spp. infection)

Giardia infects mainly mammals and is a rare parasite of birds but has been recorded in a parakeet, passerine, toucan and a few other hosts. The organism is shaped like a tennis racket without a handle and has eight flagella by means of which it swims about in the intestinal contents. It forms cysts and in this form is passed out in the faeces and transmitted to other hosts by ingestion.

Diagnosis is based on the identification of the motile organisms and/or cysts in the excreta on microscopical examination.

CLINICAL SIGNS Loss of condition, diarrhoea and death have been attributed to the parasite.

TREATMENT Strict attention should be paid to hygiene, especially avoiding faecal contamination of food. Drugs used for the treatment of malaria should prove effective.

Histomoniasis Blackhead or Infectious Enterohepatitis (*Histomonas meleagridis* infection)

This is one of the most important diseases of turkeys and more detailed information is available in books on diseases of poultry. The disease also infects the domestic fowl, pheasants, partridges, quail, peafowl and probably all species of gallinaceous birds. Birds in other Orders are not naturally infected. The parasites are carried in the ova of the caecal worm *Heterakis gallinae* (see Chapter 10) in which they can survive for long periods. Birds become infected by swallowing the infected worm eggs. The protozoa are released into the caeca when the worm eggs hatch and they then attack the caecal walls whilst some are carried in the blood to the liver. In the caeca other worms become infected and produce further ova infected with *Histomonas*.

CLINICAL SIGNS The name "blackhead" is extremely misleading because this is not a characteristic sign of the

146

disease. The usual clinical signs are drowsiness, increasing weakness, drooping wings and tail and ruffled plumage. Diarrhoea is a constant feature, the faeces usually being yellowish in colour. Occasionally the skin of the face and head of infected turkeys becomes a deep reddish-black. Young birds of all susceptible species are most commonly infected. In young turkeys mortality may reach almost 100 per cent.

DIAGNOSIS Although the disease can be suspected from the clinical signs, the presence of the infection can be confirmed only at *post-mortem* examination by finding the typical lesions in the liver and caeca. Large, round, pale grey areas of necrosis occur in the liver (Plate 3/9). At least part of the walls of the caeca are thickened and their epithelial lining is ulcerated.

TREATMENT AND PREVENTION Usually the disease can be prevented by incorporating drugs such as dimetridazole or furazolidone in the food at low dosages as recommended by the manufacturers. For actual treatment of those infected and birds in contact in the same flock, these drugs are also used, but at higher dosage rates.

Domestic fowls are less susceptible to histomoniasis than turkeys and some other species of gallinaceous birds and can be apparently healthy carriers. It is unwise therefore, to keep such birds as peafowl and ornamental pheasants on the same land as poultry or on land which has been used for that purpose. As *Histomonas meleagridis* is carried by the caecal worm, the disease can be controlled by preventing infestation with these parasites.

Avian Malaria (*Plasmodium* spp. infections)

Plasmodium causes malaria in man, other mammals and birds. The organisms are parasites of red blood cells. At this stage of its lifecycle, the parasite may produce fever and is also infective to the intermediate hosts which are various species of mosquitoes. In these insects further multiplication occurs until a stage is reached in the salivary glands when the parasites are again infectious to birds. When the blood-sucking female mosquito bites a bird, it introduces the parasites into the blood; these do not remain in the bird's circulation at this stage but invade certain cells of the liver, spleen, kidney and other organs. They reappear later, to produce attacks of the disease during which multiplication occurs in the red blood cells.

Numerous species of bird can contract malaria, both in tropical and temperate climates. Several species of *Plasmodium* exist and infect several species and families of birds. The canary is particularly susceptible to certain species of *Plas-*

modium, especially *P. cathemerium*, and is used for experimental purposes in malaria research. Although numerous species can be infected, the organisms are usually pathogenic only to penguins and the domestic fowl when these birds are kept in warm climates. Young birds are more susceptible to malaria than adults.

CLINICAL SIGNS In most species the parasites appear to be harmless under normal conditions. Heavy infections may result in a febrile disease showing as depression, ruffled feathers and incoordination, but most *Plasmodium* spp. only produce a mild illness.

DIAGNOSIS The presence of pigmented reproductive forms of the parasite in the peripheral blood on microscopical examination of blood smears. Only red blood cells are infected.

TREATMENT AND PREVENTION Mepacrine hydrochloride and other anti-malarial drugs are usually effective. Untreated birds which have recovered, may still harbour the parasites.

Mosquitoes (*Culex, Aedes* and *Anopheles* spp.) must be controlled and if necessary, the birds should be protected by mosquito-proof netting.

Haemoproteus spp. and Parahaemoproteus spp. infections

These genera are closely related to *Plasmodium* but differ in two important respects from that parasite by not multiplying in the circulating blood and by not being transmitted by mosquitoes. Multiplication is restricted to special cells in blood vessels, especially in the lungs. In the case of *Haemoproteus* the parasites are transmitted by louse flies (Hipboscids), whilst *Parahaemoproteus* is carried by midges of the genus *Culicoides* (Figure 2/9). *Plasmodium* parasites of both genera infect red blood cells and can seldom be identified and differentiated by examination of blood forms alone.

A very wide variety of birds may be infected with the parasites which are widespread in distribution.

CLINICAL SIGNS Under ordinary circumstances the parasities are harmless and rarely cause disease. In ornate lorikeets they have been reported as the cause of anaemia and congestion of the lungs leading eventually to asphyxia and there are a few indications of pathogenicity in other birds.

DIAGNOSIS The infection can be suspected by the presence of pigmented parasites showing no evidence of reproductive forms on microscopic examination of blood smears. Only the red blood cells are infected.

148

TREATMENT AND PREVENTION This is the same as that recommended for malaria.

Trypanosomiasis (Trypanosome infections)

Trypanosomes are elongated, flagellated blood parasites, some of which cause sleeping sickness and other diseases of man and domestic stock in tropical countries. Avian trypanosomes have an almost world-wide distribution, but parasites in birds are of little significance. Numerous species of birds, but especially passerines, have been found infected. Louse flies, red mites, mosquitoes and simuliids (black flies or buffalo gnats) have all been implicated as carriers.

CLINICAL SIGNS There is virtually no evidence that the parasites are pathogenic to birds, with the possible exception of canaries.

DIAGNOSIS The presence of the parasites in the peripheral blood on microscopical examination of blood smears.

TREATMENT AND PREVENTION This is unlikely to be necessary.

Leucocytozoonosis (*Leucocytozoon* and *Akiba* spp. infections)

These blood parasites (see Figure 2/9), which are confined to birds, are similar to *Plasmodium, Haemoproteus* and *Parahaemoproteus* spp. except that they do not contain pigment granules derived from the haemoglobin of the red cells. *Leucocytozoon* and *Akiba* spp. also occur in blood cells, but characteristically in the leucocytes, and unlike *Plasmodium* do not multiply in the circulating blood. *Leucocytozoon* spp. are transmitted by simuliid flies, and *Akiba* spp. by *Culicoides* midges. The life histories of the parasites with few exceptions are unknown and there is no other way of differentiating between the two genera. It is believed that the genus *Leucocytozoon* is the commoner of the two. Both organisms reproduce in various organs, including liver, heart, brain, lung and spleen.

The parasites have an almost world-wide distribution and occur in a wide variety of species, including ducks, geese, turkeys, domestic fowl, game birds, owls and other birds of prey, numerous passerines and parakeets (excluding budgerigars).

CLINICAL SIGNS *Leucocytozoon* is pathogenic to young birds of many species, especially ducks, geese, turkeys, parakeets, certain passerines such as weaver birds and probably many others. Clinical signs are not diagnostic and include anaemia. Mortality may be high and in parakeets the parasite's

149

presence in the cardiac muscle may cause heart failure. In temperate zones the disease is seasonal, occurring when the insect carriers are active.

DIAGNOSIS The presence of non-pigmented parasites in the leucocytes or red blood cells on microscopical examination of blood smears and the presence of cysts in the heart and gizzard musculature or skeletal muscles.

TREATMENT AND PREVENTION Sulpha drugs as used for coccidiosis may be effective. The disease is most likely to occur in warm weather when the vectors are active and therefore at these times, birds should be protected if possible from the insects by keeping them indoors.

Lankesterella was previously called *Atoxoplasma*. So far as is known it occurs only in birds and amphibia, inhabiting lymphocytes and monocytes. The parasites reproduce in the spleen, bone marrow, liver, lungs and kidneys. At least one species, namely, *L. garnhami*, is believed to be transmitted by the red mite *Dermanyssus gallinae*, (Figure 3/9).

Lankesterellosis (*Lankesterella* spp. infection)

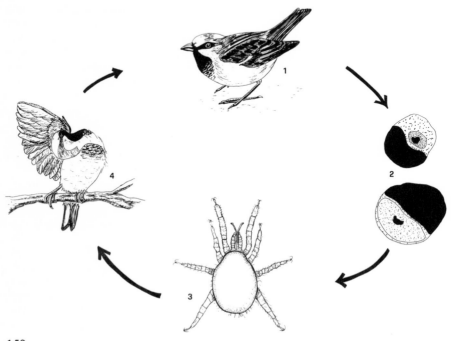

Lankesterella is widespread and particularly common in house sparrows in Great Britain. Canaries are commonly infected and the parasite has been reported in several other passerines. Young birds of all species are most susceptible.

CLINICAL SIGNS Infected canaries become listless, have ruffled feathers and show loss of appetite. The distended liver may produce a visible swelling behind the sternum. *L. garnhami* is also pathogenic to house sparrows.

DIAGNOSIS The presence of non-pigmented parasites in lymphocytes and monocytes of the peripheral blood. A prolonged examination may, however, be necessary because the organisms are usually scarce. They can most easily be found at *post-mortem* examination in impression smears of the spleen.

TREATMENT AND PREVENTION There appears to be no specific treatment for the parasite. If red mites really do transmit the infection, then it should be possible to prevent the disease by controlling these ectoparasites. Some parasitologists, however, believe that the organism may be a stage in the life-cycle of the coccidian parasite known as *Isospara*.

Other Protozoan Infections There are a few other protozoan infections which have not been included, because most of them are rare and virtually nothing is known about their pathogenicity—at least in non-domesticated birds. These include infections by *Sarcocystis* spp. toxoplasmosis, hexamitiasis and infections by coccidia belonging to the genera *Dorisiella*, *Wenyonella* and *Tyzzeria*.

Figure 3/9. Not drawn to scale. Suspected life cycle of *Lankesterella garnhami.* The infected host such as a house sparrow (1) harbors the parasite in its white blood cells (2). When the bird is attacked by blood-sucking red mites *Dermanyssus gallinae* (3) the parasites are ingested by the mite in which they survive but undergo no further development. Red mites cause irritation to their host which ingests them during preening (4). The parasite undergoes the various stages of its life cycle in the bird (1) eventually reaching the leucocytes (2). (Janet Keymer)

SELECTED BIBLIOGRAPHY

FARR, M. M. (1965). Protozoa. In *Diseases of Poultry,* p.1056–1148. Eds. Biester, H. E. and Schwarte, L. H. 5th Ed. Ames, Iowa. State University Press.

GARNHAM, P. C. C. (1966). *Malarial Parasites and Other Haemosporidia.* Oxford, Blackwell, 1114pp.

HUNGERFORD, T. G. (1969). Protozoan Diseases. In *Diseases of Poultry including Cage Birds and Pigeons,* pp.335–356. 4th Ed. Sydney, London, Melbourne. Angus and Robertson.

KEYMER, I. F. (1969). Parasitic Diseases. In *Diseases of Cage and Aviary Birds,* p.393–452. Ed. Petrak, M. L., Philadelphia. Lea and Febiger.

KOCAN, R. M. & HERMAN, C. M. (1971). *Trichomoniasis,* p.282–290. Eds. Davis, J. W., Anderson, R. C., Karstad, L. and Trainer, D. O. Ames, Iowa. State University Press.

LAPAGE, G. (1958). *Parasitic Animals.* 2nd Ed. Cambridge. Heffer. 355pp.

LAPAGE, G. (1968). *Veterinary Parasitology.* 2nd Ed. Oliver & Boyd. 1182pp.

LEVINE, N. D. (1961). *Protozoan Parasites of Domestic Animals and Man.* Minneapolis, Burgess Publishing Co., 412pp.

OLSEN, O. W. (1967). *Animal Parasites: Their Biology and Life Cycles.* 2nd Ed. Minneapolis, Burgess Publishing Co, 431pp.

SOULSBY, E. J. L. (1968). *Helminths, Arthropods & Protozoa of Domesticated Animals.* (Sixth Edition of Mönnig's Veterinary Helminthology & Entomology). London. Baillière, Tindall & Cassell. 824pp.

TODD, K. S. & HAMMOND, D. M. (1971). *Coccidia of Anseriformes, Galliformes and Passeriformes,* p.234–281. Eds. Davis, J. W., Anderson, R. C., Karstad, L. and Trainer, D. O. Ames, Iowa. State University Press.

INFESTATIONS BY THE LARGER PARASITES

Two main groups of the larger parasites are dealt with here:

Arthropods—mainly members of the insect and spider families, usually living in or on the surface layers of the body.

Helminths —the parasitic worms and flukes which live in various organs, but especially the gut.

Most pathogenic arthropods are visible to the naked eye and vary from pinpoint to about 1 cm. in size. Helminths may be fine and hair-like, short and stubby, or long and tape-like, and range from only 1 mm. or so to a metre or more in length.

Arthropods Arthropods are invertebrates which have a skeleton surrounding the body like a shell, instead of, as in vertebrates, with muscles and skin between and around the bones of an internal skeleton. The term "arthropod" means "jointed legs" and these are characteristic features of the group. Only fleas, lice, flies and bugs are true insects, bearing six legs in the adult form. Ticks and mites possess eight legs, although in the growing stage (larvae) only six legs are present. Arthropods are air-breathing animals and usually live on the outside of the body, when they are called ectoparasites. Some species, however, live in airways of the respiratory system and occasionally in other parts of the body. Few ectoparasites are lethal to their hosts, but in certain circumstances some can cause death, for example, by producing anaemia or exhaustion. Generally the parasites are little more than a nuisance, although they can weaken an already ailing bird. Owing to the irritation caused by ectoparasites, breeding birds may be prevented from settling on eggs or feeding their young.

An important feature of arthropod parasites is their mobility. They are no respector of persons (or birds), and can transmit viral, protozoan or bacterial infections by contact, by being eaten, by their blood-sucking habits and by passing from one host to another.

153

Most species of fleas are agile and, although many have been found on birds, they are not primarily avian parasites. Fleas are versatile in their choice of host and are less "host specific" than most ectoparasites, even though related species of birds are likely to harbour similar species of flea. Fleas are adaptable to an unfavourable host if the more usual one is unavailable, and may even transfer between birds and mammals. They are most common in warm climates.

Fleas may be red, brown or black and are flattened laterally, that is sideways, enabling them to run and leap rapidly in hairs and feathers. They vary from 1.5–5 mm. in length. The adults are blood-suckers, whilst the larvae feed on the faeces of adults, which are rich in blood products from the host. One species, the tropical or stick-tight flea, may embed its head so firmly in the skin that removal is difficult. Numerous stick-tight fleas may be found on the head and neck region. Incomplete removal may lead to infected wounds, irritation, and self-mutilation. Other species are more mobile and excessive preening by the bird may provoke the flea to change hosts between meals to one which is more amenable. Fleas normally lay their eggs off the host, usually in a place well supplied with animal organic matter. Eggs may hatch in four days to three weeks, but these times can vary considerably up to 18 months or even more and depend upon the environmental temperature and humidity as well as the species of flea. The larva, a maggot-like creature, eats debris in its vicinity and grows, usually moulting twice before spinning a cocoon to become a pupa. This process can take from two weeks to as much as six months. The parasites can remain in this pupal stage for even longer and are capable of breaking out, it is thought, in response to the warmth or vibration produced by a potential host. They then jump onto the bird, gorge themselves, and can mate and breed a few days later. Whilst still on the host, the females may lay eggs which eventually fall to the ground; probably more often these are laid directly into cracks or crevices nearby. A few per day may be laid up to a maximum of about 100.

TREATMENT AND CONTROL It is important to realise that eggs and pupae are not susceptible to most insecticides and so it is the adult and larval forms which must be attacked. This involves not only disinfesting the birds but also their quarters. Fleas leave their host when its body temperature falls and so a dead or dying bird and indeed one which is anaesthetised often becomes surrounded by departing fleas. This is one of the many reasons therefore why sick birds should be isolated from healthy ones at the first signs of illness and necropsied and incinerated elsewhere.

Treatment includes spraying the birds themselves, their perches, nesting boxes and quarters, with a suitable insecticide after removing and burning any loose material such as feathers, droppings, spilled seed, and old nesting material. Spraying should be repeated every 10 to 14 days until the parasites have been eradicated. Most insecticides are poisonous, especially to small birds, often indeed to mammals and man, and should be used with extreme caution. One of the safest, although shorter-acting insecticides which can be sprayed on birds is pyrethrum. Other chemicals may kill, if sprayed or painted on the bird itself. Highly toxic substances can, however, be sprayed on perches, nest boxes and floors, providing that the birds are removed from the infested cage beforehand and not returned until the parasites have been exterminated and the insecticides completely removed by washing.

The choice of parasiticide will depend on cost, ease of application, desired duration of effectiveness, and toxicity.

Special attention should be paid to the destruction of all old nests in the vicinity, whether they are actually in the aviary or are those of poultry or wild birds.

It is important to remember that reinfestation can also occur from domestic pets and other mammals, wild birds and poultry.

Lice   Lice are wingless insects and are the most common external parasites of birds. They differ from fleas in being flattened horizontally, *i.e.* from above and below, so that they can lie close to the skin (see Plate 1/10). They have hooked legs which are more widely placed than those of fleas. There is a vast number of species of avian lice, some of which are named after the bird they parasitize or the area of the body they prefer. Lice live continuously on the host, leaving it only to attack another victim. So-called sucking lice are confined to mammals, all bird lice being of the more mobile chewing or biting types. Over forty species have been found on domestic poultry alone. Many of these and numerous other species also flourish on wild and aviary birds. Lice lay sticky, triangular eggs or nits which adhere to the feathers in clusters in their favourite region of the body and after which they are popularly named —head, body, fluff, shaft and wing lice. Sometimes other adjectives in their names indicate the primary host, or their shape, *e.g.*, pigeon and narrow lice. Lice are of many shapes and sizes and vary from 1-6 mm. in length. The eggs hatch within a few weeks of being laid, the larvae feed, grow, moult their skin several times, and become adults ready for breeding. In favourable conditions, as for example when birds huddle together for warmth, lice can multiply and spread so quickly that it is possible for one pair to produce 100,000 descendants in a few months. It can therefore be appreciated how overcrowding can lead to an explosion of the louse

155

population and result in debility of the bird, paving the way for other diseases which may even lead to death. Bird lice feed mainly on the surface layers of the skin, feather vanes and skin debris, but at least one species has been found to bite growing feathers, sucking the blood from the base of young quills or even gnawing at the skin surface until blood is drawn.

Lousiness can be more than a mere nuisance; it can cause irritation, restlessness, loss of appetite and sleep. The condition of the plumage deteriorates and becomes ragged, whilst excessive preening may lead to feather-plucking or even cannibalism. Lice in small numbers, however, may be relatively harmless and most healthy birds harbour a few.

TREATMENT AND CONTROL   In spite of the diversity of species, one form of treatment suffices for all lice. Because of the relatively short life cycle and the fact that lice rarely leave one bird except to go to another in close contact, control is easy. Dusting powders, bathing solutions, and vapours have all been found satisfactory. The older and more poisonous insecticides such as sodium fluoride and nicotine sulphate, have been largely superseded by more modern ones. Solutions in the form of sprays containing pyrethrum, "Alugan", D.D.T., gammexane, and other substances recommended for eradication of fleas etc., are efficient and more persistent than dusting powders and vapours. With the exception of pyrethrum, (the least stable), they need to be used with considerable care, especially on small passerines as some are toxic to some species of birds. A binding agent is usually incorporated in insecticides which retains the insecticidal action in the plumage for some weeks, thereby killing the next generation of larvae as they hatch. Some of the eggs are also dislodged and washed away during spraying of the plumage. The owners of valuable birds are sometimes reluctant to use sprays, lest a chill or pneumonia should follow. The risk, however, is negligible provided the birds are allowed to dry in a warm atmosphere and cooled off slowly afterwards. It is wise to spray the cleaned premises at the same time as the birds, in order to remove the odd parasite which may have left its host. Regular checks of all stock should be carried out to determine when treatment is necessary.

Bugs   Bugs, of which the bedbug (*Cimex lectularius*) is the best known, can be found on various species of birds, the pigeon for example having its own species *C. columbarius*. The bedbug is a wingless insect which lays a few eggs to a total of about 200 per day in cracks or crevices of the cage or aviary. The nymphs hatch in 7-10 days and reach mature adulthood within a minimal period of about 40 days. During development, they moult five times before becoming adult. The nymphs feed on the blood of the host and, like the adults, can live up to a year without feeding. They normally stay to feed on the host for only ten minutes or so, usually at night. Affected birds give off a characteristic dirty odour. Heavy infestations are necessary before anaemia or illness results, but itching, restlessness and malaise result from lighter infestations. The insects inject saliva when they pierce the skin in order to prevent the blood clotting. This produces local skin swellings and infectious diseases may also be transferred in this way from bird to bird.

TREATMENT AND CONTROL This is similar to that recommended for lice.

The pigeon fly *(Pseudolynchia canariensis)* This is a winged insect allied to the sheep ked and one of the many species of louse-fly. It sucks the blood of nestling pigeons. Similar species also occur on other species of birds especially swallows, martins and swifts. When not feeding or mating on the host, the fly spends its time in nests or in dark crevices of buildings and nest boxes.

It is found mainly in warm and tropical regions of the world and until the advent of effective insecticides at the end of World War II was a well known scourge in pigeon lofts.

It is a flattened, stockily-built fly with strong legs and claws, a little smaller than the common housefly. It is brownish in colour, very agile and hides in the plumage, often flying off when the bird is approached. Eggs hatch inside the female and are laid as larvae almost ready to pupate. The creamy-white fat larvae are deposited in crevices and especially in nests and nest boxes; in fact any protected part of the premises will satisfy breeding females. The pupae or cocoons are also creamy-white but soon turn black. Adults emerge from the cocoons after four weeks and then suck blood from recently hatched squabs. Although only four to six larvae are produced at a time, as many as a score or more flies have been found parasitizing a single nestling. It seems that the parent birds do not eat the flies or their immature stages and the only effort on the part of the bird to reduce the annoyance is to try to remove the flies with a thrust of the beak.

Blood-sucking itself does not seem to irritate adult birds unduly, but the presence of the parasites in the plumage can cause restlessness and excessive preening. Blood loss in adults is usually inconsequential, but heavily parasitized squabs and squeakers may sometimes die from anaemia or its sequels. Viral, bacterial, or some protozoan infections may be carried between aviaries, or from wild to domesticated birds by louse-flies, as with other blood-sucking parasites.

TREATMENT AND CONTROL The most effective and safe parasiticides for pigeons is probably "Alugan". Pyrethrum, derris, and other insecticides recommended for fleas and lice seem to be less effective. The parasiticide should be used in the same manner as recommended for the control of fleas and used at three-weekly intervals until the parasites have been eradicated.

Blackflies, buffalo gnats (Simuliids) and midges (*Culicoides* spp.)

These insects (see Figure 2/9) are not commonly found on birds, being merely temporary blood-suckers. In certain freak weather conditions and in warm climates, however, swarms of some species may invade an area and large numbers attack birds. The brevity of their stay makes treatment and prevention impracticable in most cases. The flies are vectors of blood protozoa and microfilariae, the larval stages of filaria worms.

Gnats and mosquitoes (*Anopheles, Aedes* and *Culex* spp.)

Gnats and mosquitoes belonging to these genera transmit malaria (see Figure 2/9) to birds as well as certain viral infections such as equine encephalomyelitis and pox. Although exposed areas of skin in birds are relatively scanty, the head structures, eyelids and the vent region may be bitten by these insects and develop swellings.

Only the females are blood-suckers, but they are unlikely to cause anaemia unless present in large numbers. They can, however, cause discomfort and the high-pitched, threatening whine of the mosquito's wings may unsettle birds. These insects dislike intense heat and sun as much as cold weather, and choose warm places to rest that are also shady and damp. If such places also provide a food supply, so much the better from the mosquito's point of view. Tree-shaded ponds, water holes, drains and all places where stagnant water can collect are potential breeding places.

TREATMENT AND CONTROL A thin film of oil or oily insecticide over stagnant water prevents development of eggs laid on the surface. Water treated in this way, however, must not be accessible to the birds. In the premises themselves, the use of aerosol insecticides when the insects are most active is effective temporarily, but in badly affected areas it may be necessary to cover aviaries and cages with mosquito netting, especially at night.

Dipterous flies

These two-winged insects are represented by numerous genera and families. Only a few are truly parasitic but many are temporary parasites and most flourish on carrion and filth. They can thus carry disease on their feet, or inject it with their mouth parts when biting their victims. The common housefly merely vomits saliva onto its chosen morsel, dissolves it, and sucks it up again. The stable fly bites its victim. The blowflies, including bluebottles and greenbottles (*Calliphora, Lucilia, Phormia,* etc.) feed and breed mainly in decomposing organic matter, among droppings, and on dead birds, rotting food and so on. Sometimes the larval forms or maggots develop on animals, but less frequently on birds, to produce so-called "strikes". They flourish especially in hot climates and under favourable conditions a pair of flies can produce 100 to 200 offspring in two to three weeks.

TREATMENT AND CONTROL It is important to keep premises clean and ventilated and to use when necessary a safe insecticide spray such as pyrethrum.

Mites All mites belong to the *Arachnida* class of spider-like arthropods. The adults and nymphs have eight legs, and larvae six legs. There is no distinct thorax and abdomen. In fact most superficially resemble balls or discs with a small stalk-like object at the front from which project the mouth parts. The legs vary from short peg-like stumps, consisting of telescoped segments to long hairy appendages. Burrowing mites are peg-legged, spherical, slow-moving types. Non-burrowing mites have legs which usually project beyond the edges of the body. Free-living mites, such as forage or meal mites which are occasional and temporary parasites, have the longest legs. In some mites the feet have suckers, hooks, or both of these structures. The identification of mites can be difficult, even for experts.

Parasitic mites vary from between 1/10 and 1 mm. in length according to species. They are thus barely visible unless moving or on a contrasting coloured background. A powerful hand lens (x10) is suitable for mite searching. In some bird species mites are more common than is usually appreciated. Many appear to be harmless passengers, but they can nevertheless carry certain infections including some diseases well known to poultrymen, pigeon fanciers, and a few cage bird breeders. The majority of parasitic species inhabit the surface layers of the body, but some, such as the airsac mites, prefer the protected inner parts of the respiratory system.

The red or roost mite, (*Dermanyssus gallinae*) This poultry mite is a fairly common parasite of many cage birds, especially canaries and other members of the finch family (see Figure 3/9), although budgerigars appear to be quite resistant to its attacks. It affects both perching and ground-roosting birds. It is an agile, gray or brownish long-legged mite which distends and becomes bright red after

159

engorging itself with blood. It is a temporary parasite attacking the bird for short periods, usually at night. After feeding it hides in crevices in perches, the woodwork of the cage or aviary, under the droppings tray in cages, and in fact any dark secluded place. Mites may be brought in by newly acquired stock, or contracted from nearby poultry and wild birds. Apart from restlessness, caused by the nocturnal migrations, the blood-sucking habits of the mites also weaken the birds, especially the young and the old, and eventually produce severe anaemia. The plumage may become bedraggled, thin and patchy, which sometimes can lead to feather plucking. When heavy infestations occur, the wholesale desertion of young by parent birds is liable to ruin breeding plans. The anaemia often results in loss of weight and leaves the bird susceptible to chilling and infectious diseases. Other parasites such as worms and lice, often multiply under such circumstances and cause further deterioration until the bird becomes too mopey even to preen itself. Red mite infestations often remain unnoticed for months until a large population is present. At this stage, a visit at night with a powerful light suddenly switched on may show myriads of fast moving mites visible as red specks on the birds and neighbouring woodwork.

The life cycle is short, the female laying its eggs in cracks and crevices 12–24 hours after its first feed. If the environmental temperature is warm, the eggs may hatch within 48–72 hours to produce larvae. These do not feed but moult into nymphs after 24–28 hours. The nymphs feed on blood, and moult once before eventually moulting to become adults.

TREATMENT AND CONTROL Treatment of the birds alone is useless, because the mites can live away from the host for several months without a feed of blood. The premises therefore should be cleaned thoroughly. All nesting and other disposable material should be burned. Paint surfaces can be repainted with a paint impregnated with an acaricide and all cracks and crevices should also be sprayed thoroughly with a suitable acaricide. Spraying or dusting of the birds themselves may be helpful, but constant vigilance is necessary to prevent a recurrence. It is often impracticable to clean and paint the entire establishment at one time, but even if done sectionally and consecutively over 1 to 2 weeks the effect is almost as good. Acaricides, such as malathion, gamma benzene hexachloride and derris root are effective alone or in combination.

The habits, and therefore the treatment, of these mites are similar in many respects to the red mite. The former flourishes in cool, temperate regions and the latter in warm tropical

The northern feather mite *(Ornithonyssus* or *Liponyssus sylviarum)* and the tropical feather mite *(O. bursa)*

areas. The life cycle of *O. sylviarum*, however, differs from that of the other two mites in that all stages, including egg laying, may actually take place on the bird, thus making the parasite more easy to control.

The harvest mites or chiggers (*Trombicula* spp.) These mites are only parasitic in the larval stage, the adults being free-living mites which inhabit old pastures, brush or woodland areas. The larvae attach themselves to the skin and until they become engorged with blood are too minute to be seen with the naked eye. They inject an irritant which digests the skin, thus providing food and producing some capillary bleeding. An inflammatory swelling in the form of a papule or blister occurs around the point of the mite's attachment to the skin. Toxins from the larvae produce intense irritation and even illness or death, especially in small ground-living or ground-nesting birds such as quail. Because of their normal habitat, chiggers should seldom be a problem in well kept aviaries, but during hot weather the matted undergrowth of planted aviaries may attract the mites. They breed during the spring and autumn in temperate regions and at such times a careful watch should be kept in areas where they are known to occur.

TREATMENT AND CONTROL The ground in the aviary should be treated by spraying with an acaricide to control adult mites. Because of the danger of the acaricide being eaten, birds must be removed before spraying is carried out and some weeks must be allowed to elapse before birds are replaced in the aviary, unless heavy rain washes the substance to the deeper layers of the herbage after spraying. Treatment of individual birds is tedious but it is the only way to clear those which are infested. Dusting or spraying can also be carried out just before the expected chigger season as a preventive measure. When skin reaction to the bites is severe, localised treatment with sulphur ointment, iodine or antibiotic ointments is sometimes helpful. Antihistamines and corticosteroids may also be used when irritation and swellings are extreme.

The Depluming or Body Mange Mite (*Knemidocoptes laevis* var. *gallinae*) This mite does not occur on most species of cage and aviary birds, but it does occasionally infest pigeons, pheasants and poultry. It invades the feathered areas of the skin, especially around the feather bases, and causes severe irritation. Feathers break off just above the level of the skin, and fall out or become deranged. The skin may show partial or even complete baldness over the back and wings, especially in young birds. Transmission is by prolonged close contact, as for example in the nest, and when birds are overcrowded or

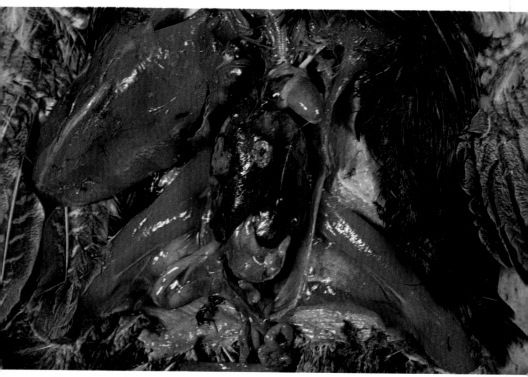

Plate 3/9. Typical lesions of histomoniasis or "blackhead" involving the liver of a pheasant. Note the large, rounded, well-defined, pale areas of necrosis. (I.F. Keymer)

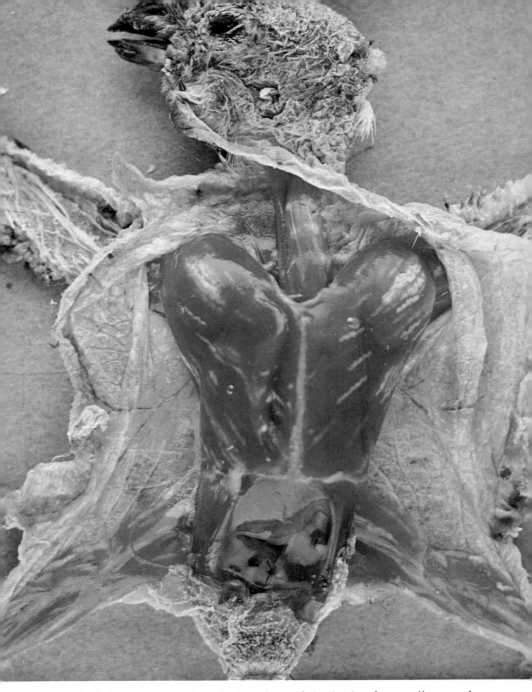

Plate 4/9. Musculature of ventral surface of the body of a small passerine bird (blue-backed chlorophonia), exposed to show pale-coloured, elongated cysts of the protozoan parasite, *Sarcocystis*. The entire musculature was infected with this uncommon parasite of birds. See Other Protozoan Infections, Chapter 9. (I.F. Keymer and T.C. Dennett, Z.S.L.)

huddle together on perches when roosting. The mites are most prevalent during the warm months.

TREATMENT AND CONTROL This is difficult. Spraying is ineffective, total immersion in a suitable acaricide being necessary to reach the embedded mites. This should be repeated at weekly intervals, but if only a few birds are affected, destruction may be preferable. Protective dipping should be carried out for any birds in contact or on the same premises as those infested. Ointments are messy and unsuitable for treatment. They may help to suffocate the mites but are less penetrating than thin, oily or spirit-based lotions. Malathion, monosulfiram, gamma benzene hexachloride, sulphur in oil and many others can be used. The efficacy of mercury, phenol and other corrosive substances in ointment bases is doubtful.

Mites of the genus *Knemidocoptes* are members of the family Sarcoptidae which includes the mites responsible for scabies in human beings and mange in domestic animals. In birds they cause the disease known as scaly leg and scaly face. The mites are microscopic, measuring only about one third of a mm. in diameter, poorly mobile, and have short stumpy legs. In most cases the life cycles are not clearly understood.

The Scaly Leg Mites (*Knemidocoptes spp.*) and the Scaly Face and Leg Mite (*K. pilae*)

Knemidocoptes mutans causes scaly leg disease in poultry and *K. jamaicensis* causes similar lesions in some passerine birds. Closely related species of *Knemidocoptes* cause similar lesions, the best known being *K. pilae* (Plate 2/10) the cause of scaly face and scaly leg in budgerigars (Plate 3/10) and also some other psittacines and the canary. The anatomical distinctions between the different species of mites are very small and difficult to detect, calling for an entomologist experienced in the taxonomy of the species. The minute differences between species need not concern us here, because what applies to *K. mutans* in poultry with regard to clinical signs and treatment applies equally well to *K. pilae* and other species which infest cage and aviary birds. Various species of birds in Britain, Europe, Australasia, the Americas, the West Indies and elsewhere have been found infested both in the wild and captive states. The author has found a few cases of infestation in old canaries with raised, thickened scales of the legs, but this usually indicates a non-parasitic senile change, perhaps related to poor limb circulation.

The way in which an isolated bird kept indoors can develop mange lesions in middle life is still something of a mystery. Possibilities include a mild, inapparent, lifelong infestation which flares up for some reason unknown. Seed may be contaminated by wild birds either at its source or in a pet store where birds and seed are kept close together. The most common method of transmission, however, is probably to nestlings from parents during feeding. A heavy infestation at this time may produce defective horn and abnormal growth of the beak to such an extent that a "scissor beak" is formed. This in turn often leads to death from starvation.

A typically affected young budgerigar shows a beige coloured deposit over one or more of the following areas: the mandibles, the fleshy angle between the mandibles, the cere, the soft skin below the beak, around the eyes and the scaled parts of the legs and feet. Long-standing infestations may spread to the feathered parts beyond these areas. In budgerigars, face lesions are far more common than those on the legs; whereas in passerines the converse appears to be true. In adults the affected areas of skin thicken to a crusty sheet and become knobbly, especially on the movable parts at the angle of the beak and around the eyes. In a few cases, horn-like growths appear from the latter areas in budgerigars and give the birds a most extraordinarily grotesque appearance (Plate 4/10). In advanced cases the nostrils may become blocked. The dry, chalk-like encrustations are composed of exudate produced by the bird in response to the irritation caused by the mites, plus skin debris thrown up by the mites whilst burrowing in the tissues. Inspection with a hand lens will show the entire area to be a honeycomb of burrows (Plate 5/10). The horny and underlying tissues, as well as the horn- and skin-producing cells, become permanently damaged. On the beak, this results in poor quality, crumbly horn being produced which is thicker than normal and fractures or flakes off when the bird dehusks its seed. Where the cere joins the beak, damage to the generative cells causes the diseased horn to grow at different rates and results in the formation of straight, upturned, deviated, wry or scissor-crossed beaks. The sideways pressure exerted by trying to eat with a twisted beak causes severe straining on the supporting bones and other tissues of the jaw. Consequently a permanent deformity of the jaw-bone may also result.

TREATMENT AND CONTROL Treatment is effective if carried out sufficiently early. Reinfestation is always a possibility, however, because these mites are very common. The usual insecticides and acaricides are rapidly effective, but even painting the lesion with a bland oil such as liquid paraffin is useful, at least in early cases. In severe cases, the encrustations should be softened beforehand with such oily preparations before applying an acaricide. Complete disinfestation is best attained by application of the chosen acaricide at intervals of a few days for up to three weeks. Bromocyclen, monosulfiram, benzyl benzoate, or indeed any of the modern acaricides are all effective. An oily or spirit base is

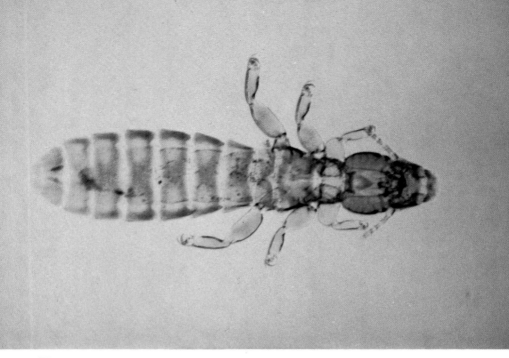

Plate 1/10. A typical biting louse of the family Philopteridae from the plumage of a common curlew. Greatly magnified.(I.F. Keymer and T.C. Dennett, Z.S.L.)

Plate 2/10. *Knemidocoptes pilae* mite. Greatly magnified. (D.K. Blackmore)

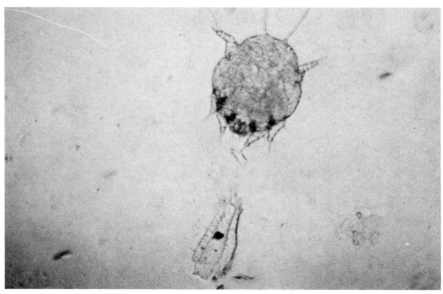

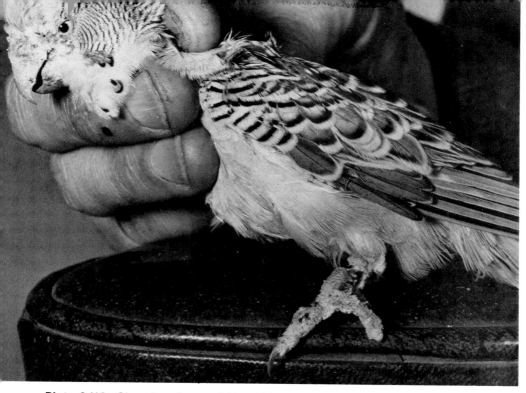

Plate 3/10. Chronic advanced Knemidocoptic mange causing Scaly Face and Scaly Leg in the budgerigar. Note deformity of the beak and thick encrustations on the foot and constriction around the leg from which the embedded identity ring has been removed. (L. Arnall)

Plate 4/10. Fleshy excrescences around eyes and beak due to chronic *Knemidocoptes* infestation. Budgerigar. See also Plate 3/24. (L. Arnall)

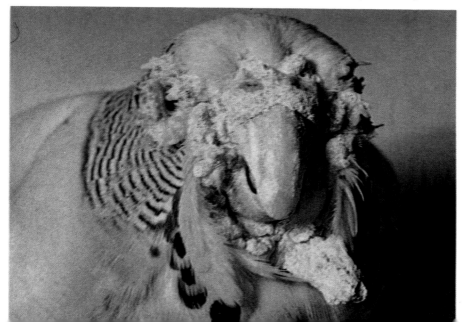

preferable for penetration and persistance, but care must be taken not to let the bird peck at the brush during application or to remove and ingest the lotion during preening. All recently acquired and fledgling budgerigars and other parakeets should be closely examined for the characteristic pinhole lesions in the skin over the sites described above. All unusual beaks should be scrutinised under a lens and not assumed to be an inherited defect or due to injury.

Other skin and feather mites

There are a considerable number of other species which occur on a wide variety of caged and wild birds and which may be encountered from time to time. Some of the species, such as those in the genera *Megninia, Rivoltasia, Protalges* and *Protolichus*, live in the plumage and seldom cause trouble unless present in massive numbers.

The species *Faculifer rostratis* is commonly found on pigeons. There are a few mites, for example *Syringophilus* and *Dermoglyphus*, which actually inhabit the feather quills and in addition to causing irritation may also produce excessive moulting.

Species of *Epidermoptes, Microlichus,* and *Myialges* produce mange on most areas of the skin which to the naked eye is indistinguishable from that caused by *Knemidocoptes*. They do not, however, appear to invade the scaly areas of the legs and feet. The life cycles of most of these mites are either completely unknown or poorly understood.

TREATMENT AND CONTROL If necessary, the feather mites can be treated in the same way as the red mites. There is no known treatment which is satisfactory for quill mites. The mange mites should be treated in the same way as the *Knemidocoptes* spp.

***Sternostoma tracheacolum* and Airsac mites**

This is the only truly pathogenic mite which has been described as occurring in the respiratory system. It has been reported from many parts of the world and occurs in all areas of the respiratory tract. Many species of birds have been found infested including the canary, gouldian finch and budgerigar. Closely related species which are almost identical to *S. tracheacolum* also occur in a wide range of hosts.

Mites such as *Cytodites nudus* although most frequently confined to the air sacs, have also been reported in various parts of the respiratory tract of the domestic fowl and other birds, but appear to be harmless.

Several other mites have been found inhabiting the upper respiratory passages of pigeons, e.g., *Neonyssus* and *Speleognathus*. Very little is known about the life cycles of any of these parasites, but they are not normally pathogenic.

Canaries and especially gouldian finches are susceptible to infestations with *S. tracheacolum*, and may show loss of condition and varying degrees of respiratory distress. Sometimes there is partial or complete loss of voice in the early stages, ruffled plumage and sleepiness. Later characteristic "sucking" or smacking sounds are made, often twice in rapid succession. Coughing, sneezing and gasping for breath result in loss of sleep, as well as loss of condition and eventually death, if no treatment is given. Without a laboratory *postmortem* examination, the disease can easily be confused with gapes due to *Syngamus* worms, the pharyngeal form of pox or aspergillosis.

Although the life cycle is uncertain, it is believed that parent birds may infest nestlings while feeding them with regurgitated food. If therefore, parents are known to be infested, nestlings should be handreared if this is possible. Affected birds should always be separated from those which are healthy.

TREATMENT
Inhalation of malathion powder has been found to be satisfactory for the treatment of *S. tracheacolum*. It is relatively non-toxic when compared with other agents. The affected bird is placed in a small sealed box or the cage is covered with a towel, after which the powder is pumped in using an ordinary puffer type dispenser. The bird should be left in the box or cage for five minutes after introducing the powder. The almost inevitable fluttering of the bird will further serve to disperse the powder. The treatment should be repeated at 4–6 weekly intervals. It is advisable to treat only one bird at a time, otherwise injuries may occur whilst fluttering about.

Ticks   Ticks are responsible for the transmission of numerous diseases of man and animals in many parts of the world. Wild birds are frequently infested and may carry the parasites for considerable distances when migrating. The fowl tick *Argus persicus* is the best known species to be found on birds. *Argus reflexus* commonly occurs on pigeons. While some have quite strict host requirements, others are satisfied with a wide range of warm-blooded creatures: man, mammals, and birds.

Different species of tick occur in different areas of the world depending upon temperature, humidity, type of vegetation and terrain. In cage and aviary birds, infestations are mainly sporadic and usually acquired from poultry, wild birds or mammals.

Ticks, like mites, are acarine arthropods. They possess eight legs except in the first larval stage of the life cycle when

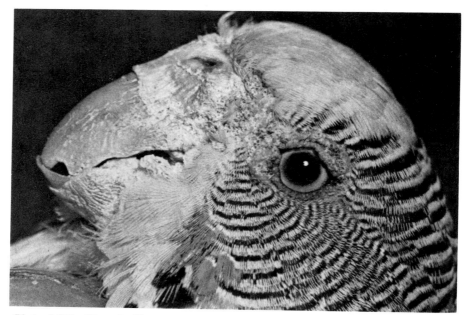

Plate 5/10. Chronic Knemidocoptic mange of the face. Note the distorted beak and the openings of mite burrows on the surface deposits of abnormal, scaly horn and skin. (L. Arnall)

Plate 6/10. Fluke *Cathaemasia spectabilis* removed from the nasal cavity of a Marabou stork. At the anterior end the mouth can be seen surrounded by a sucker, whilst the larger ventral sucker is visible posterior to it in the anterior half of the body. Situated immediately behind the oral sucker is the pharynx. The reproductive system can be seen lying along each side of the body and terminating at the posterior extremity. There is no anus. The life cycle probably involves a snail and a frog as intermediate hosts. (I.F. Keymer and T.C. Dennett, Z.S.L.)

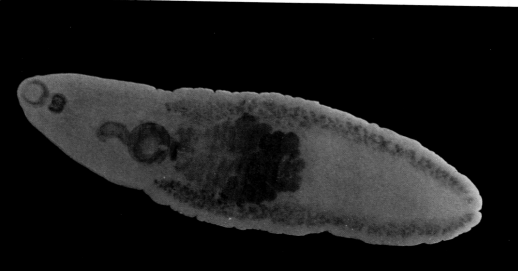

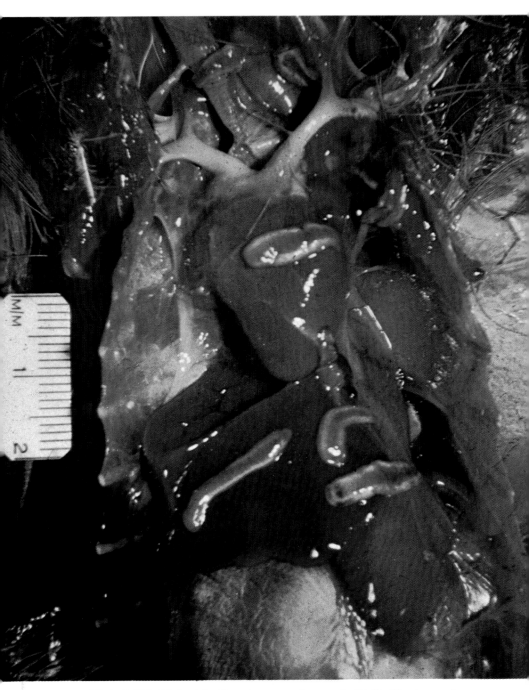

Plate 7/10. Flukes in the air sacs of a coot. (D.K. Blackmore)

they have six. They are all blood suckers and vary in size from 3–15 mm. in length being broadly oval, round or pear-shaped, according to species and whether or not they have recently fed on blood. Two main groups occur, the hard or ixodid ticks which have a horny shield on their backs, and the soft or argasid ticks. Hard ticks are parasitic, mainly as larvae or during the nymphal intermediate stages; they do not occur so frequently on birds as the soft ticks. The latter can cause considerable trouble by blood-sucking and by transmitting diseases. Important infections which they are capable of transmitting include spirochaetosis due to *Borrelia* and agyptianellosis (*Aegyptianella pullorum* infection) of poultry, the latter disease also affecting some psittacine birds.

Adult ticks may be found on birds around the head and neck, the vent and thinly feathered parts of the body and also on the limbs. When engorged they appear as small, blue to deep red coloured grape-like structures firmly embedded in the skin by their mouth parts. They are often present in bunches or small groups. When starved, for example on the ground or elsewhere, they appear as wizened, dehydrated, raisin-like objects. After feeding on a suitable host soft ticks lay about 20 to 10,000 eggs, usually in the vicinity of the bird, in cracks and crevices or under dry sand or soil. The eggs hatch within 10 days to several months depending upon the temperature, the larvae wait for a host to approach close enough to attach themselves to some part of the body. The larvae then feed for several days, moult once or twice into eight legged nymphs over a period of weeks or several months and eventually moult and become adults. The females attach themselves to hosts, sucking large amounts of blood and at least quadrupling their size in the process. They then mate and lay eggs, and the life cycle is repeated. Any stage may survive for 6 to 12 months or even more, whilst lying in wait for a victim.

Ticks must be numerous in order to cause appreciable illness or unrest and moderate infestations may be overlooked in a brief examination because the larvae are little bigger than mites. Even a few adults, however, are sufficient to produce considerable anaemia. Signs to be expected include weakness, loss of weight, reduced growth, ruffled plumage, poor appetite, restlessness and even diarrhoea.

TREATMENT AND CONTROL   As soft ticks feed mainly at night and often retreat into hiding by day, they can be checked by spraying the bird at night with suitable acaricides at two week intervals. Thorough spraying of the entire building, and especially shady areas in the flight and aviary itself, with an acaricide should be carried out whenever the accommodation can be cleared of birds for some days or weeks.

Individual adult ticks on birds are very difficult to remove. Any attempt to pull them off usually leaves the head embedded in the skin and this may rapidly become an infected wound or abscess. A chloroform or ether-soaked pad placed over the parasites will sometimes induce them to loosen their grip a little, and they may then be gently eased off or alternatively pulled away suddenly using a pair of fine-pointed curved forceps. Both young and adult stages may die attached to the skin as a result of acaricidal treatment and these too, may produce unpleasant wounds.

Suitable treatment may clear premises for a matter of months, but prophylactic spraying or painting at least every 3 months is desirable in areas where ticks are common.

Helminths   Helminths infest almost all forms of animal life including cold-blooded animals as well as invertebrates such as arthropods. They are among the most common parasites. Many are so well-adapted to their host that they are completely harmless under ordinary circumstances.

Most wild birds harbour at least one species at some time in their life and may be infested with several species at a time. Their place in zoological classification does not concern us, but four main classes or groups occur in birds. These are the Cestodes or tapeworms, the Trematodes or flukes, the Nematodes or round worms and the Acanthocephalids or thorny-headed worms.

Tapeworms   A vast number of different species of tapeworm occur in
(Cestodes)   birds, the genera *Dilepis* and *Choanotaenia* being particularly common in passerines; *Raillietina* in psittacines, pigeons and gallinaceons birds and *Hymenolepis* in water fowl. At least 18 species have been found in the pigeon alone.

Tapeworms vary in size from a few millimeters to 35 cm. or even more in length. All have a head and neck, a segmented body, and are wider than they are thick. Hence long chains of segments give the appearance of a cross-ribbed tape. The head bears suckers and/or hooks with which it attaches itself to the tissues of the host. No eyes or mouth are present. Eyes would be useless inside the dark interior of the host's body and a mouth or gut is made unnecessary by virtue of the way these unpleasant creatures feed by absorbing nutrients through their body surface. The youngest segments are nearest to the head and are short and small, whilst at the "tail" of the worm they are long and larger. The latter which are the ripe segments, are filled with many thousands of eggs produced by self-fertilization within each segment.

Male organs fertilize female organs in the middle segments of the chain. The eggs burst out of the ripe segments usually

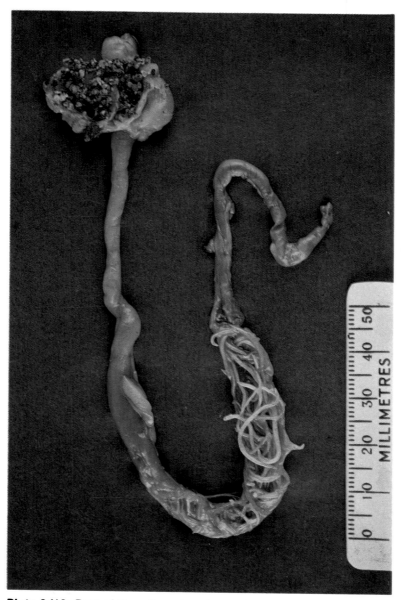

Plate 8/10. Part of the alimentary tract of a cockatiel showing impaction of the posterior half of the duodenum with a mass of roundworms, *Ascaridia* sp. (I.F. Keymer and T.C. Dennett, Z.S.L.)

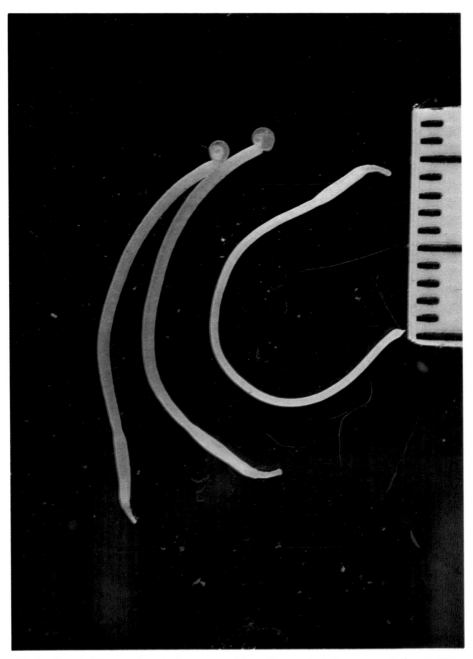

Plate 9/10. Thorny-headed worms (Acanthocephala) removed from the small intestine of a debilitated, collared, scops owl. The scale is marked in millimetres. (I.F. Keymer and T.C. Dennett, Z.S.L.)

when they are shed in the birds' droppings, because most tape worms live in the alimentary canal. Usually, eggs must be eaten by an intermediate host of another species of animal, before the first stage of development of the parasites can occur. The intermediate host may be an earthworm, snail, slug, insect, fish, or other creature which is edible to birds—the main or primary hosts. The eggs themselves are not infective to the primary host. In the intermediate host, early development into a bladderworm stage takes place in the muscle or other body tissues, and not in the cavity of the gut from which it quickly migrates after being swallowed. When the infested intermediate host is eaten by a suitable bird host, digestion of the tissues releases the bladderworm in the gut, which then gives rise to one or more adult tapeworms.

Clinical signs of tapeworm infestation are dullness, loss of appetite, sometimes excessive thirst, loss of weight, anaemia and leg weakness. The resulting debility may pave the way for infections and other diseases. Tapeworms also tend to contribute to the misery of birds which are sick from other causes. Nodules are produced in the gut wall by some species of *Raillietina* (Figure 1/10) which are reminiscent of those caused by tuberculosis, this being one of the few genera producing obvious disease changes in birds.

TREATMENT AND CONTROL Grain and seed eaters are much less likely to become infested than insectivorous birds, although at times they may eat certain types of small animal life which act as intermediate hosts. Lack of knowledge about the life histories of many tapeworms in birds is so great that it is often impossible to determine where, when, and how infestation occurred. As a result, few recommendations can be made to limit reinfestation. Attention to general hygiene may help by limiting spread of shed tapeworm ova in droppings by flies, beetles, ants and other invertebrates. On the other hand, eliminating these tasty morsels, which can be a useful source of animal protein, may be more harmful to the health of the birds than the burden of worms which they may acquire from them.

The amount of nutrients which the tapeworms absorb whilst in the gut of the host is negligible. Absorption by the host of waste products and toxins produced by the parasites is almost certainly small, although the effect they have on the bird is unknown.

Avian tapeworms are resistant to drugs. Most of those which have been tried are liable to cause more ill effects than the worms themselves and often leave the head and neck of the worm still in place, capable of growing again to maturity. Such drugs include santonin, felix mas (malefern extract) kamala and carbon tetrachloride. Stannous (tin) tartrate

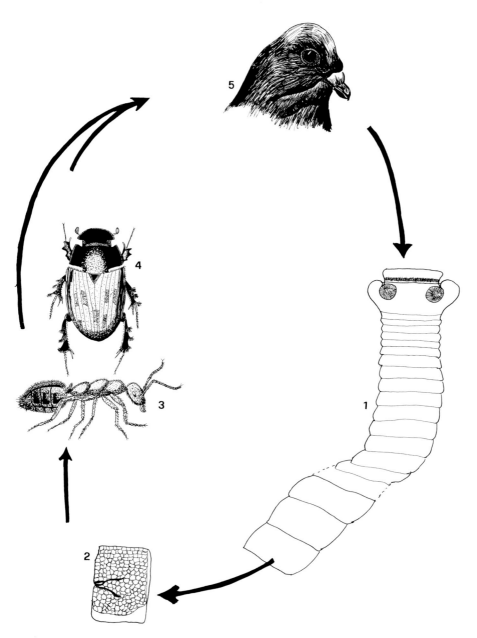

Figure 1/10. Not drawn to scale. Life cycle of a cestode (1) such as *Rail-lietina* sp. in the pigeon (5). The adult tapeworm (1) lives in the small in-testine of the host (5) and the gravid segments (2) are expelled in the drop-pings. Egg capsules released by the segment are ingested by ants (3) or various species of ground or dung beetles (4) depending upon the species of *Raillietina*. The final host which is usually a bird in the order Galli-formes, Psittaciformes or Columbiformes (as depicted here), becomes infested by eating these intermediate hosts. (Janet Keymer)

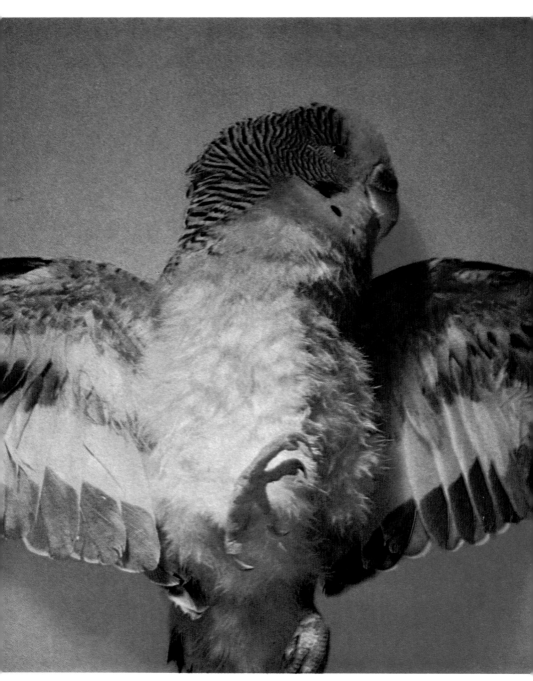

Plate 1/11. Partial loss of feathers on undersurface of wing due to self-plucking. Young budgerigar. (L. Arnall)

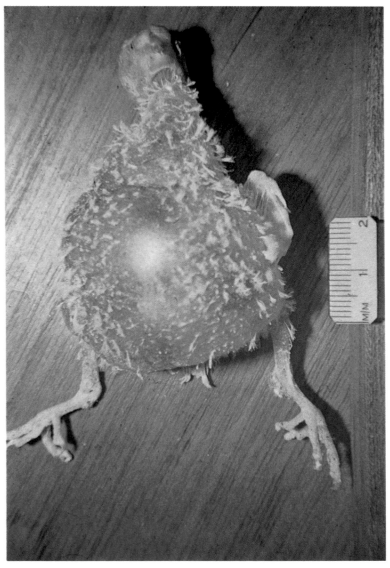

Plate 2/11. Extensive subcutaneous emphysema in nestling budgerigar causing gross distension of abdominal region. (D.K. Blackmore)

and pelleterine hydrochloride are a little better regarding toxicity and are moderately effective against *Raillietina*, whilst dichlorophen appears effective against some types of tapeworm. It is preferable, however, to rely on hygiene to reduce the possibilities of infestation and to keep birds well fed, exercised, and content, In fact, treatment should only be attempted when a veterinarian decides that it is necessary, for example following the confirmation at *post-mortem* examination of heavy infestations of other birds in the same group.

Flukes (Trematodes)

A considerable number of different species of flukes infest a wide range of birds. The incidence of infestation, however, is highest in waterfowl and other aquatic species. Nevertheless, the pigeon has been found capable of harbouring at least 28 different species of flukes. They occur in the liver, gut and many other organs.

Flukes are flat "worms" with a leaf-shaped outline (Plate 6/10), somewhat like a plaice or other flat fish (to which the name of fluke is also given). Some species are roughly cylindrical in shape (Plate 7/10). Parasitic flukes range from 3 to 25 mm. or more in length and may be 2 to 10 times longer than they are broad. The mouth is near the anterior end and usually surrounded by a sucker. A second sucker may be present on the ventral surface. Flukes feed on body fluids and in most species after digestion, the waste products are passed out of the mouth owing to the absence of an anus. Both male and female organs are present in the majority, although blood flukes are not hermaphroditic. Most flukes (blood flukes being an exception) require two intermediate hosts for their development (Figure 2/10), the first of which must be a mollusc. The other intermediate host is usually a cold-blooded creature such as another type of invertebrate, but sometimes a fish. Birds become infested by eating the second intermediate hosts, or in the case of blood flukes by being attacked whilst in water by stages of the parasite released from infected molluscs.

Flukes require moisture and warmth, and when in the intermediate host, occasional periods of dryness to stimulate reproduction. A few flourish fairly well in temperate climates, but most rapid development occurs in warm, and especially tropical areas, this being the case with many disease-producing organisms.

Clinical signs can vary considerably, ranging from general malaise, lack of appetite, thirst and diarrhoea to anaemia or jaundice. When the parasites infest the rectum and cloaca, they may interfere with egg-laying. Flukes in the respiratory tract can cause asphyxia. A heavy burden such as the pre-

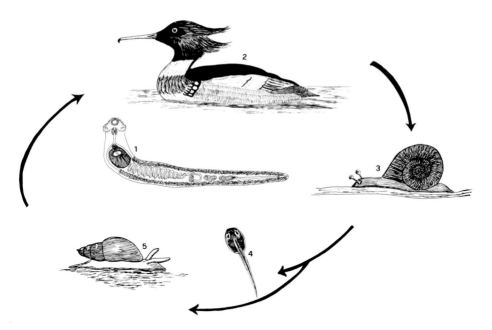

Figure 2/10. Not drawn to scale. Life cycle of the common trematode or fluke *Echinostoma revolutum* (1) in a duck such as the red-breasted merganser (2). This fluke infests numerous other species of duck as well as geese, swans, pigeons and various members of the order Galliformes. The parasites live in the intestine or caeca. The trematode eggs are passed in the faeces and the life cycle takes place in freshwater. The eggs hatch in water and release a larval stage (miracidium) which swims and penetrates an aquatic mollusc such as a ramshorn snail, *Helisoma* sp. (3), where further development occurs. A stage known as a cercaria escapes from the snail and swims in the water in search of another intermediate host such as a frog tadpole (4) or a species of freshwater snail such as a pouch snail, *Physa* sp., in which the parasite encysts. The final host (2) becomes infested by eating the intermediate hosts (4 and 5). (Janet Keymer)

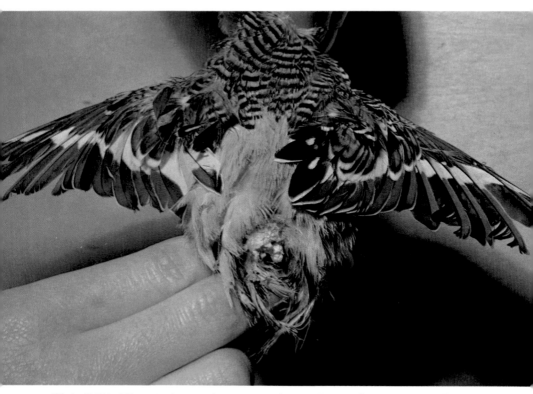

Plate 3/11. Ulcerated retention cyst and granuloma of preen gland. Budgerigar. (L. Arnall)

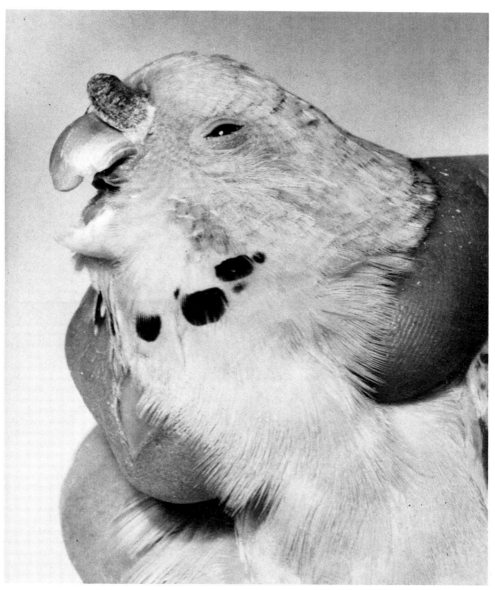

Plate 4/11. Budgerigar. Undershot lower mandible with short upper mandible 3 months after the upper was damaged. Brown hypertrophy of the cere also present. (L. Arnall)

sence of several hundred causing obstruction in the gut or in a duct may kill the host.

Flukes are regional in their distribution and if birds live in an area where they are known to occur, or if birds are acquired which have been recently obtained from the wild, samples of the excreta should be submitted to a suitable laboratory or veterinarian for examination. Diagnosis depends upon finding the typical fluke eggs in the droppings or flukes in the gut, liver, or other internal organs upon *post-mortem* examination, because clinical signs are never diagnostic in themselves.

TREATMENT AND CONTROL Flukes are well known to farmers and are common in cattle and sheep. In these animals control is effected more by removing the possibility of reinfestation than by treatment of infested animals, and in birds the same principles apply. Shady, muddy puddles and other suitable habitats for water snails should be avoided in aviaries. A copper sulphate dressing if used in a planted aviary will kill most molluscs, but it is somewhat toxic to the birds. A heavy shower of rain or the use of a water-can will help to wash the dressing down to the grass roots and to reach the snails. Treatment of individuals using carbon tetrachloride, tetrachlorethylene, or hexachlorethane, although suitable for farm animals, is extremely toxic to birds and liable to kill them more quickly than the flukes themselves.

Roundworms (Nematodes)

These are probably the most common parasites of all and include the gapeworms, threadworms, proventricular and gizzard worms, caecal and filarial worms. The worms are cylindrical, smooth and unsegmented with tapered ends. In birds they are usually well-adapted and therefore non-pathogenic to their host so that the presence of small numbers is not suspected by the owner. The parasites have no eyes, heart or lungs, but a simple tube-like alimentary tract running the entire length of the worm from the mouth to the anus. A reproductive tract capable of producing thousands of eggs daily, liberally ensures future generations of worms in spite of the great hazards awaiting eggs and larvae in the outside world. Roundworms of birds are mainly small and thread-like, the largest being a few centimetres long and about 2 mm. thick. The habits of roundworms vary greatly and their life cycles may involve an intermediate host or be direct. Most can only exist as adults inside the host's body. Just as size, shape, and habits vary, so does the shape, size, and form of the eggs, although large groups of worms produce identical eggs.

Although some roundworms are harmless in moderate numbers, they are undesirable because they are always liable to multiply rapidly, especially if the condition of the host is lowered in some way, such as by the presence of an infectious disease or due to incorrect feeding.

The Gapeworm (*Syngamus trachea*) This worm, long recognized in poultry, has been found in a very wide range of avian species. Transmission is either direct from the soil by eating infective eggs or larvae, or by eating earthworms or snails which act as transport hosts for the parasites encysted within them (Figure 3/10). On arrival in the alimentary canal of the bird, the parasite migrates to the upper respiratory passages where it breeds. The female attaches itself to the epithelial lining of the trachea and is characteristically seen with the much smaller male, permanently attached to it and giving the pair of worms the appearance of a "Y". The presence of adults in the windpipe causes irritation, excess production of mucus, and often frenzied bouts of coughing or sneezing as the birds attempt to dislodge the parasites. In this way the eggs are coughed up, swallowed, and passed out in the droppings. After an incubation period as short as 1 to 2 weeks, the eggs become infective. Small species are worst affected, because large numbers of the worms can block the windpipe. Throwing forward of the head, head-shaking, and gasping (or gaping) for breath is frequently seen in infested birds. Exhaustion, loss of weight, loss of appetite, and death may result from gradual asphyxiation and starvation. On opening the mouth, worms may actually be seen through the larynx in the opening to the windpipe.

TREATMENT AND CONTROL Adult birds bearing a few gapeworms are a serious danger to nestlings and if possible should therefore be prevented from eating infective larvae in transport hosts such as earthworms. The aviary should be shielded from the droppings of wild birds and should never be built outside in the vicinity of free-ranging poultry or game birds such as pheasants.

An old treatment was the inhalation of barium antimonyl tartrate powder puffed into a large cardboard box containing the birds. A more modern treatment is the oral administration of thiabendazole. This drug appears to be quite effective, but the birds may have difficulty in coughing up the worms. In birds larger than a mynah it is sometimes possible to remove the worms mechanically from the trachea by using a cotton and wire pipe cleaner. The bird's beak is prised open and the cleaner pushed gently through the opening of the larynx and into the trachea. As it is withdrawn it is twisted round two or three times when the worms should stick to the

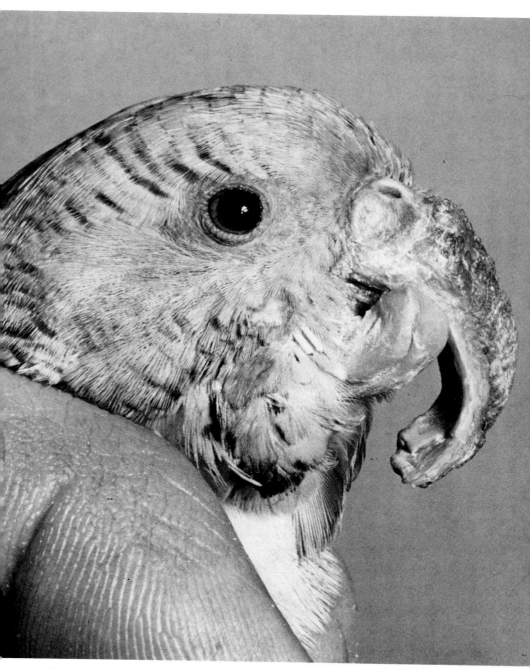

Plate 5/11. Carcinoma of upper beak with secondary wrybreak. Budgerigar.
(L. Arnall)

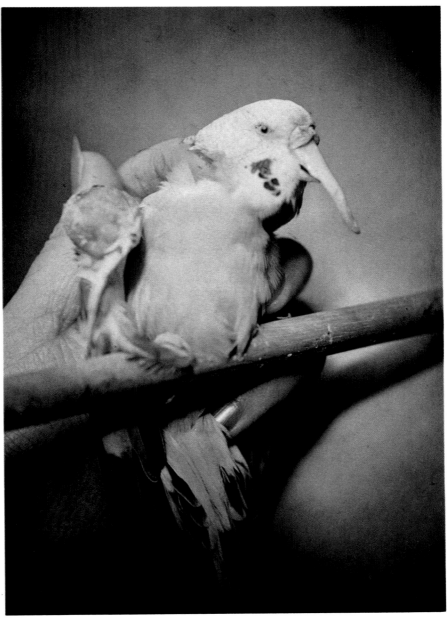

Plate 6/11. Budgerigar with long straight overgrown beak and lipoma of carpus. (L. Arnall)

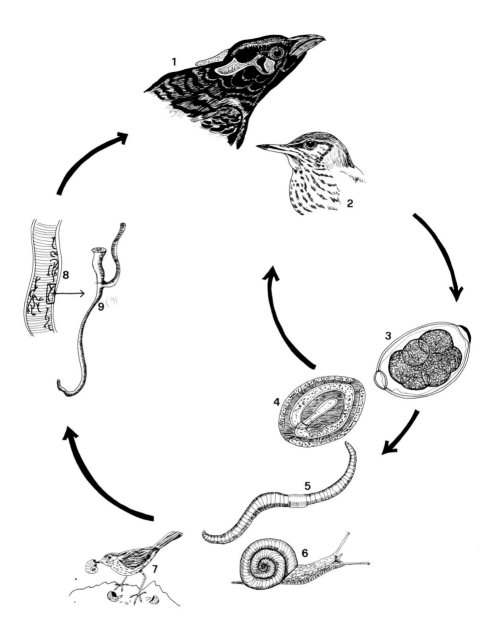

Figure 3/10. Not drawn to scale. Life cycle of gapeworm *Syngamus trachea* depicting hosts such as a hill mynah (1) and a song thrush (2). The worm eggs (3) are passed by the birds and then after embryonation (4) are either eaten by the bird or ingested by transport hosts such as earthworms (5) or snails (6). When a transport host is eaten (7) the worms reach maturity in the bird and become attached to the lining of the trachea (8) where they live in pairs (9). (Janet Keymer)

soft cotton surface. This must be done quickly or else the bird may be asphyxiated.

Threadworms
(*Capillaria* spp.)
These are hair-like worms of the intestinal tract, parasitizing various levels from the crop to the small intestine.

There are many species of *Capillaria* and these vary from only 1 to 8 cm. in length, most being at the lower end of the range, with males smaller than females. The eggs, which are roughly oval with a plug at each end, pass out in the droppings and develop in about a month to a stage infective to other birds. An intermediate host may be required for some species. The worms can flourish in most climates and have a worldwide distribution.

A light infestation is tolerated well by adult birds of most species. Under favourable conditions for the parasites, such as bad sanitation and overcrowding, heavy populations of infective larvae can build up and mild or serious outbreaks of disease can occur. Light infestations may present signs of indigestion, dullness, poor appetite, regurgitation of food, and soft droppings. In severe cases, the inflammation of the gut may be so severe that parts of its lining mucous membrane may separate, producing slimy, yellow or bloody diarrhoea. Such birds· rapidly become mopy, emaciated and anaemic, and are likely to die.

Many wild birds harbour *Capillaria* worms and by perching on the netting over the aviaries, contaminate the aviary floor with their droppings. However, close attention to hygiene can limit infestations to a low level. Severe outbreaks may occur in pigeons, which is understandable since they have more access to food and land outside their home premises. Gamebirds and waterbirds are also commonly affected and occasionally birds of prey kept by falconers. The more "natural" the aviary, the more liable are the inmates to become infested owing to the build-up of parasites in the soil and vegetation.

TREATMENT AND CONTROL As with all roundworm infestations, strict attention to hygiene is essential to stop build-up of the parasites. It should be remembered that helminth ova require damp and warm conditions in order to develop. In heated indoor aviaries therefore, it is particularly important to prevent leakage or spillage on the floor from drinking vessels. Damp areas around water receptacles contaminated with droppings provide ideal conditions for the parasites.

Capillariasis can be treated with levamisole hydrochloride or tetramisole by mouth.

189

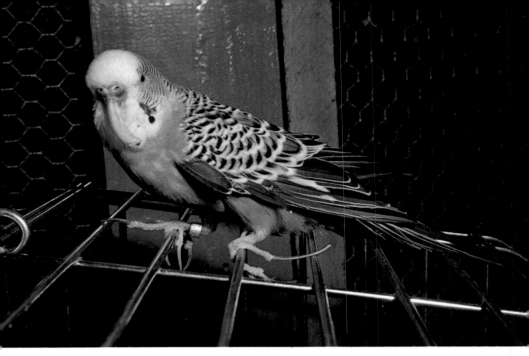

Plate 7/11. Budgerigar with laterally deviated upper mandible and straight grossly overgrown claws. (L. Arnall)

Plate 8/11. Budgerigar with crossed mandibles, so-called wrybeak or scissorbill. (L. Arnall)

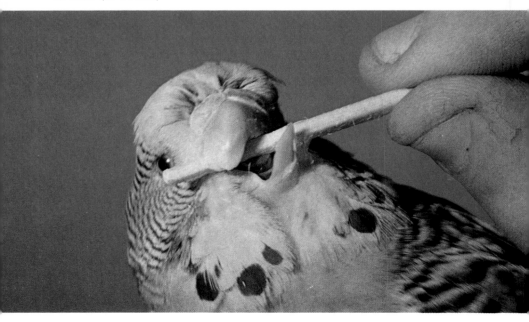

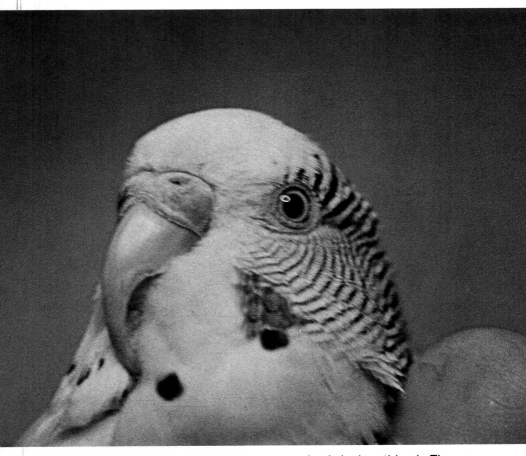

Plate 9/11. Budgerigar with overgrown upper beak (epinagthism). The curvature is near normal. (L. Arnall)

These worms, depending upon the species, occur in the walls of the forestomach, beneath the horny lining of the gizzard, and to a lesser extent the small intestine and oesophagus of many species of gallinaceous, psittacine and passerine birds in various parts of the world.

Proventricular and Gizzard Worms (*Acuaria* and *Spiroptera* spp.)

They burrow deeply into the mucous lining where they cause inflammation or severe ulceration with chronic thickening of the lining layers, depending upon the degree of infestation. Severe infestations cause digestive disorders, loss of weight and even death. In all species the life cycle is indirect. The eggs after being eaten by an arthropod, produce larvae in the intermediate host before becoming infective to birds (Figure 4/10). Although not commonly reported parasites, more thorough *post-mortem* examinations of mysterious deaths in aviary birds may show these and similarly sited worms to be more common than is realised.

TREATMENT AND CONTROL No satisfactory method of treatment is known; control measures similar to those advised for gapeworms and threadworms should be used.

These are primarily poultry parasites, but peafowl, game-birds and other gallinaceous species are commonly infested. The worms are approximately 0.5–1.5 cm. in length and are usually confined to the caeca. Eggs pass out in the droppings and usually become infective in about two weeks. The eggs are frequently taken in by earthworms so that birds may also become infested by eating these invertebrates.

Caecal Worms (*Heterakis* spp.)

Although the worms are usually harmless, very heavy infestations especially of *Heterakis isolonche* in pheasants, do sometimes cause pinpoint haemorrhages and nodules on the epithelial lining of the caeca. The importance, however, of the caecal worm, *Heterakis gallinae* of the domestic fowl and other species, is its capacity to carry the protozoan parasite *Histomonas meleagridis* which causes the disease known as blackhead.

TREATMENT AND CONTROL Infestations can be treated if considered necessary with tetramisole. Control measures should be on the same lines as those recommended previously for other roundworm infestations.

These delicate, pink-coloured worms are vicious bloodsuckers, which occur in the proventriculus and small intestine of pigeons in Europe, North America, Africa and Australia. The worms measure approximately 1–2.5 cm. in length. Eggs passed out in the droppings hatch within approximately two days; then becoming infective to another or the same host.

Ornithostrongylus quadriradiatus

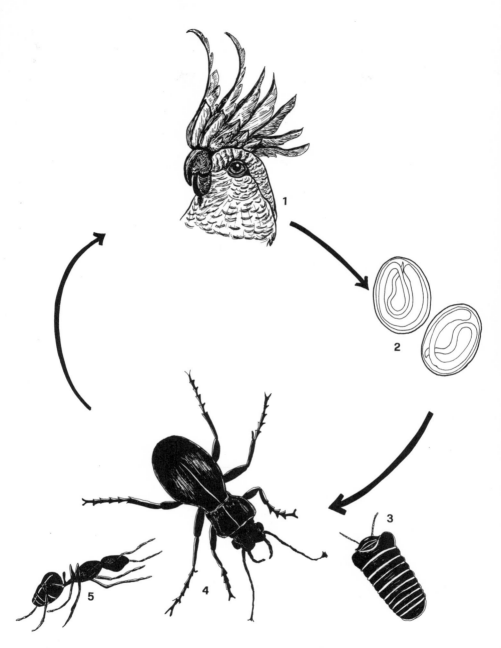

Figure 4/10. Not drawn to scale. Life cycle of proventricular and gizzard worms such as *Spiroptera* spp. The infested host, for example, a sulphur-crested cockatoo (1) passes the worm eggs (2) containing larvae in its faeces. These are eaten by arthropods such as pillbugs (3), beetles (4) and ants (5). Birds become infested by eating the invertebrates. (Janet Keymer)

The worms can cause serious trouble in pigeons when infestations are heavy, producing high mortality, especially in squabs. Illness or death are accompanied by mucoid enteritis and anaemia as the result of severe haemorrhages in the intestinal tract. The clinical signs of the disease include depression, weakness, loss of appetite, regurgitation of bile-coloured fluid, loss of weight and green, slimy diarrhoea containing flakes of mucous membrane. Breathing becomes rapid due to the anaemia.

TREATMENT AND CONTROL As with other roundworms, treatment resolves around three factors, namely, cleanliness, good nutrition and removal of the parasites at a vulnerable stage of their life cycle, thus preventing opportunities for fresh infestation.

Methyridine either by subcutaneous injection or in the drinking water has been recommended. Thiabendazole and phenothiazine have also been suggested, but there is little information available concerning their efficiency.

Large Roundworms (*Ascaridia* spp.)

Ascaridia hermaphrodita and closely related roundworms are common in psittacines, especially the larger Australian parakeets. Their importance as a cause of disease in these birds has only recently been realised. The very similar *Ascaridia columbae* is common in pigeons and *A. galli* in gallinaceous birds. The worms, which are probably cosmopolitan in distribution are easily visible to the naked eye on *post-mortem* examination or when they are passed in the faeces. They can measure as much as 10 cm. in length, are whitish in colour and round in cross section, being about as thick as an ordinary pin.

The life cycle of the worm is direct (Figure 5/10). The eggs are passed in the faeces and the larvae develop in the egg outside the body of the bird. Within 1 to 2 weeks the eggs become infective to the host, but they can remain viable for over three months under suitable conditions of warmth and moisture. Direct sunlight kills the eggs, however. When the eggs are ingested by a suitable host the larvae are released in the small intestine. The larvae live in the gut and also penetrate the wall of the intestine. After moulting they reach the adult stage, produce eggs and the cycle is repeated.

Young birds of most species are more susceptible to infestation than adults, but in parakeets this is not necessarily the case. Parakeets lose condition and may develop apparent paralysis of the legs, because the worms in these birds most frequently cause trouble by impacting and blocking the small intestine (Plate 8/10). In a small parakeet, only a few worms may produce trouble, since they are relatively large and often

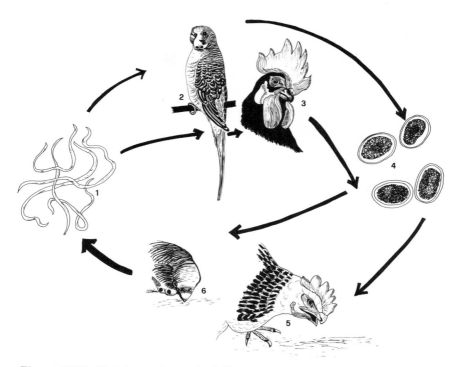

Figure 5/10. Not drawn to scale. Life cycle of roundworms *Ascaridia* spp. (1) in birds such as a budgerigar (2) and domestic fowl (3). Infested birds pass the worm eggs (4) in their faeces. After embryonation these are infective to other birds (5) and (6), which eat them. Within the bird the larvae develop into the adult worms (1). (Janet Keymer)

difficult for the bird to pass; this is because the diameter of the lower part of the small intestine is smaller than that of the duodenum where the worms are most frequently found.

TREATMENT AND CONTROL In pigeons and gallinaceous species which normally drink liberally, the worms can be successfully treated by the addition of piperazine adipate to the drinking water. Parakeets, however, need to be dosed individually with piperazine or tetramisole by mouth, using a stomach tube. It may also be necessary to administer an intestinal lubricant such as liquid paraffin (NOT paraffin oil or kerosene) to help the passage of the paralysed worms through the gut.

Prevention and control of infestations is based on the same principles as those recommended for other worms such as *Capillaria*.

One species, *Porrocaecum ensicaudatum* , of these small roundworms is particularly common in passerine birds, whilst another, *P. crassum*, occurs in ducks. Unlike their relatives, *Ascaridia* and *Capillaria*, these worms always have an indirect life cycle requiring an intermediate host such as an earthworm.

Not much is known about the capacity of the worms to cause disease, but it is likely that young birds are most susceptible and that light infestations, especially in adults, are relatively harmless. Ruffled feathers and inability to maintain balance have been attributed to the worms. It is virtually impossible, however, to diagnose the disease except at *postmortem* examination, when the worms may be found beneath the horny lining of the gizzard or attached to the epithelium of the small intestine where they may produce fibrous tumours on the external surface.

TREATMENT AND CONTROL   No treatment has been described. Control mainly depends upon avoidance of intermediate hosts, using similar methods to those recommended for gapeworms.

Adult filarial roundworms are long, thin nematodes measuring several cms. in length depending upon the species. They occur mainly in the air sacs or thoracic and abdominal cavities of a wide variety of birds. The larvae of many species, known as microfilariae, occur in the blood. *Diplotriaena* is common in passerines, and *Serratospiculum* is frequently encountered in various species of birds of prey.

The life cycle of filarial worms, although well understood in man and some mammals, is mainly unknown in birds. It is very likely, however, that in most cases microfilariae in the blood are taken up by blood-sucking insects such as midges or "punkies" (*Culicoides*) and buffalo gnats or black flies (*Simulium*) (Figure 6/10). They undergo development in the insect intermediate host, and eventually infective larvae are introduced back into the blood stream of the bird when the insect bites. The larvae in the bird develop into the mature adult worms, which produce numerous eggs; these in turn give rise to the larvae (microfilariae) which enter the blood.

There is evidence that the life cycle of at least one species of *Serratospiculum*, (*S. tendo* of birds of prey), is not transmitted by biting flies. The hosts become infected by eating certain insects such as those in the order Orthoptera, for example, locusts (*Locusta migratoria*) which have ingested ova passed by infested birds (Figure 6/10).

Pneumonia, inflammation of the air sacs and fits have all been attributed to filarial worms, but it is likely that they are harmless except in heavy infestations.

196

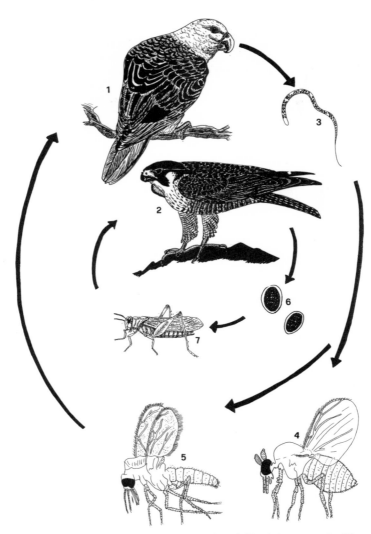

Figure 6/10. Not drawn to scale. Life cycle of filarial worms in (1) a parrot and (2) a diurnal bird of prey. Psittacine birds become infested with a species of filarial worm which produces larval stages known as microfilariae (3) found in the blood. The microfilariae are taken up by blood sucking insects such as buffalo gnats, *Simulium* spp. (4), and midges, *Culicoides* spp. (5), in which they undergo development. When these insects bite a suitable host such as a psittacine or passerine bird, infective larvae enter the blood stream. They develop into the adult worms which are most frequently found in the air sacs. At least one species of *Serratospiculum* filarial worm of birds of prey which also inhabits the air sacs, produces eggs (6) which are passed in the faeces of the bird. The eggs are ingested by insects belonging to the order Orthoptera, *e.g.*, locusts, *Locusta migratoria* (7). Suitable hosts become infested by eating these intermediate hosts. (Janet Keymer)

TREATMENT AND CONTROL No satisfactory treatment is known. If there is evidence from the results of *post-mortem* examination or microscopical examination of blood, that the parasites are troublesome in an aviary, then steps should be taken to control possible insect hosts by the use of insecticides. Transferring birds to an indoor aviary may also be necessary if *Culicoides* midges are suspected carriers, because they are so small that they can easily penetrate ordinary mosquito netting.

Gizzard Worm of Waterfowl (*Amidostomum anseris*)

This small, thread-like worm measures up to nearly 2.5 cm. in length and is common in many species of geese and ducks, including domestic breeds, as well as species of ornamental waterfowl. It most frequently occurs beneath the horny lining of the gizzard, but may also be found in the proventriculus and oesophagus. The life cycle is direct. The eggs are passed out in the faeces of infested birds and larvae develop to the infective third stage actually within the egg. Both eggs and larvae are destroyed by drying, but remain active for several weeks in water and under moist conditions. Susceptible birds become infested by swallowing the infective larvae, which reach maturity in the alimenary tract of the bird after about 40 days.

The worms can do considerable damage to the gizzard lining, especially in young geese, and cause heavy losses. Affected birds show loss of appetite and weight, leading to lethargy, prostration and death. Sometimes diarrhoea occurs.

TREATMENT AND CONTROL Unfortunately, treatment is often unsatisfactory. A combination of tetramisole and levamisole are likely to give the best results. Control largely depends upon hygiene. Where possible keep the surroundings dry in order to destroy the infective larvae. Adult birds which may be symptomless carriers should be treated before the breeding season.

Thorny-headed worms (Acanthocephalids)

These parasites are closely related to the roundworms or nematodes. The adults also occur in the intestines of other vertebrates as well as birds. Waterfowl are common hosts, but the worms also infest many species of passerines and birds of prey.

The adult worms are elongated or roughly cylindrical in shape (Plate 9/10) and have a head armed with numerous hooks with which the worm attaches itself to the intestinal mucosa of its host.

Probably all species require one or more intermediate hosts before reaching the stage which is infective to the final host (Figure 7/10). The intermediate hosts of water birds are commonly aquatic invertebrates such as freshwater shrimps and other crustaceans, whilst those worms infesting passerines are usually terrestrial insects and other invertebrates.

Heavy infestations with these worms, especially in young birds, can cause enteritis, debility and even anaemia.

TREATMENT AND CONTROL Satisfactory treatment is difficult, although thiabendazole has been recommended. When infestations occur, attempts should be made to restrict the birds' access to possible intermediate hosts, and thus interrupt the life cycle of the parasite.

Figure 7/10. Not drawn to scale. Life cycle of a thorny-headed worm (1) such as *Polymorphus boschadis* which occurs in the small intestine of many species of aquatic birds, especially members of the order Anseriformes, *e.g.* the pochard (3) and less frequently passerine birds such as thrushes (2). The spindle-shaped eggs (4) are passed in the faeces and the larval stage develops in the freshwater shrimp, (*Gammarus pulex*) and possibly other crustacea (5). The final hosts (2 and 3) become infested by eating the crustaceans. (Janet Keymer)

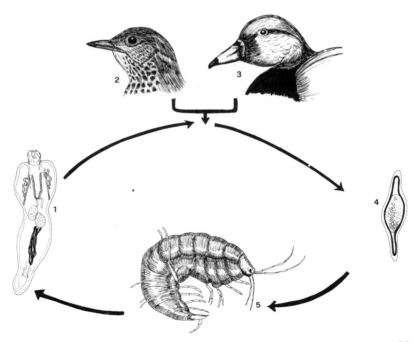

SELECTED BIBLIOGRAPHY

BENBROOK, E. A. (1965). External Parasites of Poultry. In *Diseases of Poultry,* p.925–964. Eds. Biester, H. E. and Schwarte, L. H. 5th Ed. Ames, Iowa. State University Press.

HUNGERFORD, T. G. (1969). Internal Parasites of Poultry. In *Diseases of Poultry including Cage Birds and Pigeons,* p.483–529. 4th Ed. Sydney, London, Melbourne. Angus and Robertson.

KEYMER, I. F. (1969). Parasitic Diseases. In *Diseases of Cage and Aviary Birds,* p.393–452. Ed. Petrak, M. L., Philadelphia. Lea and Febiger.

LAPAGE, G. (1958). *Parasitic Animals.* 2nd Ed. Cambridge. Heffer. 355pp.

LAPAGE, G. (1968). *Veterinary Parasitology.* 2nd Ed. Oliver & Boyd. 1182pp.

OLSEN, O. W. (1967). *Animal Parasites: Their Biology and Life Cycles.* 2nd Ed. Minneapolis. Burgess Publishing Company, 431pp.

PRICE, F. W. (1965). Trematodes of Poultry. In *Diseases of Poultry,* p.1035–1055. Eds. Biester, H. E. and Schwarte, L. H. 5th Ed. Ames, Iowa. State University Press.

ROTHSCHILD, M. &. CLAY, T. (1952). *Fleas, Flukes and Cuckoos. A Study of Bird Parasites.* New York, Philosophical Library, 304pp.

SOULSBY, E. J. L. (1968). *Helminth s, Arthropods & Protozoa of Domesticated Animals.* (Sixth Edition of Mönnig's Veterinary Helminthology & Entomology). London. Baillière, Tindall & Cassell. 824pp.

WEHR, E. E. (1965). Nematodes and Acanthocephalids of Poultry, p.965–1005, and Cestodes of Poultry, p.1006–1034. In *Diseases of Poultry.* Eds. Biester, H. E. and Schwarte, L. H., 5th Ed. Ames, Iowa. State University Press.

WEHR, E. E. (1971). Nematodes. In *Infectious and Parasitic Diseases of Wild Birds,* p.185–233. Eds. Davis, J. W. Anderson R. C., Karstad, L. and Trainer, D. O. Ames, Iowa. State University Press.

THE SKIN AND ITS APPENDAGES

The Skin Diseased avian skin presents different problems from mammalian skin. This is because of its high flexibility and low elasticity, its poor glandular content and its relative thinness. Additionally, a bird often inflicts further injury to itself with its own beak (Plate 1/11), possibly because of its poor response to pain. The bird in fact seems to find pecking and scratching its own damaged skin a pleasant, rather than a painful process.

Inflammation of the skin is known as dermatitis and may involve a single patch or numerous and extensive areas. These areas, depending on the causal agent, have different appearances. The skin may simply be reddened, show papules (red pimples), pustules (pus-filled, conical pimples), vesicles (blisters), exudations (oozing of body fluids resulting in scabs), puffiness due to subcutaneous oedema, or emphysema (see Plate 2/11 and Chapter 21), induration (chronic, rubbery or leather-like thickenings), ulceration (craters with jagged edges) or show areas of haemorrhage. Of these lesions, pustules and induration are the least common lesions encountered in birds.

Skin reaction varies with the cause, the tolerance of an individual or species, the area of skin affected, climatic factors and other aspects of health and environment. In thin birds the lack of subcutaneous fat may allow deeper tissues, especially muscle, also to become diseased.

Avian skin is not prone to pus formation as the result of infection with pyogenic or pus-forming bacteria. The most common reaction is congestion of blood vessels and slight swelling, leading to fissuring, exudations and the production of scabs. This usually appears to cause irritation and may lead to further inflammation as the result of pecking.

Parasites frequently cause skin lesions (see Chapter 10). Blood sucking insects inject irritants and anticoagulants to prevent clotting of blood at the site of the bite. Biting lice feed on the dead skin debris, while blow flies salivate in wounds before sucking up the dissolved exudates and dead tissues. Some species of mite eat the feather roots in the follicles and can cause feather loss with surprisingly little skin reaction. Red mites (*Dermanyssus* and *Ornithonyssus*), ticks, fleas, lice and insects such as the pigeon fly, black flies and others can cause local and generalized dermatitis in addition to restlessness and anaemia leading to loss of condition. Ectoparasitism can also result in self-inflicted wounds as the result of irritation from the parasites.

Pox viruses cause vesicles, general skin swelling and later copious scab formation (see Chapter 6) and the favus fungi (*Trichophyton*) can produce lesions on the head and less frequently in the axillae and other tender areas of skin (see Chapter 8).

If sufficiently diluted, some disinfectants may cause dermatitis, especially of the feet; abrasive sandpaper floors, roughened perches, frost bite and wet, unhygienic conditions can have a similar effect, predisposing bumblefoot granuloma.

Certain discharges or exudates from the nostrils or vent, as well as discharging, ulcerated tumours or abscesses, may cause dermatitis of varying severity in the areas of skin near these lesions.

Areas of skin where the blood supply is relatively poor and where the skin is tense and often subject to pressure, such as over the ventral aspect of the breast-bone (so-called "keel" of the sternum), often develop thickenings which may become ulcerated. Such lesions of the breast are most likely to occur in perching birds with arthritis of the leg joints. Often the only remedy is complete surgical removal of the entire lesion, including part of the underlying prominence as well. Arthritic birds, however, are best painlessly destroyed.

Hereditary defects of the plumage such as *hypopteronosis cystica* of canaries are dealt with in Chapter 25.

Specific treatments are given elsewhere and can be located under the appropriate headings (see Index), *e.g.*, abscesses, allergies, burns, contusions, favus, French moult, gangrene, granulomas, haematomas, lacerations, mite infestations, mosquito bites, pox, scalds, subcutaneous emphysema, etc.

The Skin Glands

The largest skin gland is the uropygial or preen gland above the root of the tail; others are the meibomian glands of the eyelids, the mucous glands of the conjunctivae, the cells which produce the waxy varnish of the cere in birds such as the budgerigar, and cells which produce the horny structures of the beak and claws.

The uropygial gland, which is absent in a few species, produces an oily secretion, which until recently was thought to be of value in preening, lubricating and waterproofing the plumage (see Chapter 2). As an active and prominent organ it may be damaged occasionally, impacted with secretion or become the site of granulomatous lesions (Plate 3/11). Tumour formation, however, is rare. Its removal or partial

202

destruction does not appear to give more than a temporary check to the well being of the plumage.

The secretion of the meibomian glands is both a protection against infection and a lubricant. When the consistency of the secretion is abnormal it causes minute swellings and even small abscesses along the margins of the eyelids; it is sometimes associated with purulent discharge due to secondary bacterial invasion. Cheesy masses of pus may develop under the upper eyelids. These lesions are not uncommon in debilitated parrots and mynahs. Tetracycline ophthalmic ointment applied to the eye two or three times a day, after bathing away all discharges from beneath the lids, is often the only treatment required.

The cere is prone to inflammation associated with nasal discharges, injuries and, especially in budgerigars, *Knemidocoptic* mite infestation. An abnormality of the cere which is not uncommon, is that known as brown hypertrophy (Plate 4/11). This is characterised by a considerable increase in the keratin layers overlying the fleshy part of the cere. It is usually a sign of mild, chronic, ill health or senility. The heaped-up keratin debris can be picked off or scraped away, but usually it accumulates again slowly, unless the general condition of the bird improves, when it subsides. No treatment or change of diet improves the abnormality to any great extent.

The Appendages   Wattles, combs, caruncles and other featherless, fleshy protuberances of the head region are richly supplied with blood vessels and are vulnerable to injuries. They are also prone to frost bite and attack by biting insects. Large haematomas or blood blisters often form as the result of fighting and in some infections such as pasteurellosis, gangrene of the wattles can occur.

The Beak   Most birds are unable to adapt to new feeding habits after damage to the beak (Plate 4/11 and 5/11). In humming birds, the beak and tongue occasionally become fixed into one single structure, if the consistency of the food is unsuitable. Prompt trimming of the dying or necrotic area will allow normal feeding to be resumed. Sometimes the beak may be shattered when a bird flies into a window or wire netting as the result of being frightened. This often leads to death from starvation unless the beak can be mended with a splint or wire suture.

Distortion of the beak occurs in chronic, advanced *Knemidocoptes* infestations or "scaly beak" of budgerigars, and occasionally other pstittacines. The beak, in addition to becoming distorted, becomes powdery and flakes. It often becomes overgrown or badly deviated and therefore wears irregularly.

203

Even after successful treatment of the mites, good quality horn is seldom produced again and euthanasia is often the only choice. The various effects of mite infestation on beak structure are discussed in Chapter 10.

It is probable that certain deficiencies in the diet such as those of vitamin A and D, and minerals, especially calcium, give rise to poor development and quality of the beak. Similarly amino acids, such as methionine, may also be important for healthy horn.

Overgrown straight (Plate 6/11), recurved or sometimes excessively curved, deviated (Plate 7/11) or crossed mandibles (Plate 8/11) of good quality horn are sometimes congenital or even hereditary in origin; the former are possibly due to dietary deficiencies, while hereditary deformities are of course independent of nutrition, whether pre- or post-hatching. Many beak deformities, however, are due to injury of the horn-producing tissue on one side of the beak only. The injury interferes with growth, while the other side develops normally. Regular trimming will enable the bird to eat, but it will not effect a permanent cure. Care must be taken not to cut the corium or "quick" and cause pain and haemorrhage. It is also important not to file away the shiny surface layer, otherwise the beak will become friable.

Epinagthism (Plate 9/11) and prognathism are the names given to an over-developed upper and lower beak respectively. They can be either hereditary or acquired defects, and cause grotesque profiles often leading to difficulty in feeding. Badly affected birds should be destroyed, and if the deformity is thought to be hereditary they should never be used for breeding. In budgerigars, a form of prognathism can follow an upward deviation of the upper beak. The latter can be caused by pressure from layers of unsuitable, especially sticky food impacted over the inner surface of the hard palate and inside of the beak. Parrots and cockatiels also seem prone to suffer in this way. Similar impaction between the tongue and sides of the lower mandible can cause lateral bulging and deviation of the horn, so that the edges of the lower mandible jut out beyond the edges of the upper mandible. Similar impactions may also occur in nestlings, especially when there are unhygienic conditions in the nest box and the parents feed sticky or excessively soft food to the young. Disorders of the beak are also discussed in Chapter 13.

The Claws or Toes

The shape of the claws varies widely according to the habits of different species. Birds are seldom incapacitated by the loss of one or two of these digits, even in the free-living state. Perching birds, however, are more prone to breast sores, or even arthritis and respiratory troubles, if damage to the feet is sufficiently severe to prevent perching. In birds of prey, damaged or painful feet are a severe handicap because these birds use the feet to hold food such as meat and carcases while tearing the flesh with the beak. Seed-eating birds, on the other hand, can manage quite well with several damaged toes or even an amputated foot because the claws are not used for feeding.

The health of the horn in claws, like that of the beak, depends on an intact, generative tissue or corium of smooth, regular contour. The bulk of this horn or keratin is produced from beneath the claw by ridges or laminae which deposit support struts of keratin. The polished, hard surface of the claw is produced by a line of cells at the junction of the claw and skin. These two horny layers are constantly being renewed and in the wild state they seldom overgrow because of normal wear and tear.

Overgrowth of claw horn, especially in weak birds, leads to strain on the flexor tendons of the toe producing a flattening of the claw's curvature. Sometimes an affected bird walks on the side of its toes and the deformity becomes spiral or corkscrew in shape (Plate 10/11). In a few cases, the claw becomes so curved that there is little opportunity for normal use and wear. Such birds are sometimes found weak or dead in the cage or aviary, trapped on the wire netting and exhausted from panic and inability to reach their food.

The most common cause of deformity of a single claw is an injury of some kind; this includes fractures, infection of the claw bed due to pecking, constriction by a human or animal hair, or damage due to the claw becoming trapped in wire netting or hinges. Claws may also be injured as the result of burns, both thermal and chemical. Usually the bird suffers little inconvenience from such injuries, except when clasping or holding down food in its claws. When all the claws and parts of the toes have sloughed or become deformed, perching may be difficult.

Perches should preferably be oval and not round. Those which are too small for the species having to use them, are commonly blamed by breeders for many claw deformities. Certainly an oval perch of abnormally wide diameter does seem to help in the treatment of some foot contractures. Large diameter perches are better than those which are two small, and which cause the tips of the forward and backward facing claws to meet or overlap. Wide perches are particularly important for birds of prey which have sharp pointed talons, because these can puncture the fleshy part of the ball of the foot, and often introduce infection leading to "bumblefoot".

Scales of Feet and Legs   The distribution, shape and pattern of scales differs according to the type of bird. Some, such as the *Strigidae* and cer-

205

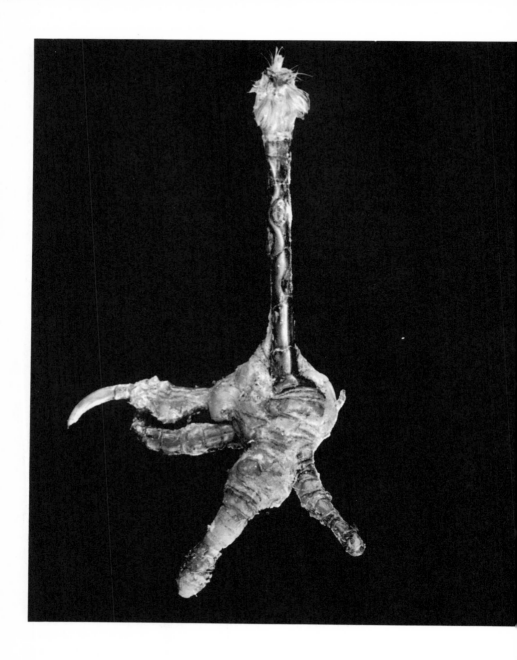

Feet and legs of a short-tailed thrush (*Chamaeza campanisona*) showing loss of nails and digits and marked swelling of the joints. The cause was localised bacterial, *Staphylococcus pyogenes*, infection resulting in bursitis, synovitis and arthritis. See Chapters 12 and 7. (I.F. Keymer and T.C. Dennett, Z.S.L.)

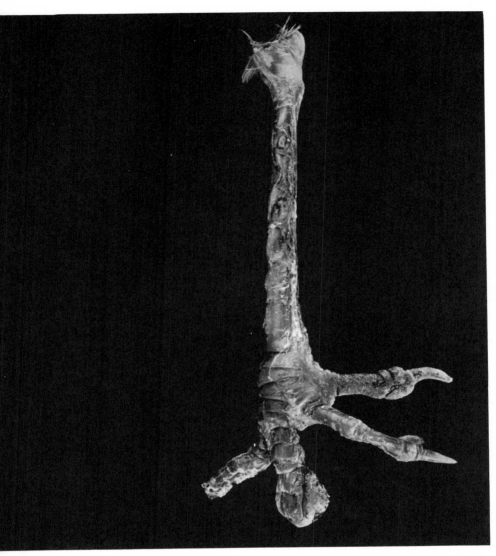

tain members of the *Columbidae* and *Phasianidae*, are feathered down the shanks and even on to the toes.

The major abnormalities of the scaled areas are caused by chronic inflammatory and degenerative processes. These are characterized by raising of the scales due to deposits beneath and between them, or as the result of thickening of the scales themselves. Often the thickening and roughening is over all the scaled areas. In the early stages of knemidocoptic mange in budgerigars, however, only part of the leg or feet may be covered with the typical honeycombed deposit (see Plate 3/10 and Chapter 10).

In old or middle-aged canaries, various finches, many other passerines and also gallinaceous birds, the scales become elevated to give a serrated appearance like armour plate. This mostly occurs on the shanks, and in aged canaries may be associated with varicose veins (Plates 10/11 and 11/11). In advanced cases there may be beige, crumbly deposits containing keratin, dried serum, and sometimes chalky material or dried blood. Usually no cause can be found and the lesions merely seem to indicate senility. Septic arthritis is sometimes a sequel to productive shank and toe lesions of this type. The possibility of deficiences of vitamin A and D, fats or oils, thioamino acids (as the result of feeding food of low or poor quality protein) or of dietary imbalances should be considered. Secondary low-grade bacterial infections may sometimes be a complication, especially when the enlarged scales abrade the skin near joints and cause fissures or ulcers. Occasionally the thickenings can become so gross that they can be broken off in lumps or flattened flakes. The latter type of lesion has given rise to the term "tassel foot" (Plate 12/11), but in passerines such as canaries this is nearly always due to *Knemidocoptes* infestation.

Except with knemidocoptic mange, no specific treatment is available. Symptomatic treatment consists of chipping off the thickest scales and debris and gently massaging olive oil into the scales and skin: this of course is in addition to ensuring that the diet and environment are suitable. A simple disinfectant can also be used such as proflavine cream or the newer dexamethasone or betamethasone preparations containing neomycin or other antibiotic. Such treatment serves to soften, lubricate, counteract inflammation and prevent the entry of bacteria.

Deposits of urates beneath the scaly areas of skin, especially around the joints, may be visible as pale yellow or cream coloured swellings. These lesions appear to be very painful and sometimes ulceration of the overlying skin occurs. The lesions, however, are not strictly skin lesions but gout, which is discussed elsewhere (see Chapter 15).

The Plumage— Abnormalities of the Moult

Prolongation of moulting or so-called "stuck-in-the-moult" may occur, especially in canaries. Particularly heavy, out of season moults and baldness or alopecia (see Plate 13/11) affect a number of species. The same factors are probably also involved in perpetual chewing, pecking and self-plucking syndromes, which so often ruin the general health and value of birds, particularly of pet parrots kept in isolation. The causes attributed to moulting abnormalities are numerous.

NUTRITIONAL   Protein, vitamin and mineral deficiencies (see Chapter 23).

ENVIRONMENTAL Extremes of temperature, especially sudden changes of temperature. Excessive humidity or dryness. Excessive artificial light or insufficient illumination during the daylight period.
Poor hygiene.
Draughty quarters.
Boredom; particularly common with parrots kept in small cages lacking objects to investigate and especially when a bird is kept in isolation.
Frequent disturbance by strangers at irregular periods, particularly after dark.
Frequent disturbances by such marauders as cats, dogs, rats, mice, or owls, leading to "night frights" and other forms of stress.
Parasites such as red mites, pigeon flies, mosquitoes, blackflies and heavy louse infestations causing restlessness and skin irritation.

PHYSIOLOGICAL Thyroid deficiency or lack of dietary iodine causing retarded moult and the production of defective feathers. Thyroid excess induces moult and the production of a new and lighter plumage, but the condition is rare.

The above list is not exhaustive but covers the main suspected causes of plumage defects. The precise cause of most feather disorders is unknown and many are completely intractable to all forms of treatment, including changes of management. Nevertheless, after the factors in the above list have been considered and appropriate measures taken without effect, it may pay to analyse the problem even further.

Imagine an imported foreign bird, which is used to plenty of space for escape and vegetation in which to hide. In the wild, the bird is fully occupied physically and mentally in its search for food, for safety and rest. In captivity, the same bird is placed in an enclosed cage or aviary, but the bird probably feels insecure because it is unable to hide when it feels the need to do so. Food is always readily available and therefore the minimum of activity is necessary to obtain it. Under such conditions many birds, especially the more intelligent types such as parrots, other psittacines and members of the Corvidae, gradually sink into an apathetic state. The muscles are inadequately exercised, but the adrenals are probably continuously over-stimulated. Eventually the bird shows signs of becoming neurotic, indulging in purposeless activity, such as shifting from one foot to another, pecking its claws, excessively preening, bobbing up and down, weaving, bowing or screaming at the slightest provocation. If a minor injury to the skin or appendages occurs, instead of being too preoccupied to notice it, the bird will idly scratch at the area or investigate it with its beak or tongue. To relieve the irritation from the skin reaction a feather may be plucked out with the beak and then the real trouble begins. This activity soon becomes a habit and then obsessional. Any attempt at repair or other treatment of the area is unlikely to keep pace with the constant interference.

Occasionally a recovery can be brought about by placing the bird near some companions, and later introducing them into the same cage or aviary if they prove to be compatible. Transfering the bird to a colder environment such as a large established planted aviary full of new features to investigate also sometimes helps. Where transference to a planted aviary is impractical, head scratching and body pecking can sometimes be prevented by placing a flat or conical stiff Elizabethan collar around the neck (see Chapter 21). This protection gives time for new feathers to become well established if kept in position for about three weeks and may break the habit if some dietary and/or environmental changes are made at the same time. An alternative type of collar is cylindrical, to prevent the neck flexing. These collars, however, effect a permanent cure in only a minority of cases and not infrequently create frustration and initial loss of balance as well as a degree of local dermatitis and damage to feathers where the collar is in contact with the plumage. Plucking out damaged feathers also sometimes helps to promote the growth of new ones.

French Moult is an abnormality of the feathers of young budgerigars and occasionally other small psittacines. Its main features are excessive moulting and feather deformities. Feather growth is stunted at an early age and quills fall out before they reach full size.

Probably more has been written about this disease of budgerigars than any other cage bird problem. In no other field has more research been carried out with less return. In spite of the inability to find the cause, or more important, a cure, we have now a much better understanding of the disease than previously and the ability to reduce its incidence and severity.

Most fanciers who have bred budgerigars, even for a short time, will have seen the disease and will have noticed at least some of the following points:

1. Cases occur unexpectedly, sometimes being bred from the better, sometimes from the poorer stock.

French Moult

2. Some birds are mildly, and others seriously affected in the same clutch.
3. Early or late season and out of season clutches are often the first to be affected. First year breeders and old birds seem to be more prone than others.
4. Repeated breeding from pairs which have produced affected offspring is likely to produce a higher proportion and more severe cases.
5. Mildly affected birds are less likely to breed than normal ones, and severely affected birds usually fail to breed.
6. Affected birds which do breed, produce a higher incidence and severity of French Moult.
7. The feeding of food supplements, vitamin, mineral and amino acid additives has little if any effect on the frequency or course of the disease.
8. Except in severe cases, French Moult does not affect the general health, although the birds are reluctant to mate.
9. Severely affected birds are smaller than normal and may have virtually no primary or secondary wing feathers or tail quills. Such birds are unable to fly and are referred to by fanciers as "runners" or "bullets".
10. Fleas, lice, mites, ticks, or other parasites are not normally associated with French Moult.
11. No bacteria, fungi or viruses have been isolated from cases of the disease except as secondary invaders.
12. Stopping the complete breeding programme for the rest of the season greatly lessens the severity and frequency of the disease.
13. Certain strains of buderigars are more prone to French Moult than others, although none appear to be immune.

POSSIBLE CAUSES The experience of breeders and information derived from research projects has established fairly well what the disease is *not* and produced some strong pointers as to what it is.

It is not:
(a) a simple infection by bacteria, viruses or fungi;
(b) a simple infestation by ectoparasites;
(c) a deficiency of any one vitamin, mineral or amino acid, or of fat, oil or carbohydrate;
(d) a single hereditary factor;
(e) a simple hormone deficiency or imbalance;
(f) a single reaction to environmental factors such as light or overcrowding.

The following circumstances appear to favour French Moult by increasing its incidence and severity:

(i) Stress due to overbreeding, also early breeding, and out-of-season breeding.
(ii) Selection of birds for show points at the expense of health.
(iii) Poor hygiene.
(iv) Infectious agents, dietary deficiencies, etc. as listed (a) to (f) and (i) and (ii) above, although not capable of causing the disease on their own, may by increasing stress cause a more severe outbreak or hasten its development.
(v) Strains with a history of French Moult more readily produce young with the disease.
(vi) Feeding excess cod liver oil greatly increases the incidence of French Moult.

CLINICAL SIGNS Young birds, especially those which have just left or are about to leave the nest, show excessive moulting and occasionally breakage of wing and tail quills. The quills may be fully developed but are usually shorter than normal. The feather shaft becomes fractured at its base and a dark shadow caused by blood clots is often seen when the quill is held against a strong light. In many cases, the secondary as well as primary quills are affected, and in the most severe, also the covert feathers. Indeed, almost all feathers may be lost as soon as or even before, they reach full development. In mild cases only one or two tail feathers may be lost, usually symmetrically. Some breeders believe that these mildest cases can recover completely. Feathers nearest the mid line of the body tend to fall first. Dark spots of dried blood are often seen at the points where the feathers have fallen out, indicating that the feather is still a living and therefore developing organ, unlike a true moulted feather, which is shed like a dead branch from a tree.

PATHOLOGY Although French Moult affects the plumage primarily, other pathological lesions occur.

Microscopical examination of the skin reveals no inflammation or abnormality, except involving the feather follicles. The blood, however, has a much reduced proportion of circulating red cells, and the bone marrow shows great activity as if attempting to replace the blood cells. The red blood cells are particularly fragile and it is believed short-lived. The capillaries in the region of growing feathers are fragile. Both the blood capillary and red blood cell fragilities are, according to one authority, the result of excess vitamin A and a relative or actual deficiency of vitamins E and/or K.

By feeding excess vitamin A in oil, it has been found possible to double at least the incidence of French Moult. Nevertheless, it cannot be reduced below 35 per cent in the progeny of established French Moulters even by an almost total suppression of the vitamin.

The disease appears to pass through the egg, because it will appear in young birds reared by foster parents which have never bred an affected bird. Recently the view has been put forward that the primary cause of French Moult may be a virus. There the matter rests until funds are available for a virologist to investigate this theory. It is readily seen that the disease is very complex and some authors have suggested it represents several diseases. I believe, however, that it is a single disease caused by several different factors.

SELECTED BIBLIOGRAPHY

ALTMAN, R. B. (1969). Conditions involving the Integumentary System. In *Diseases of Cage and Aviary Birds,* p.243–254. Ed. Petrak, M. L., Philadelphia. Lea and Febiger.

KEYMER, I. F. & BLACKMORE, D. K. (1964). *Diseases of the skin and soft parts of wild birds.* Brit. Birds 57, 175–179.

PECKHAM, M. C. (1965). Conditions affecting the skin and integument. In *Diseases of Poultry,* p.1179–1190. Eds. Biester, H. E. and Schwarte, L. H. 5th Ed. Ames, Iowa. State University Press.

TAYLOR, T. G. (1969). French Molt. In *Diseases of Cage and Aviary Birds,* p.237–242. Ed. Petrak, M. L., Philadelphia. Lea and Febiger.

ARNALL, L. (1965). *Conditions of the beak and claw in the budgerigar.* J. Small anim. Pract. 6, 135–144.

STARTUP, C. M. (1970). The Diseases of Cage and Aviary Birds, (Excluding the specific diseases of the Budgerigar), p.46–58. In *Rutgers, A. & Norris, K. A. Eds. Encyclopedia of Aviculture, Vol. I.* London. Blandford Press.

THE MUSCULO-SKELETAL SYSTEM

Fractures and Dislocations   Bone is a brittle material. In birds it is more porcelain-like than in mammals and the areas of porous or spongy bone form a much smaller part of the skeleton. In small flying birds, many bones are little thicker than egg shells but they have internal reinforcing struts. Avian bones are therefore very prone to fracture.

When a bird collides in flight with a solid object, it frequently fractures the skull, limb bones, or spinal column. Most fractures are quite easy to locate, although fractures of the skull are difficult to diagnose and liable to be made far worse by the probing of inexperienced fingers. Shock, cranial haemorrhage and concussion may be just as severe in the absence of a cranial fracture, as they are when one is present.

Dislocations are much less common than fractures and generally produce obvious deformities. They can be rectified by gentle pressure and manipulation of the dislocated joint. Quite often the bones will click back into place quite readily. Dislocations with fractures near the joints are more difficult to diagnose and to treat, and an x-ray may be necessary to establish accurately the nature of the damage.

Fractures are dealt with in detail in Chapter 29 and dislocations in Chapter 21.

Periostitis   Bone is produced mainly by the thin sheet of cells or periosteum which covers its surface. When this covering is injured it tends to separate from the bone beneath, because of the presence of haemorrhage or oedema. New bone then develops in the fluid-filled cavity and forms a hard lump, which may be felt through the skin if the cavity is large. If the wound becomes infected, and especially if a major blood vessel is cut and the vitality of the tissues greatly lowered, periostitis may result. When the invading bacteria are of low virulence, nodular masses of bone will be deposited. If more virulent bacteria are involved, they may cause the periosteum to be underrun with pus, so that large areas are stripped away from the bone. This can be a very painful condition. Sometimes infection may spread through the existing bone into the marrow cavity and cause osteomyelitis, or disperse outwards between the muscles and tendons causing myositis and tendonitis. If the joints become infected, arthritis and synovitis result and lead to severe lameness.

Treatment involves the use of anaesthesia by a veterinarian, and the scraping out of diseased and necrotic tissue. The wound must be packed with antibiotics or other drugs as indicated, to assist the healing process. Administration of antibiotics by injection or by mouth for several days, however, is also necessary. Most birds nevertheless will remain chronically ill for a while or may die. Luckily periostitis and its associated lesions are not commonly seen in birds.

Inflammation of the bone marrow is almost invariably **Osteomyelitis** caused by infectious agents such as bacteria. Most of these gain entrance through dirty wounds, associated with severe tissue bruising which impairs the blood supply. It is most likely to occur when broken ends of bone project from a wound, as happens in compound fractures. In a few cases infection may reach the bone marrow via the bloodstream. It is quite amazing, however, that even in such injuries osteomyelitis is relatively rare. When infection does become established, pockets of pus may form and become surrounded by granulation tissue. This may allow the fracture to heal to a certain extent, although in some areas no bone formation occurs. In other areas it becomes excessive and grossly irregular in distribution. Although the skin and muscle layers over such bone will heal in a week or so, the limb never returns to full use and sooner or later pus is likely to work its way through a weak area of the bone. The pus may then spread between the granulating replacement tissue, and up or down the affected limb between the sheets of connective tissue which bind the muscles and tendons. Eventually it emerges through a hole or sinus to the external surface of the skin. Such a sinus is likely to ooze pus mixed with blood and serum either continuously or intermittently until the bird is satisfactorily cured or dies. Various distortions of the limb result from lesions of this kind. There may be thickening of the bones and wastage of muscles due to disuse as the result of pain. As the result of adhesions caused by infection, the muscles and tendons may become incapable of functioning and this immobility can lead to crippling deformity. When such an advanced stage is reached treatment is not likely to be of much avail, because the fibrous sealing-off of the diseased tissues will prevent antibiotics reaching the area via the bloodstream and combating the infection. In any case the bacteria will probably be resistant to all available antibiotics by this late stage. Similarly, the long tortuous sinus tract cannot be adequately cleansed and packed with suspensions of antibiotic in sufficient quantities to reach inside the bone itself.

Injections of chymotrypsin (in a form suitable for local and intramuscular use) help to digest and liquefy dead tissue and aid access to the infected area by antibiotics. Hydrogen peroxide ("20 volume" solution) can be used with beneficial effect in larger birds to flush out the sinuses.

Surgery is the last resort, amputation of the affected limb well above the suspected highest point of infection being the only treatment which is likely to succeed. Clearly this procedure is the province of a veterinarian.

Arthritis Inflammation of joints or arthritis can arise in several ways. Mechanical injuries are probably the most common cause, although a popular unproven belief is that arthritis may arise from standing or sitting in cold or damp places. Infection is often introduced through puncture wounds or scratches of the skin in the region of a joint. Joint infection which is borne by the blood may also arise in birds with a septicaemia.

Traumatic lesions or localised infections will often resolve quite quickly, especially if the bird rests the affected joint. Such lesions are characterized by swelling, as the result of congestion and oedema, associated with varying degrees of lameness or other disability, depending upon the joint affected. The swollen joint feels warm as the result of the increased blood flow to the area. Severely infected joints are most painful in the early stages, when there is an increase in the amount of synovial fluid or "joint oil". Pressure from the excess fluid confined by the joint capsule is responsible for much of the pain.

As the early acute stage passes, the excess synovial fluid is slowly absorbed, providing that the infection has been overcome by the defence mechanisms of the body. When pus has been produced this is gradually reduced by organizing granulation tissue which eventually forms a scar, immobilizing the articular surfaces of the joint. Although this chronic stage is less painful, it usually restricts joint movement. Eventually, actual bone may be deposited in or around the joint, causing osteoarthritis and ankylosis, or immobility of the joint. This is rather more painful, especially when the joint can be moved a little and the spiky deposits of bone press on the soft tissue. The cartilages covering the joint surfaces may be eroded irregularly and produce clicking, scraping and creaking sensations when the joint is manipulated. When there is arthritis of the leg joints, or several toes, the bird usually shuffles about on its hocks, and then the under surfaces become covered with infected corns or thickened pads of skin or scales. Arthritis involving the wing usually results

217

in it being held away from the body in a dropped position because this is less painful than when the wing is held normally. Arthritis involving the vertebrae of the spine (spondylitis) is quite common in the sacral, lumbar, posterior and thoracic regions, but only occasionally affects the neck. It often results in consecutive vertebrae becoming fused into a solid single piece of bone with large irregular masses underneath the vertebrae. This state is referred to as spondylosis. It occurs most commonly in older budgerigars and senile parrots. No real clue as to its cause has been found in birds, although increasing age or mineral and vitamin imbalance may be contributory factors.

Spondylosis does not respond to any form of treatment. Acute septic arthritis of the limbs caused by bacteria such as *Staphylococci* is best treated with broad-spectrum antibiotics in the acute stages, given either in medicated seed, drinking water, by dropper, or preferably by subcutaneous injection for five to 10 days according to the response.

In the chronic stage after infection has been controlled, treatment consists of lessening the pain and freeing the fibrous tissue which is restricting movement of the joint. This can be done by the use of various salicylates (aspirin), the cortisone group of drugs such as hydrocortisone, as well as other drugs only available to veterinarians. Such drugs may also be used in conjunction with anabolic steroids.

Defects of Bone Development and Maintenance—Rickets, Osteomalacia, Osteofibrosis and other Osteodystrophies

Rickets, or more precisely rachitis, is a disease of young growing animals. Young birds of prey, reared by hand on a purely meat diet, soon develop this disease; but all young birds are susceptible, especially long-legged species, which grow rapidly and need large amounts of calcium and phosphorus. A high level of vitamin D_3 is also needed at this stage. This is available in fresh food and can even be formed in the skin of the bird itself, provided adequate sunlight is available to stimulate its manufacture. Absorbable calcium and phoshorus, in the ratio of between 1.5:1 and 3:1, are essential. Adequate intake of vitamin D_3 is also essential for the absorption of calcium and phosphorus. Small amounts of magnesium and other trace elements are also required. Even if all these minerals are present in adequate amounts and balanced, bone formation may be impaired by illness. If the appetite falls or diarrhoea results from a change of diet or a chill, these raw materials are not used in sufficient quantities, or they are lost by excretion in diarrhoea. Additionally, an adequate output of parathyroid and other hormones is necessary to regulate blood levels of minerals and their rate of deposition in developing bone.

A rickety bird is small, bow-legged, with a large head,

ungainly feet and knobbly joints, and is more prone to fractures of the wing and lower limb bones. X-ray examination shows a shortening of many bones of the skeleton, and the long bones with thin external surfaces. The ends of these long bones, called epiphyses, which articulate together, show spreading or "mushrooming", with thick irregular layers of cartilage instead of the usual thin line separating epiphyses from the shafts of the bones.

In behaviour, the bird is subdued, walks and moves its wings reluctantly, rests on its hocks and is reluctant to perch. It eats little, has loose droppings, and appears to be waiting for death. The latter will soon occur if the bird remains untreated, especially as such specimens have little resistance to disease.

Vitamin D_3 is essential in the treatment of rickets, either by injection or by mouth. A varied, fresh and interesting diet should be provided, together with warm, dry and if possible sunny quarters. Calcium lactate or gluconate tablets can be ground to a powder and mixed with fruit or gentles, according to the feeding habits of the affected bird. Calcium gluconate (with or without magnesium or phosphorus) in a 20 per cent or 40 per cent solution, as used for injecting cattle with "milk fever" can be used at a dilution of one part to 10 or 20 in the drinking water. It can also be injected in 10-20 per cent solution under the skin of the neck. A general vitamin and mineral tonic in the drinking water is also recommended.

Osteomalacia is the name for rickets in the adult bird. It is sometimes associated with diseases, injury or tumours of the parathyroid gland and occasionally occurs in old parrots. Most frequently it is a result of prolonged egg laying when the bird is receiving inadequate amounts of calcium. Signs of the disease are often inapparent until some trivial accident results in a fractured limb, because the shafts of the bone have become thin and fragile. The deeper, spongy type of bone in the vertebrae for example, becomes softer than usual. When bone or osseous tissue releases its calcium salts it leaves behind pre-bone or osteoid tissue. Fortunately this process—which occurs in the laying bird—is reversible once the young are fledged, providing the diet is satisfactory.

Treatment consists of removing the cock to stop breeding and if possible to foster any young onto another hen. Close attention must be paid to the diet and intake of calcium, phosphorus and vitamin D_3. Fortunately parathyroid lesions are rare, as they are generally untreatable.

Osteofibrosis is the replacement of bone with fibrous tissue. This can happen in small areas as the result of local inflammatory reactions or it may be generalized. It may be associated with liver dysfunction and kidney disease, the latter resulting in failure to discard urates which build up in the tissues, causing gout. Another important effect is the loss of calcium by excretion and the retention of phosphorus. Since calcium is not conserved by the kidney, more of it is mobilized from the bone in order to maintain adequate blood levels, without which severe nervous signs would result. In the process, an excess of phosphorus accumulates in the body tissues and bone becomes replaced by fibrous or scar tissue. There is consequently a softening of all layers of bone, which is most noticeable in the pelvis and limbs and the facial bones supporting the beak. The advanced and clinically apparent disease is seldom recognized, however, but the signs of renal disease may be, and it is this which is responsible for death.

There is little hope of cure or even of easing the clinical signs for any length of time. A simple bacterial infection is seldom responsible for the renal disease and usually the cause cannot be found.

Other osteodystrophies are poorly understood in birds. A skeletal abnormality which is characterized by thin walled and soft long bones, which buckle or fracture without external violence of any sort, is sometimes seen in parrots, macaws and other large psittacines. It is probably a dietary deficiency of a similar kind to osteomalacia. It is referred to as osteoporosis (porous bone) because calcium salts are sparsely scattered throughout the osteoid tissues, leaving unmineralized spaces containing soft tissue.

A skeletal deformity associated with disturbances in oestrogen production and known as hyperostosis is discussed in Chapter 19.

Ligaments and tendons are seldom affected by disease, although occasionally they do become cut or torn. They are composed of parallel bundles of cords of fibrous and sometimes elastic tissue, which contain few cells and have very little blood supply. When damaged, the healing process produces a less springy scar substance which is composed of criss-crossing fibres that are not as strong as the original tissue. Such areas are the weak link in the ligament or tendon and are prone to further rupture which results in the formation of bigger and bigger scars. In small birds, the joints are so small that it is almost impossible to diagnose these tears unless a whole group of tendons or ligaments is torn.

Diseases of Ligaments and Tendons

Treatment consists of immobilizing the limb by the application of sticking plaster or, for birds over 200 grammes in weight, a gypsona plaster. The limb should be restrained for $1\frac{1}{2}$ to 3 weeks until the repair is achieved and the swelling has largely disappeared. As tendons are liable to pull apart at the level of the tear, healing is often slow and incomplete. Where an entire group of tendons is cut through on one face of a limb, the joint supplied by those tendons is liable to drop. When the gastrocnemius tendon of the hock is cut, the bird drops onto its hocks and loses all power of extending the leg. Surgical repair of tendons is difficult, especially in birds weighing less than 200 grammes. Surgery is hampered by the fact that immediately above the hock joint the limb consists of little more than skin, bone, tendons, blood vessels and nerves. A slight error with the scalpel can therefore result in a necrotic or a paralyzed foot if the blood or nerve supply is damaged. The original injury may produce similar results, so a delay of one to three days between accident and operation is preferable to be as sure as possible about the vitality of the lower part of the limb.

Perosis or slipped tendon is a disease of poultry produced mainly by a deficiency of manganese, but other elements may be involved. In turkeys the disease is sometimes called "spraddle legs" or "hock disease". In captive, mainly seed-eating birds, such as budgerigars, canaries, Java sparrows and probably other species, a similar clinical disease occurs, but no conclusive evidence of dietary deficiency has yet been found in these species. Perosis is first noticed soon after youngsters leave the parents. The hocks become broadened; they bow outwards or inwards and appear to be mechanically weak, the bird soon becoming content to rest on its breast and hocks. Corns, in the form of thickened pads of skin, develop at these pressure points. The large gastrocnemius tendon which extends to the under surface of the toes normally runs over the back of the hock in a deep bony groove, but in perosis the broadening of the bones comprising the hock results in the groove becoming shallower and incomplete. The tendon therefore easily slips out of the groove and forward onto the inside of the hock, so that the toes of the foot, instead of tightening when the bird sinks down on its perch, stay loose and flaccid and are unable to grip.

The clinical signs superficially resemble some forms of arthritis of the hock. An arthritic joint, however, tends to be a cylindrical or spindle-shaped swelling and the tendon cannot be displaced with the fingers as in perosis. The lesions of perosis are irreversible in the advanced stages and cannot be cured by feeding the minerals or vitamins which prevent the disease.

Bursitis and Synovitis

Bursae—which are specialized synovial membranes surrounding and lubricating tendons and ligaments where they pass over bony prominences—are prone to mechanical damage. This may occur, for example, when a cage bird is released into an aviary to which it is unaccustomed, and gets a direct injury by colliding with obstructions. It may also occur as the result of a blow or peck, or by being trapped in a cage door or the wire netting, etc. Depending upon the degree, direction and nature of the injury, inflammation of muscles, tendons, ligaments, synovial membranes, or even of nerves, bone and cartilage may result.

After a period of rest these tissues usually repair themselves, and unless the damage is very severe, normal functioning is soon re-established. A torn tendon or ligament, however, may so alter the action of muscles around a joint, that the resulting abnormal wear produced in the joint, causes a painful condition. Muscles may then no longer function correctly and cause deformity of the affected limb, resulting in so-called "rheumatism" or "cage paralysis".

The damaged limb should be immobilized in a comfortable semi-flexed position using an adhesive, plaster support with or without stiffening splints. After two to three weeks, assisted by the application of skilful dressings, nature will usually have repaired the damage.

Apart from simple injuries, such as cuts and sprains and infected wounds, skeletal muscles suffer little from specific disease. Certain deficiencies such as vitamin E, sometimes in conjunction with methionine, are thought to produce muscle dystrophy. This is manifested by muscle weakness and in severe cases leads to wasting of the affected muscles, particularly the most powerful ones such as those of the thigh and the pectoral muscles.

Diseases of The Skeletal Muscles

Birds do not suffer from rheumatism as far as it is known. The various types of lameness and impairment of muscles seen in birds are usually caused by temporary or permanent loss of nerve function to the affected limb and may be due to a variety of causes. When loss of nerve supply is complete, and in other circumstances when there is disuse of muscles for some weeks, the muscles become flabby and smaller, eventually being replaced by fibrous tissue. This decrease in muscle size is called atrophy. In the absence of a nerve supply an atrophied muscle cannot regain its normal size. Atrophy from other causes is, however, usually reversible if the cause is removed.

SELECTED BIBLIOGRAPHY

ALTMAN, I. E. (1969). Disorders of the Skeletal System. In *Diseases of Cage and Aviary Birds,* p.255–262. Ed. Petrak, M. L., Philadelphia. Lea and Febiger.

THE DIGESTIVE SYSTEM

The Beak The beak, in addition to being a vital organ for grasping food, is also important for investigating the bird's environment, for preening, carrying nesting and other material and as an offensive or defensive weapon.

Hereditary defects of the beak are sometimes seen (see Chapter 25), although it is often impossible when presented with a young bird showing a deformity of the beak to establish whether its nature is hereditary. This is made less difficult when a breeder notices that some of his birds periodically produce chicks with abnormal beaks. It is not sufficient for him to destroy these freaks and carry on breeding as if nothing has happened, because he is liable to intensify the character in his stock, since it is liable to be a recessive factor.

There are numerous other causes of beak deformity. In the nestlings, sticky food presented by the parents tends to coat the palate and lower jaw or accumulate under the tongue. Most parents clean the food material away at regular intervals, but if they are disturbed the young may be neglected and the food will then build up into thick plaques in the mouth. The constant pressure of the tongue on these plaques can slowly elevate, or deviate the position of the beak until the whole mechanism of its movement is deranged, resulting in uneven growth and distortion of both mandibles. Quiet, methodical methods of management, close attention to hygiene and diet, and regular checks on the cleanliness and progress of young stock help to prevent such deformities.

Caking of food in the mouth may be complicated by secondary fungal infection in adult parrots and some "soft-billed" birds. The primary cause is usually feeding soft and mushy scraps of food and is therefore most common in pet birds which are sometimes fed incorrectly in this way. The fungi *Candida* and *Aspergillus* are secondary or contributory causes. In such cases, a mass of hard material is found impacted under the tongue, firmly attached to the lower beak. Sometimes the tongue is ulcerated due to pressure or friction and infection, and slight distortion of the beak may occur.

A lack of inclination or the disability to eat is the main sign, with a tendency to pick up and drop food as if playing with it. Dribbling from the beak is another sign, the odour from

223

the mouth being sour or cheesy. Picking out the mass with a sharp-hooked instrument brings immediate relief, and no further treatment is usually necessary.

Knemidocoptic mange of the cere of nestling budgerigars is common in some establishments. Often the early stages are missed and only when the thickened, spongy horn of the upper beak begins to spread over the face do some owners suspect abnormality. In this disease deformities occur in adults as well as in nestlings and growing stock, resulting in a wide range and degree of deformity (see Chapter 10).

Injuries to the beak may occur when the bird flies into a door or snaps its beak in the framework of its cage. Soft-feeders can manage to eat if adequate supplies of food are available and if there is the minimum competition for food. Nut- and grain-feeders, which shell or dehusk seed are less able to adapt to the resultant deformity, but can manage if a stump of beak is left, on which to crack the seed. However, repeated trimming of the unopposed beak is necessary to prevent its overgrowth. Birds with long, slender beaks, such as sunbirds (Figure 2/AP; Chapter 31), rapidly succumb to necrosis of the tongue under these circumstances so that the tongue projects and cannot be withdrawn. It is therefore liable to become dry and its tip shrivel and die so that feeding becomes impossible. Similar lesions can be caused by giving insufficiently diluted honey or sugar water to nectar-feeders; in such a case the tongue sticks to the beak and cannot be withdrawn. Rinsing the mouth is usually sufficient to free the tongue, but when the beak is broken, more drastic treatment is necessary, such as trimming the undamaged part of the beak and the tongue to the length of the broken mandible. This is of course a task for a veterinarian. Wading birds with long, slender bills (see Figures 8/2 and 12/2) are completely unable to seize and swallow food and therefore soon starve to death if the beak is badly injured.

The Mouth

Simple congestion of the mucous membranes in the mouth is difficult to see, because birds lack soft, fleshy gums and a soft palate comparable with that in mammals. Inflammations accompanied by exudates or discharges are more obvious. Excessive salivation can result from injury, ulceration, or an impacted foreign body in the buccal cavity. Infections of the upper respiratory tract may also sometimes over-stimulate the salivary glands. An excessive amount of bubbly saliva may indicate infestation with gapeworms.

Thick, white or cream-coloured material adhering to the mucosa of the mouth, oesophagus, pharynx, larynx or trachea denote a possible deficiency of vitamin A. In pigeons, however, the most common cause of these lesions is trichomoniasis. The one-celled parasite, with flagellae or whiplike processes, is readily found by microscopical examination of fresh exudate (see Chapter 9). Other species may contract trichomoniasis, but the disease is most important in young pigeons when a high proportion of birds may become affected. *Candida* and less frequently *Aspergillus* may produce similar deposits in the mouth. In "sour crop", oesophageal or crop obstruction, or in general alimentary tract inflammations, a tenacious bubbly fluid may be produced in the throat and mouth, and this usually contaminates the face as well. Regurgitation of crop contents, especially in budgerigars during courtship display, leads to similar signs, so that care is needed before a diagnosis can be made.

The Oesophagus and Crop

Carnivorous birds, especially those which habitually swallow whole carcases such as fish or the heads of rats and mice or other mammals, occasionally suffer from impaction of the cervical part of the oesophagus. Such obstructions can be gently manipulated into the mouth. The oesophageal walls of these birds are tough, but if tearing or other damage is to be avoided, the manipulation must be carefully and slowly carried out. Obstruction of the oesophagus beyond the crop will sometimes induce a bird to carry on eating until the greater part of the oesophagus is a dilated mass of food. This can sometimes be broken down by the fingers through the intact tissues of the neck and squeezed upwards in small quantities at a time through crop and oesophagus to the mouth, using intermittent pressure only, to obviate the danger of asphyxiation.

Impaction of the crop is also a common occurrence in birds which eat an omnivorous diet, including hard shelled seeds. The impacted crop can assume the consistency and size of a golf ball or be even larger and almost as hard. In predominant seed-eaters, a less durable impaction may result from lack of sufficient saliva to lubricate and soften the seed, or when a highly, absorbent, glutinous material such as oatmeal is incorporated in the diet. Usually, however, only debilitated birds are affected by such crop impactions, which should be treated as previously described. It is sometimes necessary to operate in cases where starvation or other serious sequelae are imminent.

It must not be assumed that every swelling at the base of the neck is an impacted crop or oesophagus, because tumours in this area and enlargements of the thyroid gland are easily confused with distended crops. Tumours and cysts of the thyroid, however, usually have the consistency of sponge rubber and are smooth in outline. If too great a pressure is applied to cysts of this type they may rupture and give rise to

225

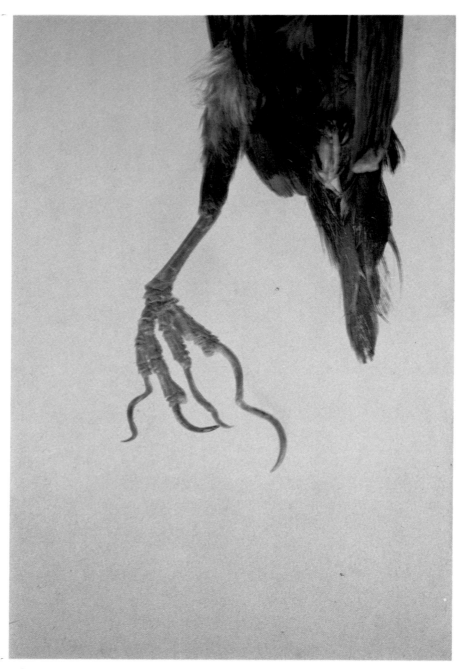

Plate 10/11. Tricolored Nun with spiralled overgrown claws. (L. Arnall)

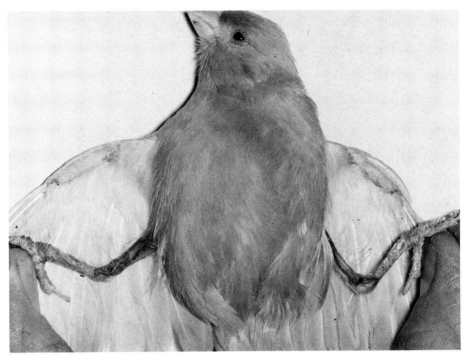

Plate 11/11. Hyperkeratosis of scales of feet and legs and varicose veins in an aged canary. The latter are visible overlying the medial aspect of the tibiotarsal region. (L. Arnall)

internal haemorrhage. Death then will occur fairly rapidly. If a skin incision is inadvertently made over such a cyst, the deep, red colour of the swelling should be sufficient to discourage further surgery and the skin wound should be sutured or the bird destroyed.

On rare occasions a concretion or stone develops in the crop of budgerigars (Plate 1/13) but the cause is obscure. It has been suggested that when the primary constituent is urate the cause may be due to eating excreta from the floor of the cage: such a theory, however, would not account for the composition of the calculus illustrated here.

Occasionally, the subcutaneous fat stored on the breast is displaced forward to the crop region and this hinders digital examination. Large fatty deposits of this type can also be easily mistaken for a full or impacted crop. Infected injuries of the crop wall occasionally develop into granulomas which appear as hard tumour-like masses and these may also affect the skin.

Regurgitation, or vomiting as it is so often referred to by bird fanciers, is very common in many species. Caged budgerigars kept alone frequently regurgitate at their reflection in a mirror with apparent enjoyment, this probably being an abnormal form of courtship display.

The regurgitation of crop contents may also indicate an inflamed or ulcerated crop, or so-called "sour crop". The crop contains evil smelling fluid, which may result from ingestion of poorly nutritious, stale or mouldy food. Irregular feeding, chilling, or some infection or other disturbance lower down the alimentary canal may also be contributory causes. "Sour-crop" may often be associated with vitamin or protein deficiencies, infections such as candidiasis and trichomoniasis, or with liver or kidney disease. Another possible cause is pressure from growths inside the body cavity which may hinder the flow of intestinal content, causing backflow into the proventriculus and crop. Sometimes it is possible that destruction of mucous- or enzyme-producing glands in the proventriculus may stimulate the return flow of acid into the crop and in poor health this alone may be sufficient to cause "sour crop" with erosion of the crop epithelium.

Sometimes the crop becomes flaccid, as a result of the muscles of the crop wall losing their tone or contractibility. This results in food being held up in the crop because of its inability to force the food further down the oesophagus into the proventriculus. There is often no actual obstruction, but when the crop becomes full the food material begins to overflow into the upper part of the oesophagus and this may eventually lead to true obstruction. The circumstances leading to crop obstruction and "sour crop" are similar.

Mild inflammations may be checked by intermittent

"milking out" of the crop contents or removing them with the aid of a wide-bored, hypodermic needle and syringe; the latter method being less likely to interfere with the breathing. An antifermentation liquid may then be given by dropper or by using the hypodermic syringe and drainage needle. A harmless antiseptic or an antibiotic should be added if infection is suspected. Gentian violet, hexamine, potassium permanganate, or one or two drops of 1 per cent formaldehyde are suitable to check fermentation. When irritation is suspected, a bland fluid such as liquid paraffin, lime water, egg albumen, barley water, kaolin or aluminium hydroxide may suffice. The diet should consist solely of liquids every hour or two for the first 24 to 36 hours after emptying the crop, gradually followed by semi-solids, finely chopped and softened solids, and finally the normal diet after 3 to 5 days. A multivitamin and mineral tonic should always be added to the drinking water during the recovery phase.

If there is no response to such treatment in budgerigars, it will indicate the presence of a specific type of necrosis or ulceration of the crop (Plate 2/13). With this disease death often occurs within a few days. Early cases sometimes respond to treatment with oxytetracycline or chloramphenicol by mouth. Experiments have failed to prove that the disease is infectious, in spite of the fact that many birds in a flock may become affected. In addition to vomiting, greenish diarrhoea is usually present. Theories that allergic, deficiency or stress mechanisms produce the disease have not been supported so far by convincing evidence. At *post-mortem* examination the crop lining shows elevated, parallel ridges or finger-like projections, which are yellowish in colour and consist of necrotic material. Death is probably the result of impaired digestion, and loss of fluid due to vomiting and diarrhoea.

The Proventriculus or glandular stomach

Food passes through the oesophagus and crop to reach the proventriculus, which it tends to traverse relatively easily. When the normal passage of food is interrupted by irregular feeding, it may interfere with the outflow of proventricular juices. The normal peristaltic or squeezing onward movements of the oesophagus and crop, may then be reversed (antiperistalsis) resulting in souring of the crop contents by proventricular secretions, and producing irritation of the crop lining and vomiting. Deficiencies in the diet, for example of vitamin A, and certain bacterial and possibly viral infections, may lead to ulceration of the epithelium of the proventriculus. Candidiasis is also capable of producing lesions in the proventriculus. Abnormal fermentation, as in the crop, can also result in distension of the proventriculus with gases.

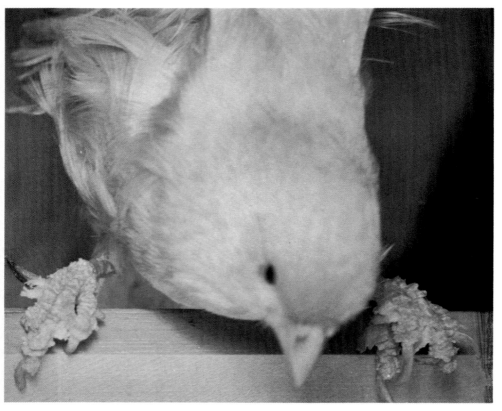

Plate 12/11. Canary with advanced "tassel-foot" caused by *Knemidocoptes* sp. (L. Arnall)

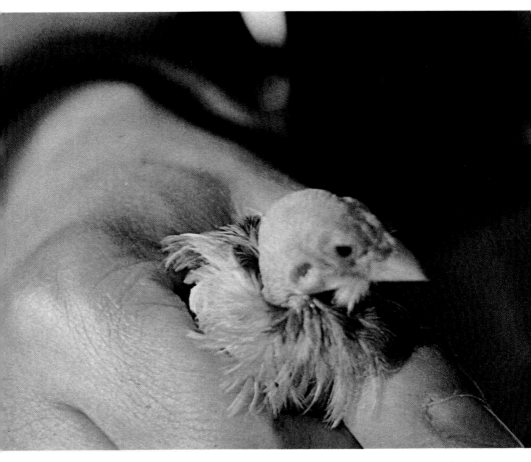

Plate 13/11. Canary with alopecia of head region. Cause unknown. (L. Arnall)

The gizzard is a tough structure and resistant to the enzymes **The Gizzard**
and acids produced by the proventriculus. In the gizzard of
omnivorous and seed-eating birds a great deal of pummeling
and grinding of food occurs aided by grit which is normally
present in this organ. The ingesta or partially digested food
emerges as a pulp of fine particles of gruel-like consistency
and is still strongly acid. In weak, debilitated birds the ingesta
may be incompletely pulverized on entry into the duodenum,
where it is then liable to irritate the openings of the bile and
pancreatic ducts thus leading to digestive disturbances. If a
foreign body, such as a coin, button, nail, staple or small piece
of wire is swallowed, it may cause no trouble until it reaches
the gizzard, where it tends to be retained, in the same way as
grit. Round objects cause a mild, chronic "gastritis" or ven-
triculitis, which may not prevent the bird from living a
relatively healthy life, but may cause occasional brief bouts of
indigestion. Sharp or hooked objects tend to bury their ends
into the gizzard wall during contraction of the organ, probably causing pain and perhaps resulting in loss of appetite and
consequently weight. Sometimes a sharp object will perforate
the gizzard wall and cause peritonitis and death. Unfortunately x-ray examination does not always differentiate between
foreign bodies and the shadows cast by grit in the gizzard.
When a foreign body is strongly suspected an operation for
removal is not to be embarked on lightly, even by an experienced veterinarian, because this is usually very difficult and
the chances of success are low.

Erosion of the horny lining of the gizzard does not appear
to be as common in cage and aviary birds as it is in poultry,
but it may result from a lack of vitamins such as vitamin A.
In waterfowl and occasionally other species, gizzard worms
produce severe erosions. Gizzard erosion can be suspected
in vague illnesses accompanied by indigestion and loose,
greenish, mucoid and intermittently bloodstained droppings.

Distension and flabbiness of the gizzard musculature occurs
mostly in debilitated birds, especially when the exit into the
small intestine is impacted with hard fibrous ingesta. Such an
obstruction soon causes depression, loss of appetite, and
soft droppings which rapidly become smaller in amount,
and are passed progressively less frequently. If the condition
is not relieved, death can result from toxaemia even before
the effect of starvation is felt. Birds affected in this way are
generally those kept in planted aviaries or where little food
and an abundance of coarse fibrous material is present. Liquid
paraffin given slowly by mouth in liberal amounts using a
dropper (10-20 drops per 100 gramme body weight) is the
most effective and safest treatment. This tends to ease and
soften the obstruction, and soothe the mucous membrane of
the gut. Diagnosis is difficult and has to be based on careful
observation, and consideration of all the circumstances.

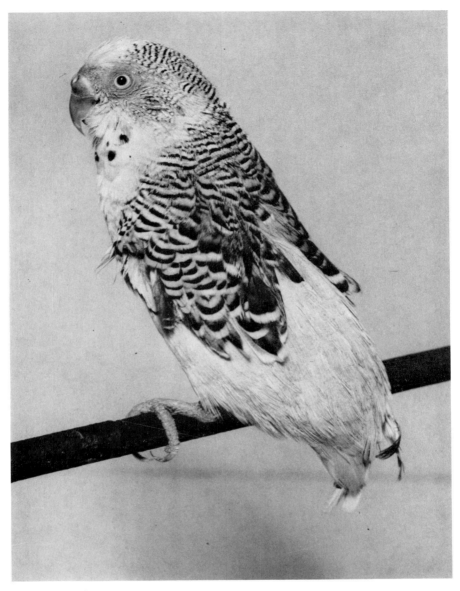

Plate 14/11. Young budgerigar with French Moult. Note complete loss of tail and larger wing feathers. (L. Arnall)

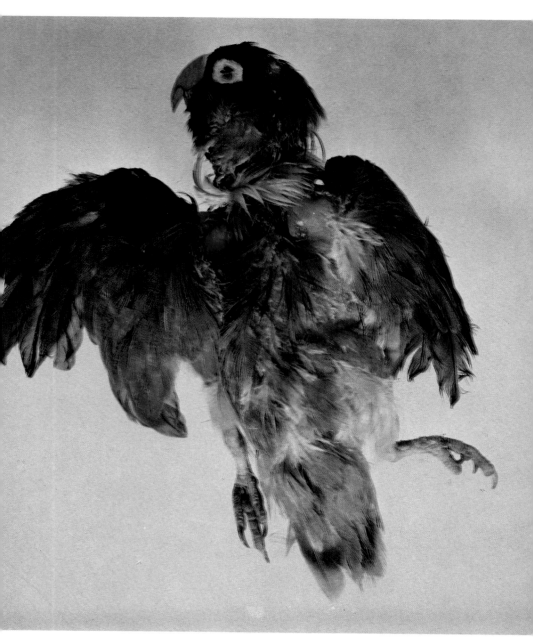

Plate 15/11. Masked lovebird with extensive areas of alopecia. Both sides of body, ventral aspect of thorax, abdomen, legs and to a lesser extent the back, were all affected. Most tail and primary wing feathers were missing. The bird had the typical appearance of a French Moult "runner". (I.F. Keymer and T.C. Dennett, Z.S.L.)

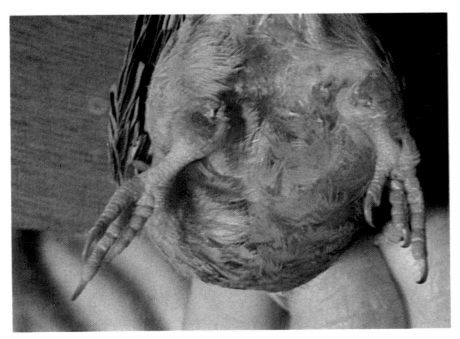

Plate 1/12. Budgerigar showing ankylosis (fusion) of both hock joints with secondary "corns". See "Arthritis". (L. Arnall)

Plate 1/13. Calculus from crop of budgerigar. On an analysis this contained potassium phosphate and oxalate, also cystine. (L. Arnall and G. Dibley)

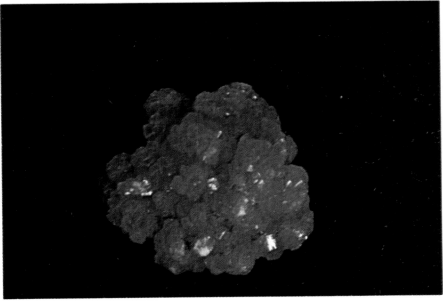

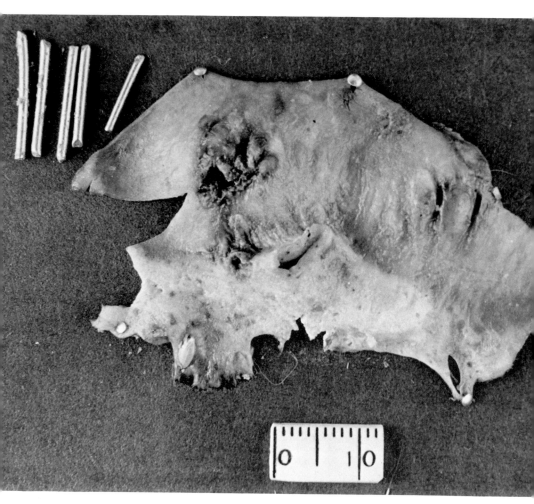

Speckled pigeon (*Columba guinea*). Gizzard showing perforations caused by pieces of wire which had been dropped inadvertently in the aviary when the netting was being repaired. See Chapter 13. (I.F. Keymer and T.C. Dennett, Z.S.L.)

These organs are erroneously believed by many avicultura-lists to be the seat of over half of the ills that affect birds because loose droppings are a common sign in digestive disorders and many diseases which are not confined to the digestive tract. These diseases are frequently lumped together, being referred to as "diarrhoea" or more often as "enteritis", the two words being used interchangeably by bird keepers.

Diarrhoea is not a disease but a clinical sign. It simply refers to the voiding of fluid faeces. It can be caused by irritation or infection of the gut resulting from eating unaccustomed or contaminated food and drinking excessive amounts of milk or oily liquids. The watery urate fraction of the droppings is often mistaken for diarrhoea. Excessive amounts, however, indicate urinary upset and not alimentary disease.

Enteritis is the inflammation of part or all of the gut behind the gizzard. Although a specific gut infection or other localized inflammatory change may be responsible, much more likely causes of diarrhoea are the results of a septicaemia; pressure from a tumour of a gonad or kidney; liver damage; visceral gout; parasitism; a localized bacterial infection elsewhere, causing a toxaemia or even a change of environmental conditions or feeding routine.

The first step towards a diagnosis is to establish that true diarrhoea and not watery urine is being excreted. Both fractions of the droppings, urinary and faecal, are often affected simultaneously when a generalized disease is present, but in the early stages one fraction usually alters before the other. In order to diagnose the cause and significance of diarrhoea many factors have to be considered, for example, whether or not the disease is contagious; the ages of those affected; the significance of other clinical signs; the diet; general management, and all factors known to influence disease. It is thus an exercise for the veterinarian. In an isolated pet bird, the cause of diarrhoea can be undiagnosable, when it is the only or main sign of illness, even with the full services of a laboratory at one's disposal. Although *post-mortem* examinations do not always reveal the cause, carcases of any dead birds should always be submitted to a laboratory, as well as samples of excreta from live birds.

In the case of illness in only one bird, factors such as impactions, foreign bodies, large abdominal tumours and abdominal rupture should be considered. When a bird suddenly becomes ill, and is well fleshed, but huddles, shivers, or pants, an acute infection or poisoning must be suspected. In such acute cases the administration of a broad-spectrum antibiotic to both the affected and the other birds may be indicated. A veterinarian should be consulted as soon as possible since unscientific treatment can merely mask deadly diseases until the cause is well and truly established in the premises and stock. Diarrhoea without significant depression or illness

237

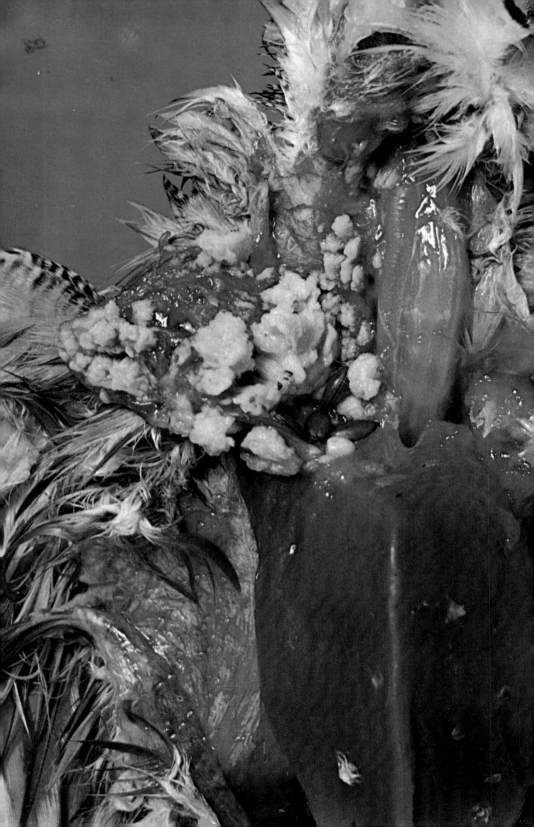

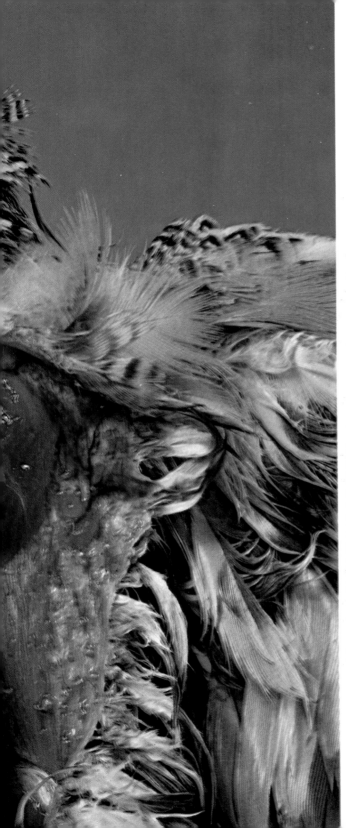

Plate 2/13. Crop and oesophagus of a budgerigar opened to show advanced lesions of necrosis involving the epithelium. Cause is unknown. The yellowish, caseous, necrotic material is mainly in the form of parallel ridges which reached a maximum width of 0.5 cm. in thickness. The lesions involved the crop and the entire length of the cervical part of the oesophagus. Note the prominent keel bone and wasting of the pectoral muscles on either side. (I.F. Keymer and T.C. Dennett, Z.S.L.)

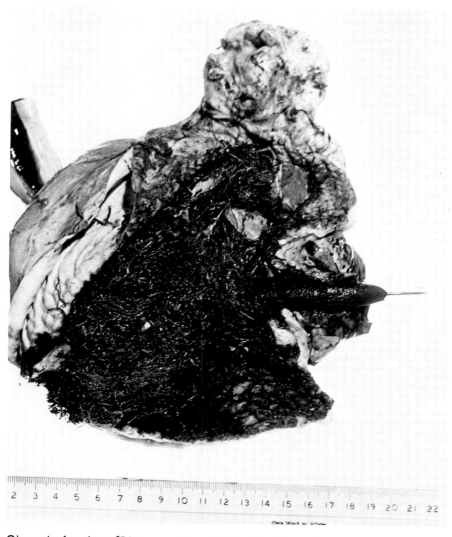

Gizzard of a rhea (*Rhea americana*) showing impaction with coarse grass and perforation of the wall by a dart. See Chapter 13. (I.F. Keymer and T.C. Dennett, Z.S.L.)

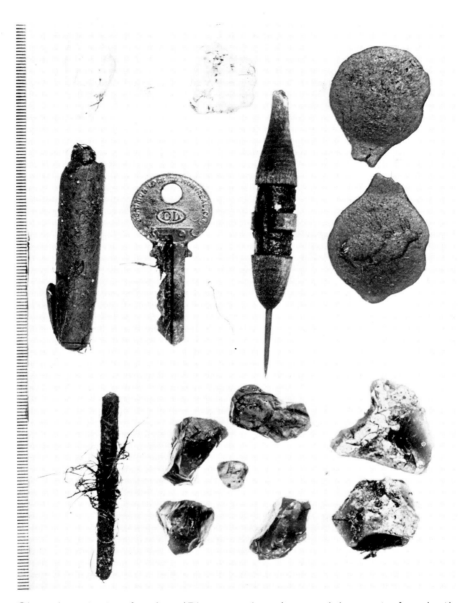

Gizzard contents of a rhea (*Rhea americana*) comprising part of a plastic ball pen, door key, end of a dart, two plastic identity discs, broken nail and large pebbles. See Chapter 13. (I.F. Keymer and T.C. Dennett, Z.S.L.)

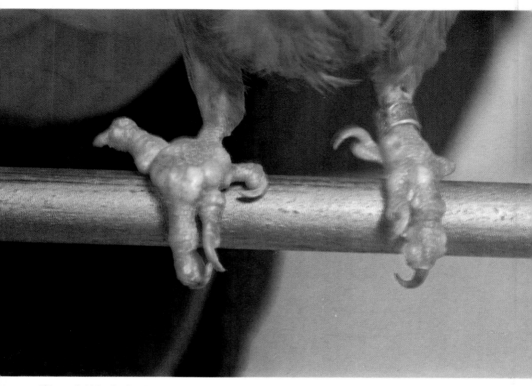

Plate 1/15. Articular and peri-articular gout involving the feet of a budgerigar. (L. Arnall)

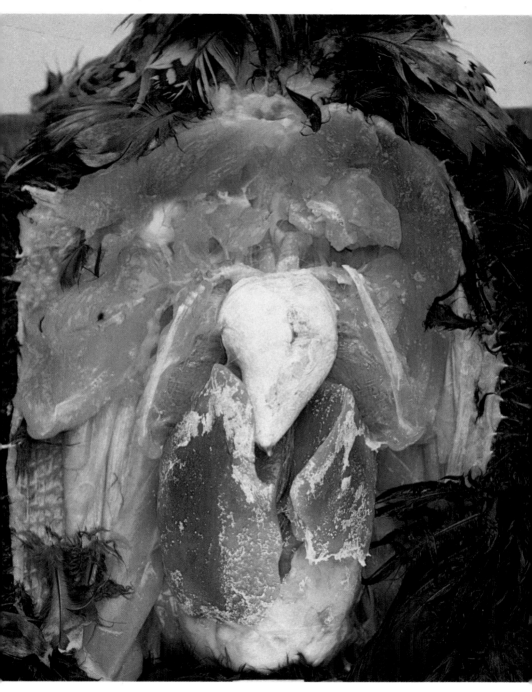

Plate 2/15. Ventral surface of body cavity opened to show visceral gout in a black-bellied sandgrouse. Note the "chalky" white deposits of urates thickly covering the pericardial sac and to a lesser extent the ventral surface of the liver. (I.F. Keymer and T.C. Dennett, Z.S.L.)

in one or several birds may have a dietary origin; so this possibility should be checked. When appetite is reduced, a multi-vitamin/mineral/amino-acid elixir given by dropper is most useful. It aids recovery in most diseases, increasing the appetite and vitality, especially if vitamin B_{12} is included. It also temporarily alleviates most dietary upsets, including deficiency of various food factors. When marked loss of breast muscle and fat is noticed, this suggests a chronic type of disease. Aspergillosis, nephrosis, large tumours of internal organs and certain slowly developing bacterial infections such as tuberculosis come into this category.

A true inflammation of the duodenum and/or small intestine can be a serious matter. An inflamed gut is more permeable than normal; it allows poisonous substances and bacteria to pass through more easily, even though its increased blood supply brings an army of defending white cells with it. The increased blood flow causes swelling of the gut wall, in particular its lining mucous membrane. Mucous outflow is increased, and digestive juices are unable to function properly because the increased gut movements hustle the ingesta on towards the cloaca before digestion is complete. The swelling of the mucous membrane may be so marked as to close the openings of glands, and also involve the bile or pancreatic ducts, causing damage to the liver and pancreas and leading to infection of these organs. An acute hepatitis or pancreatitis (the latter fortunately appears to be rare) causes more severe illness than an inflamed duodenum. If the pancreas is damaged it tends to digest itself, and because its enzymes are so potent, it partly liquefies; this results in a local or generalized peritonitis with dire results. If the liver is infected first in a septicaemia, the flow of bile may cease and this in itself interferes with digestion, causing a duodenitis and enteritis. It can be appreciated therefore that little can happen in a single tissue or organ of the body without it having effects in the neighbouring or distant organs.

Probably a further result of intestinal inflammation is the liberation of certain substances into the bloodstream which may produce shock. This results in lowered intake of food and weakness. The excessive loss of water, acids, enzymes and mineral salts also has a rapidly weakening and debilitating effect. In birds, with their high metabolic rate, this rundown is rapid and soon becomes serious.

The type of treatment depends upon the cause but is usually a matter of trial and error.

The Liver

The liver features in many diseases, especially infections, mainly because it is a kind of sieve, a factory and a scrapyard for the various products reaching it via the bloodstream.

Degenerations, especially of a fatty type, are common and usually associated with unsuitable food, lack of exercise or certain poisons. Fatty infiltration of the liver is common in otherwise healthy budgerigars, parrots and cockatoos. Later stages lead to fibrous replacement of liver tissue (cirrhosis) which, when advanced has widespread effects, especially on the heart, kidneys and digestive functions. Tumours of liver tissue, and metastatic, multiple tumours originating from cancerous growths elsewhere, are quite common in budgerigars and seriously interfere with metabolism. Single, large, benign tumours and cysts of the liver produce effects mainly by pressure—destruction and replacement of liver substance as well as pressure on neighbouring organs. Clinical signs develop more slowly in these benign cases, and usually only when the lesion has reached a considerable size.

It is virtually impossible to diagnose liver disease in the live bird.

The Pancreas   This organ is remarkably free from localised inflammations and degenerations, although it can readily be inflamed or otherwise damaged in many generalized affections. Pancreatitis, either acute or chronic, is occasionally found at necropsy, but can rarely be diagnosed in life. Diabetes does not appear to have been reported in birds. Tumours of the pancreas are uncommon.

Atrophy of the pancreas has recently been reported for the first time in budgerigars. An affected bird loses weight in spite of the fact that its appetite increases markedly. At the same time the amount of faeces produced also increases greatly. The general condition of the bird gradually deteriorates and the abdomen becomes distended. The faeces are a light grey in colour and a little greasy on the surface. Eventually the faeces become hard and chalky obscuring the white urate part of the excreta. The faeces stain dark blue with iodine owing to the presence of undigested starch. The cause of the disease is at present unknown and it is incurable.

The Caeca or   Most birds have two caeca lying at the junction of the long,
blind guts   small intestine and the short, large bowel. In a few species, only one caecum is present. Large caeca occur mainly in species which eat bulky, vegetable food such as grain, but the organs are by no means vital and their surgical removal causes little or no departure from normal health. Only in the large, flightless birds, gallinaceous species, and some seabirds, do the caeca have a major function, and even in these species removal does not seriously impair health, although digestive processes are less efficient.

245

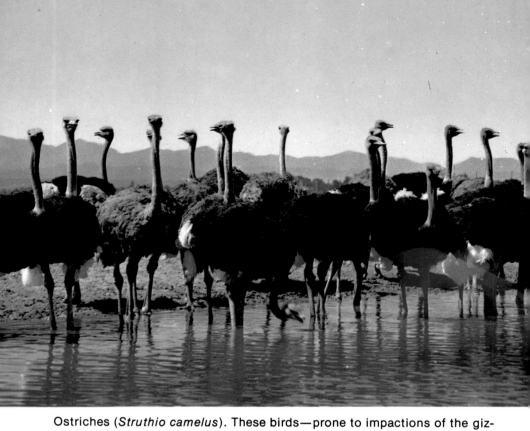

Ostriches (*Struthio camelus*). These birds—prone to impactions of the gizzard with fibrous grass and foreign bodies—have an intestinal tract in which the large intestines and caeca are unusually long (Chapter 2). Ostriches also lay the largest egg of all birds. Unlike most birds, they are susceptible to anthrax (Chapter 31).

Common peafowl (*Pavo cristatus*). This beautiful but noisy bird is commonly kept loose in parks and seem to be particularly susceptible to tuberculosis, pseudotuberculosis (Chapter 7) and "blackhead" (Chapter 9).

246

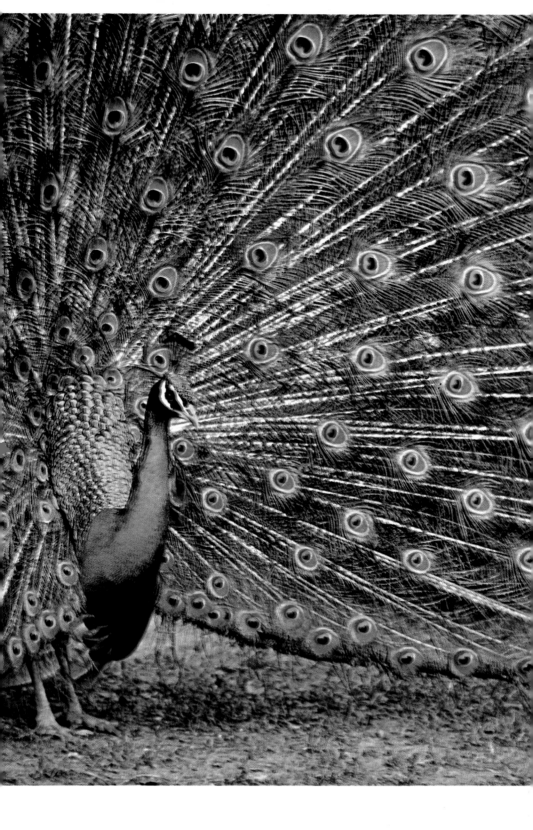

The larger caeca of gallinaceous birds, like the appendix of human beings, can be the site of trouble and become infected by pathogenic bacteria such as *Salmonella* or *Escherichia coli*, causing inflammatory changes. In these species too, certain nematode worms, coccidia and *Histomonas* can flourish in the caeca. Most passerine birds have vestigial caeca which cause no trouble, while budgerigars and a few other species are without them. In those species possessing caeca fermentation may produce gas, causing marked distension if the exit into the large bowel is obstructed by swelling of the mucous membrane, or by solid ingesta. Such distension appears to cause pain, depression, and loss of appetite, and spread of the inflammatory process to neighbouring parts of the gut may cause diarrhoea. Caecal disease is not generally diagnosable in the living bird although specific bacterial infections or parasitic infestation of the gut, including the caeca, can be diagnosed on laboratory examination of faeces. An operation for the surgical removal of caeca in turkeys has been devised, but although this prevents certain diseases, mortality from the operation is high and it probably has no useful place in the surgery of cage birds.

The Rectum and Cloaca

The large bowel or rectum (colorectum) is a short, straight structure, whose main function is reabsorption of water and all useful digestive soluble materials; it is helped in this by the proctodeum of the cloaca. The useful materials include bile, mineral salts, used enzymes, sugars, fatty acids, amino acids and vitamins. If an inflammatory process occurs higher up the digestive tract, not only will the flow of ingesta be quicker than can adequately be dealt with by the absorptive powers of the rectum, but also the inflammation may eventually spread to the rectal wall itself. An enteritis seldom remains limited for long to a short portion of the tract. Both acute and chronic inflammations interfere with absorption from the rectum, and diarrhoea results.

Tumours of the gut wall are not common in birds, abdominal tumours which press on the gut or liver being more frequently seen. These may cause irritation, increasing the flow of gut contents, or more usually causing partial obstruction. In the case of a large tumour, retained egg, or cyst of the oviduct or other structure in the posterior half of the abdomen, pressure on the rectum or cloaca results in partial or complete obstruction of the gut. When there is a slowly developing structure such as a tumour, the muscles of the gut above the growing obstruction tend to enlarge in response to the extra work. The obstruction to the lumen of the gut results in impaction with faeces anterior to the obstruction, and soon leads to general abdominal enlargement. When straining

248

occurs, the abdominal wall is liable to rupture and the power of the abdominal contraction is lost. This stage usually causes obvious respiratory difficulty. The rate of breathing may increase, panting may occur, and abnormal, fluid-like clicking sounds may be heard in the chest on auscultation. Complete constipation may occur or faeces may be passed in small amounts and be infrequent, depending upon the severity of the obstruction. Sudden obstruction causes considerable straining and distress. Successful palpation of the obstruction is often impossible. Continuous pressure must be avoided because it will kill the bird by causing interference with respiration and blood circulation.

Sometimes the masses of faeces in the cloaca become very sticky owing to the absorption of moisture. The impaction then becomes difficult to void and may cause pressure on the gut, reproductive or urinary tracts. Liquid paraffin by mouth is the most useful simple remedy.

"Pasting of the vent" is the result of a disease causing diarrhoea or excessive excretion of urates, and is not a disease in itself. The "paste" can be composed of abnormal faecal or urinary products. Excessive brooding, incubating in wet or dirty nests, poor diet and hygiene, can all play a part in producing this unpleasant condition. At best it is a sign of some defect in diet, hygiene, or other aspects of husbandry, but in most cases it is a portent of disease about to show itself in some other way. First, one should eliminate the simpler and less harmful possibilities and then consider the various infections. In uncomplicated cloacal inflammations and diarrhoea due to dietetic disorders, all that may be necessary is simple bathing of the vent, liquid paraffin by mouth, the use of an enema (under professional advice only), and attention to diet and hygiene. In other cases, the causal agent must be found and appropriate treatment given. Further information is provided in Chapter 15.

"Vent gleet" is a chronic inflammation of the vent or cloaca, particularly in the laying domestic fowl and occasionally in the male. It is characterised by necrosis of the mucous membrane which becomes covered with a yellowish layer of dead epithelium. The lesion gives rise to a very unpleasant odour and starts with swelling and reddening of the mucosa. The exact cause is not known, but since the greatest number of victims are laying birds, metabolic or stress factors may be involved. Although various bacteria may be isolated from affected vents, none are apparently capable of producing the disease without a predisposing cause. Only a few birds at a time usually become affected. Diarrhoea with "pasting of the vent" may occasionally be a contributory factor. Although this is primarily a disease of poultry, cage birds sometimes develop clinical signs which are indistinguishable.

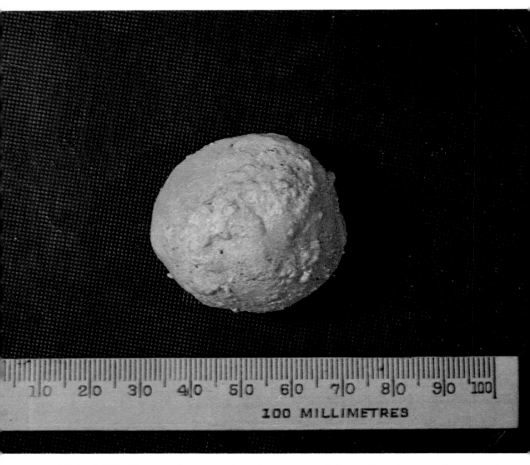

Plate 3/15. Rounded mass of urates removed from the cloaca of an aged Verreaux's eagle affected with chronic and severe kidney disease. (I.F. Keymer and T.C. Dennett, Z.S.L.)

Plate 1/16. Egg peritonitis associated with the bacteria *Escherichia coli* in a Japanese quail. The thorax and abdomen have been opened to show large masses of yolk material in the peritoneal cavity. A soft-shelled egg had passed up the oviduct and ruptured so that it was resting near the opening of the fallopian tube. The ovary is active and contains numerous large yolks, some of which have ruptured. These yolks are visible between the lungs and the egg material in the peritoneal cavity. They are covered by a thin vascular and congested layer of tissue. Numerous fibrinous adhesions were present between all parts of the intestinal tract, ovary and oviduct. In addition, the posterior extremity of the oviduct was grossly distended with necrotic egg material. (I.F. Keymer and T.C. Dennett, Z.S.L.)

250

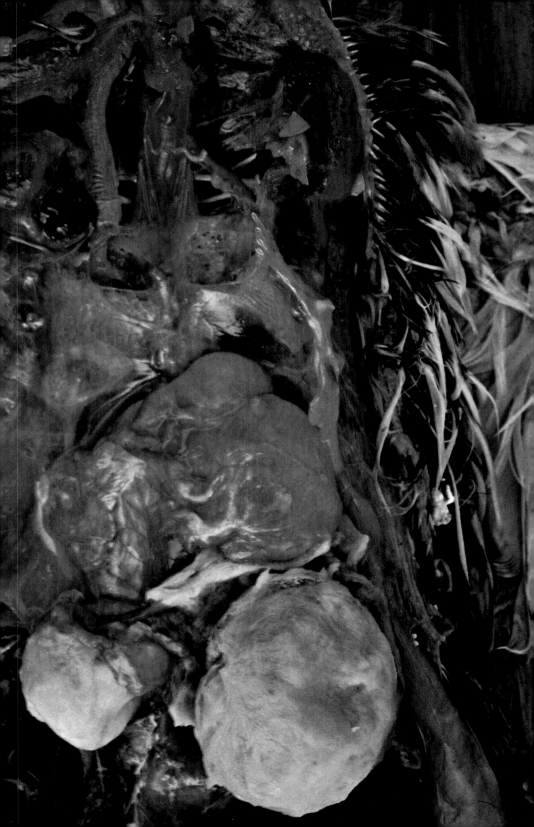

"Constipation" is the name given for the excessive dehydration of the faeces in the rectum and cloaca which causes partial or complete retention. Contrary to common belief, this seldom occurs to a serious extent, unless a mechanical obstruction has held up the faeces in the first place. In other cases the cause may be due to an excess of fibrous material or grit in the diet, poor tone of the muscles in the bowel wall due to inactivity or obesity, or "pasting of the vent". Prevention and treatment are self-evident, an oily laxative being most helpful.

Prolapse of the Rectum

Prolapse of the rectum is usually the result of, or in association with, enteritis of some severity or duration, which produces straining. In some cases the pressure from an enlarged organ or an abnormal structure such as a retained egg, tumour, cyst, or a ruptured or distended abdominal wall is the cause of the straining. This may result in the cloaca being turned inside out and either the oviduct or rectum, or both, also being partly everted and visible. The treatment requires the services of a veterinarian and is usually surgical in nature.

SELECTED BIBLIOGRAPHY

MINSKY, L. & PETRAK, M. L. (1969). Diseases of the Digestive System. In *Diseases of Cage and Aviary Birds,* p.303–311. Ed. Petrak, M. L., Philadelphia. Lea and Febiger.

PECKHAM, M. C. (1965). Conditions affecting the digestive system. In *Diseases of Poultry,* p.1174–1179. Eds. Biester, H. E. and Schwarte, H. L. 5th Ed. Ames, Iowa. State University Press.

THE RESPIRATORY SYSTEM

Obstructions and Local Inflammations The upper air passages, except for the nasal sinuses, are relatively long in birds. The nostrils are generally quite small holes or slits and can readily be blocked by various types of foreign material. In several chronic affections involving discharges from the specialized parts of the head, eyes, mouth and nostrils, these exudates dry and cake around or across the nostrils. This results in noisy breathing through the mouth. Chronic infection by bacteria, perhaps following a viral infection, is the usual cause of such a discharge. Seeds held in the sticky, mucous exudate sometimes find their way into the nostrils and cause sneezing. In budgerigars deep-seated abscesses or granulomas of the cere or of the horn-generating layers of the upper beak are also occasionally involved. Tumours are seen on the head from time to time, involving and even closing the nostrils. Treatments depend on the cause and these are dealt with elsewhere under the relevant headings.

In budgerigars, a brown-coloured thickening of the cere occurs sometimes, this being made up of dead cells, keratin and waxy material. This so-called "brown hypertrophy" may be likened to catarrh of a mucous surface and occurs in many types of chronic ill health. Apparently it is not caused by local infection, and ideally treatment consists of finding and treating the underlying cause. The cere should be treated also by picking away the heaped-up material and applying a little oily lotion, cod liver oil or bland ointment.

Obstructions of the larynx and trachea due to the production of yellow, necrotic material occur in vitamin A deficiency. Similar deposits are seen in trichomoniasis (canker) of pigeons, birds of prey, some species of passerines and possibly other birds. Candidiasis in some types of gallinaceous birds and in parrots, also causes obstructions and similarly chronic pox infections in pigeons. Gapeworms (*Syngamus*) may cause obstruction of the trachea in many species. All these conditions are accompanied by loss of appetite and weight or retarded growth. Examination of the mouth, pharynx and larynx, supported by laboratory examination of exudates help to differentiate the various infections. For further details see the relevant chapters.

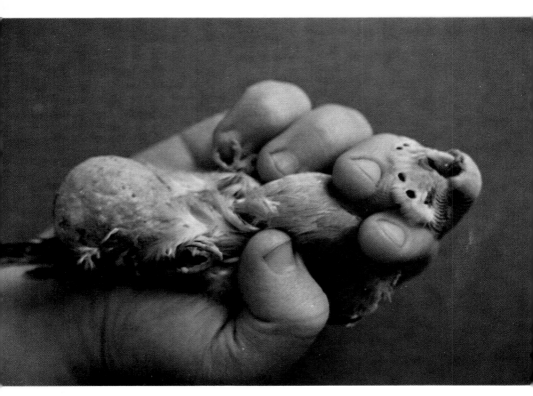

Plate 2/16. Abdominal distension due to muscular degeneration and rupture associated with a dilated atonic oviduct. Budgerigar. (L. Arnall)

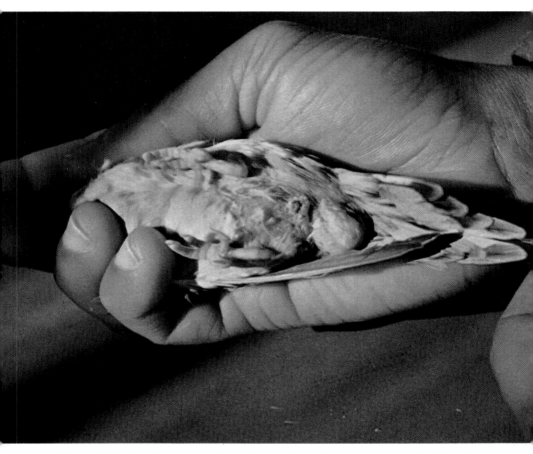

Plate 3/16. Budgerigar with prolapsed swelling above and behind the cloaca. It contained a dilated oviduct, egg material, some small intestine and adhesions. (L. Arnall)

"Asthma" is a term used by many people associated with birds to denote a condition involving rapid, heaving, noisy breathing. Under this heading the processes of disease in many parts of the body can be included, some being quite unrelated to the respiratory tract.

In true asthma, bouts of partial closure or spasm of the smaller, bronchial tubes occur. The air is therefore unable to pass freely through to the lungs. Sneezing, coughing or gasping in order to achieve passage of air, increases the blood flow to the lungs and congestion and oedema result. This further embarrasses the breathing as well as the heart's action, and hinders the interchange of gases. In man there seems to be a hereditary predisposition to asthma, while a nervous or worrying nature also favours it. Chemical irritants, and allergies can bring on an attack in some people. Certainly a mental or emotional problem, a city fog, contact with pollen or animal hairs, eating or drinking certain substances, have all been shown to bring on bouts of asthma. There is no real evidence, however, that true asthma occurs in birds, although some of these factors may play a part in some of their respiratory troubles. Badly polluted air and irritant fumes will certainly affect or even kill a bird, but not necessarily produce signs of typical asthma as it occurs in man.

Another affection which may be considered here is so-called "cardiac asthma". With a failing heart, the pulmonary blood pressure is so low that it is insufficient to overcome the resistance of capillary and venous blood accumulating in the lungs. Since the right ventricle cannot adequately force blood into the lungs, the right auricle cannot receive blood from the body. The slowing of the blood flow in the lungs allows tissue fluid to leave the arteries but not flow back fast enough into the veins. The congested lungs therefore become water-logged and cannot function properly in oxygen and carbon dioxide exchanges. The poorly aerated blood creates an "air hunger", which in turn leads to panting and gasping. Wheezy lung sounds can be heard on holding the side of the bird's breast or its back against the ear. Loud clicking sounds which may also be heard are almost certainly pieces of loosely attached exudate or airsac walls expanding and closing with each respiration. If no improvement occurs damage to the brain rapidly follows owing to lack of oxygenation from the blood.

Obese birds are most commonly affected, but difficulty in breathing soon causes loss of weight and in some cases leads to emaciation. Treatment is unlikely to have much effect but should be along the lines indicated for circulatory disease.

Sinusitis and Blepharitis

The inflammations of the eyelids and sinuses which are known as blepharitis and sinusitis, lead to watery discharges from the nostrils and eyes. The condition is known as coryza and is quite common in gallinaceous birds, parrots, birds of prey, canaries and other small passerines. It is generally complicated by bacteria flourishing in the inflamed, mucous membranes. The primary cause is sometimes a virus or bacterialike organism such as *Mycoplasma* or *Chlamydia*. If neglected, the watery discharges may develop into thick, purulent exudates causing obstructions to the nasal passages and thus choking, wheezing and other difficulties in breathing. The airsacs slowly fill with exudates and pneumonia or even septicemia may result. Coryza is often a flock problem and frequently infectious.

Infection occurs by inhalation of infected aerosols and less often by eating or drinking contaminated food or water. So long as one bird in a flock has this infection the other birds are at risk. Infections may result in debility or death from septicaemia or pneumonia. Even after recovery, the birds may still harbour the causal organisms.

Treatment with antibiotics is helpful in controlling the bacterial secondary invaders and the *Mycoplasma*, but is useless against viruses. If ornithosis or psittacosis (*Chlamydia* infection) is present, it is usually advisable to destroy the bird.

Bronchitis, Tracheitis, Syringitis and Laryngitis

Inflammations of the upper parts of the respiratory tract from the larynx to syrinx do occur, but they are usually associated with sinusitis and coryza or pneumonia and inflammation of the airsacs.

Bronchitis is a term which is frequently misused by bird owners to describe any condition affecting the voice or respiration. Although the bronchi may be involved in many respiratory diseases or in a septicaemia, bronchitis is seldom the only lesion present. Therefore the use of the term is almost always a great over-simplification of the situation. A tracheobronchitis usually accompanies gapeworm infestations and can be very severe in infectious viral laryngo-tracheitis, the bronchi also sometimes being involved. The latter infection, however, is confined to the domestic fowl and pheasants.

Syringitis is also a common inflammatory change in several respiratory infections, causing loss of voice, or croaking, squeaking and whistling sounds according to the degree of swelling which is present. In budgerigars, pressure on the syrinx from thyroid enlargement or tumours in the confined space at the entrance to the thorax is the commonest cause of voice change. Generally the pitch is raised and a squeak is made before the bird produces other sounds. As the pressure increases, the distorted vocal cords vibrate with each respiration, producing a rhythmical squeak which continues day and night. No treatment, except surgical removal of the mass (a hazardous procedure) or in the case of some thyroid enlargements, administration of potassium iodide or thyroid extract, will have any effect. When bacterial infections are present, antibiotic treatment should be helpful.

Pneumonia, or more correctly pneumonitis, is a term used to describe any inflammatory change in the lungs. True asthma is non-inflammatory and is therefore not included. Pneumonia can be a response to chemical, mechanical or infectious challenge. Pneumonic changes in part of a lung are rarely diagnosed in the live bird, being found only at *post-mortem* examination. Many diseases called "pneumonia" by the public are more often a type of respiratory embarrassment due to oedema or water-logging of the lungs caused by circulatory disease or, in the case of budgerigars, due to thyroid enlargement. Pressure on the lungs by tumours, other abdominal masses, or lesions in the airsacs are other causes of respiratory distress. "Pneumonia," like "asthma," is therefore a much over-used term and frequently an inaccurate diagnosis.

Pneumonia

Important types of pneumonia are those caused by infections. Organisms which have been incriminated include various pus-forming germs such as *Streptococcus* and *Staphylococcus*. Sometimes the lungs are affected in septicaemias due to organisms such as *Pasteurella, Yersinia, Erysipelothrix, Salmonella* species and *Escherichia coli. Mycoplasma* or so-called pleuropneumonia-like organisms are occasionally involved. Sometimes, ornithosis (psittacosis) or a viral infection may be the original cause of the pneumonia.

The fungi *Aspergillus* and more rarely *Candida* cause lesions in the lungs as well as in the airsacs.

There is no ready means of detecting the causal organism in the live bird because swabs taken from the nostrils, mouth or droppings do not necessarily contain it, therefore treatment in most cases is a matter of trial and error.

The best course of action is to use a broad-spectrum antibiotic which has an effect on a wide range of bacteria. Tetracyclines are safe and most likely to be effective, but sometimes sulphadimidine may be useful. These drugs can be given by mouth if the respiration is not too difficult, or preferably by subcutaneous injection. If a fungous disease is suspected, a nystatin aerosol may be tried, or oral administration of potassium iodide. Response, however, is frequently poor. Affected birds should be isolated, and if a group is at risk by direct contact, the preventive or prophylactic dosing of all birds with an appropriate drug is strongly advised.

These changes are responses to a number of factors such as chills, poor circulation, pressure on the lungs or their blood supply, or obstruction to the flow of air to, from or within the

Congestion and Oedema of the Lungs

258

lungs. Congestion and oedema often lead to pneumonia and are therefore found in the early stages of airborne or septicaemic infections of the lungs. As with pneumonia, "congestion of the lungs" is another vague term used by bird keepers and applied to many differing types of respiratory distress. The cause, whether infectious or mechanical, may be very difficult to determine.

Treatment with antibacterial drugs should be given early since an infectious disease is the most likely cause and could rapidly be fatal if treatment is delayed.

Inflammation of the Airsacs or Airsacculitis

Several species of bacteria, fungi (especially *Aspergillus fumigatus*) and some mites are capable of producing exudates which cause the walls of the airsacs to adhere to each other. In some instances, masses of cheesy, yellowish material are formed. Visceral gout may also produce whitish deposits on the walls of the airsacs, but this cannot be diagnosed during life. Obstruction of the airflow by adhesion of the opposed walls of the airscas or by accumulation of exudates severely interferes with the mechanism of respiration. Although the bird may not appear to be very ill and may eat well and be lively, its breathing becomes heavy, its tail pumps noticeably up and down, it loses weight, and clicking sounds during breathing may be heard some distance away. After quite brief exercise, particularly flight, respiration becomes very distressed for a time and the heart rate greatly increased. Unless there is also a generalized infection present, the bird usually recovers within a few minutes. In the live bird the cause of airsacculitis is rarely ascertained. It is usually chronic, and respiratory trouble can exist for months or even years before causing death. If such an affected bird contracts pneumonia or an acute infection, it is of course serious and frequently fatal.

Treatment seldom has any effect on chronic airsac disease.

Pressure Factors as a Cause of Respiratory Signs

In species such as the budgerigar, mechanical causes are of considerable importance in the production of respiratory signs and they frequently originate in the body cavity. This is because there is no clear division between the thoracic and abdominal organs in birds, and any increase in size of an organ therefore produces pressure, not only on neighbouring organs but eventually on all the viscera. Causes include tumours or cysts of the ovary, testes, kidney, or liver; chronic congestion of the liver; retention of eggs or egg material in the oviduct; abdominal dropsy (ascites) and excessive deposition of abdominal fat or the accumulation of faeces in the gut, causing impaction. Very careful examination of the bird must be made if the cause is to be found and appropriate treatment carried out.

SELECTED BIBLIOGRAPHY

ARNALL, L. A. (1969). Diseases of the Respiratory System. In *Diseases of Cage and Aviary Birds,* p.263–289. Ed. Petrak, M. L., Philadelphia. Lea and Febiger.

THE URINARY SYSTEM

The kidneys of birds have the particular property of being able to deal with richly nitrogenous waste material and concentrate the watery fluid which filters through the renal glomeruli, so that the "urine" is semi-solid on excretion.

Specific infections of the kidney are uncommon, but bacteria are sometimes present, either as the result of a septicaemia or by direct spread from an adjacent diseased organ such as the intestine or reproductive tract.

Gout It may seem strange that birds are prone to this disease which is traditionally associated with the well-to-do of bygone days who were given to consuming inordinate quantities of venison and claret! Gout is due to failure to eliminate nitrogenous waste products from the bloodstream through the kidneys. As a result, insoluble material, mainly in the form of urates and related substances is deposited in certain areas of the body. In birds, an excessive appetite, especially for an unbalanced diet, combined with inactivity, are undoubtedly predisposing causes. Renal disease of different kinds including nephritis (inflammation of the kidneys) can produce gout.

Two types of gout occur in birds, named according to the distribution of the lesions: articular and visceral gout. They are most frequently seen in gallinaceous birds, budgerigars and waterfowl, to a lesser extent in parrots, and less frequently in pigeons and canaries. Sporadic cases or even outbreaks of gout can occur in many species.

In articular gout, which is much less common than the visceral form, urates are deposited around the joints, the tendons sheaths, tendons, ligaments and periosteum (Plate 1/15). Accumulations of these deposits produce cream-coloured, shiny swellings which bulge up through the overlying skin and subcutaneous tissues. The swellings seem to be intensely painful especially when the affected joint is touched or manipulated. The lesions may distort and cripple the limb. If a swelling is incised, the contents are found to be of a creamy, pasty or gritty consistency, according to the amount of fluid accompanying the urates. The creamy and pasty

261

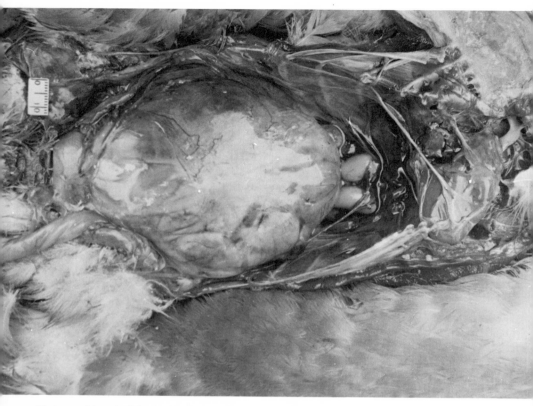

Male ruddy shelduck (*Tadorna ferruginea*) with grossly enlarged kidneys. The enlargement was caused by chronic inflammation (nephritis) and cyst formation, resulting in slow haemorrhage and the formation of blood clots. (I.F. Keymer and T.C. Dennett, Z.S.L.)

types may easily be mistaken for abscesses, though in fact they rarely take this form. In the early stages, gout is easily mistaken for a type of acute, infective arthritis.

Visceral gout is more insidious and lethal than the articular type, although probably less painful. The two types often coexist. In visceral gout (Plate 2/15) the deposits are to be found in almost any organ of the body cavity, but the liver, kidney, pericardium, heart and air sacs are most frequently affected. Beige, white, or occasionally, pale, yellowish deposits are seen on the peritoneal or serous surfaces of the organs. Sometimes the deposits infiltrate into the organs themselves and a few important diseases may be confused with this form of gout, such as aspergillosis or other infections affecting particularly the abdominal or thoracic air sacs. Egg peritonitis may give rise to similar lesions, but the deposits of yolk can more easily be scraped off the surfaces of the organs and they are more yellow in colour.

Gout has long been associated with overeating, especially of protein foods, but it also occurs as a result of malnutrition. The "Poor man's gout" of past ages was a scourge of people on the breadline who also drank a large amount of alcohol. In such cases there was doubtless a protein deficiency. Instead of an otherwise healthy liver and kidney overworked and damaged by excessive metabolism of rich food, these organs are striving to function by converting a low-protein, low-vitamin and high-carbohydrate diet into utilisable body substances, while their mechanisms are badly impaired by dietary deficiencies. This may explain why in birds, a low diet, even more than one high in protein may result in nephrosis (kidney disease) and gout. As an example the author can recall a female budgerigar kept by a schoolmistress for her children, which bred over 20 offspring in two seasons on a diet of only 80 per cent millet, 20 per cent canary seed, plus a little grit. At $2\frac{1}{2}$ years of age it was a lean but still lively bird, with large gouty swellings affecting both hocks and feet. The teacher, however, was very careful to follow instructions about diet, and the bird recovered in about six weeks. It remained clinically normal for at least a further two years, when it received treatment again for quite a different reason.

Treatment depends upon establishing whether the gout is due to overeating, a high-protein or low-protein diet, or if there is an amino acid or vitamin deficiency or imbalance in the diet. The fact that so few birds respond well to dietary adjustments is probably mainly due to the fact that the kidneys have become permanently damaged, and partly due to the inability of many people to persevere with a new diet for several weeks, when this at first is usually rejected by the bird leading to initial loss of weight. Having assessed the protein intake, it can be increased by adding egg, grubs or insects, or reduced by adding cereal products to the diet. At the same time, a mineral and vitamin supplement must also be given. A caged bird should be put into a flight or planted aviary if at all possible, because muscular activity stimulates the circulation and the thirst, both of which should help in the dispersal and excretion of urates. Water intake can also be increased by placing a pinch of salt in the drinking water. Green food and fresh fruit should also be given. With many species perseverance is necessary to ensure that the bird eats a satisfactory diet.

Renal Impactions

Birds have no urinary bladder, and urine is temporarily held in the cloaca. The flow of urine down the ureters is normally almost continuous. Sometimes, however, it may be interrupted; for example, when there is excessive water reabsorption in the kidneys, as may occur when drinking water is not available. The urine then becomes thickened or pasty and it is only slowly excreted. If it is witheld too long, irreparable damage occurs in the kidney, waste products build up in the bloodstream and rapidly poison the bird. When sudden deaths occur with little or no previous signs of illness, these accumulations of solid, pasty, urate material are often found in the kidney tubules or ureters. Normal urine in these structures is of a translucent watery consistency.

Nephritis and other types of renal disease

Kidney disease (nephrosis) including inflammation of the kidneys (nephritis) may be due to irritation of the glomeruli, tubules or ureters by infection or toxic substances, including over stimulation by certain drugs. These may be an alteration of the rate of filtration, reabsorption or ureteral flow of urine during its production. Increased blood flow to the kidneys increases the rate of filtration. According to the cause, this may be followed by increased or decreased reabsorption of water, salts, sugar and other useful commodities. The same causes may produce swelling of the lining membranes of the tubules and ureters, interfering with the absorption and flow of fluid respectively. At *post-mortem* examination especially following sudden death, these sort of lesions are quite frequently found, and are associated with congestion of the kidneys and with no other significant disorders. Whether the primary cause is due to a virus, a poison, allergy, chilling or shock can seldom be established, even after exhaustive laboratory tests which may take several weeks to perform.

"Pasting of the vent"

"Pasting of the vent" is a clinical sign which causes considerable concern among cage bird owners and is sometimes taken to be a specific disease. It is often a sequel to nephritis, some other type of renal disease, intestinal or generalized infection, and occurs mainly when the droppings are sloppier and more sticky or mucoid than normal. The tenacious droppings cling to the feathers around the vent and can even block it completely. If this occurs, both faeces and urine are held back, distending the cloaca inwardly and eventually causing visible distension of the abdomen. Intermingling of the two products can result in gut bacteria entering and infecting the urinary tract and in the female, also the oviduct. The so-called "paste" which may form into a hard, rounded mass (Plate 3/15) can either be faeces from the intestinal canal or urine from the kidneys, or a mixture of both. If the affected bird shows huddling, depression, weakness or abnormal breathing, the prognosis is extremely serious, these signs being strongly indicative of kidney involvement.

264

It is imperative, when attempting to diagnose the underlying trouble, to differentiate between the two fractions of the droppings. In seed eaters, normal faeces can vary in colour being black, brown, fawn, slate grey, khaki or green. In birds feeding on fruit, green food, insects, carrion or other foods, the colour range is even wider. Yellow, orange, light grey, red or bright green faeces can usually be regarded as abnormal, especially if watery or mucoid in nature. Consistency, however, also varies with the species and diet. The urinary fraction of the droppings which is normally a white to light yellow colour and almost solid in most birds, varies only moderately in consistency. A translucent greyish-white fluid is likely to be abnormal. Sudden changes of diet, water intake or environmental temperature can cause fairly marked but temporary changes in the colour and consistency of the urine. Care must be taken to learn the normal appearance for each species kept. Indian mynahs, for example, have watery faecal and fairly watery, urinary fractions in their droppings. Hummingbirds and sunbirds (unless also taking insect or other solid food) pass little faeces, the greater part of their droppings consisting of the urate fraction.

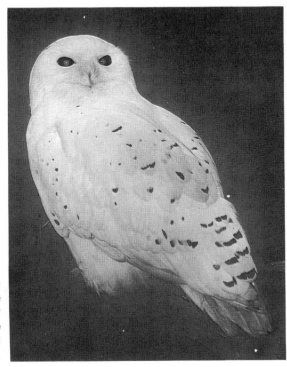

Snowy owl (*Nyctea scandiaca*). This handsome species breeds quite readily in captivity. Diseases of the kidneys are quite common in captive owls.

Treatment consists of first establishing which tract is primarily affected and if possible establishing a cause. In all cases, treatment involves clipping the feathers around the vent, washing away the caked mass with a 5 per cent solution of salt water and (under the direction of a veterinarian only), irrigation of the cloaca, rectum, or possibly the oviduct. The latter is performed by using a small funnel or syringe connected to a length of 20 to 50 cm. of bicycle valve rubber, or other soft, flexible tube of a diameter appropriate for the bird concerned. The bird should be held on its back and the free end of the tube lubricated with vaseline and gently inserted into the cloaca, after which a solution of 5 per cent saline, glycerine, liquid paraffin, or antibiotic solution as required, is slowly introduced. The liquid will percolate through the mass of blocked material, softening it and allowing it to be voided. If an infection is suspected then appropriate antibiotic or other treatment must be given.

SELECTED BIBLIOGRAPHY

HASHOLT, J. (1969). Diseases of the Urinary System. In *Diseases of Cage and Aviary Birds,* p.313–320. Ed. Petrak, M. L., Philadelphia. Lea and Febiger.

PECKHAM, M. C. (1965). Diseases affecting the kidneys. In *Diseases of Poultry,* p.1198–1201. Eds. Biester, H. E. and Schwarte, H. L. 5th Ed. Ames, Iowa. State University Press.

THE REPRODUCTIVE OR GENITAL SYSTEM

The Testes The testes show variations in size and structure, depending to some degree on the bird's maturity, the time of year and the opportunities for breeding. Inflammatory changes are uncommon except as part of a generalized infection or other disease. A shrivelling-up or atrophic degeneration of both testes occurs in starvation and after certain hormonal disorders. Only one testis may be affected under some circumstances. Tumour formation and damage by infection, such as a septicaemia, can inhibit sperm production and make the bird temporarily or permanently sterile, although this seldom occurs. Sterility is more likely to result from damage to the genital tract in certain deficiency diseases or hormonal imbalances.

The testes in budgerigars are one of the commonest sites for tumour formation, but other species are relatively little affected. Since the testis has two major functions, namely to produce sperms and to produce the hormones which create the sexual urge or libido, neoplastic lesions can seriously affect fertility. Most cases of sterility are, however, attributable to the female. Atrophy of both testes is occasionally seen, with total loss of sexual desire and secondary male sex characteristics such as plumage colour, and it is assumed that the pituitary or other endocrine dysfunction is responsible. Chronic orchitis or inflammation of the testes, seems to be quite rare in birds.

Attempts to tread other males, especially by young birds, can be assumed to be normal, especially if the assaulted male is small, dull-coloured, non-assertive or deformed in some way.

The Vasa Deferentia From the testis, sperms pass through the epididymis in which they mature and are prepared for fertilization and then into the vas deferens. The latter is rarely affected by disease except if its lumen is occluded by swelling from inflammatory changes or if it is involved in abdominal tumours, when only one vas deferens may be affected. The usual site for obstructions of these types is at the emergence of the ducts into the cloaca near the sexual papilla or rudimentary penis, inflammatory changes here usually being brought about through contamination by the faeces.

The age of sexual maturity may be reached in the off-season winter months, but it is only in the normal breeding season that the testes become fully functional. These seasonal changes depend on the length of daylight and for birds in the temperate climates this is usually the summer months.

Variation in Sexual Function

Some domesticated species such as the budgerigar, bred for generations in captivity, can mate and produce young in the winter months. This unnatural state of affairs, which is utilized by some breeders to take advantage of the higher prices commanded at this time of year, brings its attendant troubles. Weakly youngsters, French moult, and a high proportion of dead-in-the-shell chicks and deaths among nestlings are some of the penalties for this unwise practice. By supplying extra light or artificial daylight, to lengthen progressively the shortening winter days, it is possible to stimulate the pituitary gland and induce breeding out of season in several species of birds. This practice, however, should be considered an experimental exercise only; it is not advocated as a recommended method of avian husbandry.

Libido, the urge to court and mate, is a strictly seasonal affair with male birds of most species. In many species in the wild state courtship starts on almost exactly the same date each year, although a particularly cold period just before this time may cause some delay. In the case of captive, wild birds brought from other climates, it is not surprising that even in the most natural of planted aviaries breeding is often extremely difficult to achieve. Breeding a species successfully for the first time in captivity is an attainment of which to be proud, and a tribute to the breeder. In addition to luck and much patient observation and study of the habits and diet of the birds in captivity it is also necessary to apply knowledge based on the habits of the species in the wild. Many of the rarer species have of course not yet been bred, in spite of many attempts, and it may be wondered why this should be so. In the first place, the selected pair stubbornly refuse to mate and no sexual interest is shown. This may be because the birds are in a perpetual state of fear in their new surroundings and cannot escape beyond the wire netting from threatened danger. In many cases, the effects of unsatisfactory methods of transport when hundred of birds are crammed into boxes like sardines in a tin, must have a considerable and long term effect on some individuals. Incorrect

Sterility of the Male

diet, violent changes of temperature and humidity, and other privations increase susceptibility to infections and parasitic burdens, and may permanently impair health and fertility. Birds with the best chance of surviving to breed are those which are flown rapidly from source to ultimate destination, or those brought over by ship singly or in small numbers by an attentive bird-lover who acclimatizes the birds gently to human handling, a modified diet and to their new environment. The absence of this type of attention is probably the most important reason for loss of libido in the less-studied, delicate and rarer species. In species which have been bred for generations in this country such as budgerigars and the hardier species of parakeets, lovebirds, Java sparrows and pigeons, these factors are less important. In such species, although good health is still a major factor, free accessibility to daylight and exercise, an adequate food supply and freedom from persecution by other aviary birds and marauders, play an important part in successful breeding.

Sufficient space, lack of disturbance and a correct diet are the three most important inducements to breeding. Other causes of sterility are anatomical defects which prevent the production, maturation, passage or ejaculation of active living sperms. Orchitis, testicular degenerations, tumours, obstructions or alterations in the chemical constituents of the fluid portion of the ejaculate may be at fault. In poultry, ejaculation can be produced by electrical stimulation, but so far this technique has not been developed for the smaller cage birds; consequently an ejaculate cannot readily be obtained for microscopic or other examination. A practical means of determining fertility in a male which is seen to mate satisfactorily is to mate the cock with a series of females. If all hens lay infertile eggs then the male is likely to be sterile. Unfortunately this test is not possible with birds which pair with one hen for a season or for life.

Homosexuality In males, if mounting or being mounted by members of the same sex persists, it can be taken as pathological. Sometimes organic evidence of a cause is lacking, but usually one or both testes show neoplastic or other abnormal growth, including the production of ovarian tissue. Homosexuality is sometimes brought about by the administration of thyroid or oestrogenic hormone for the treatment of plumage disorders. When it occurs spontaneously, testosterone given by mouth in liquid form, or powdered thyroid gland, can be tried for two to three weeks. Little permanent effect usually results, since pathological changes in the testes, unlike physiological ones, are generally irreversible.

The female genital tract is an asymmetrical structure in almost all species, only the left of the two primitive gonads and ducts persisting. Inherent in this atrophy of the right and hypertrophy of the immature left ovary and oviduct is a tendency to certain metabolic or hormonal diseases, as will be seen later.

The ovary of a mature female is at first small and consists of numerous minute cysts or follicles which contain undeveloped ova or egg yolks. Between the follicles is the glandular tissue which produces oestrogenic hormones. At the approach of the breeding season, the glandular part develops and the follicles enlarge one after the other so that there is always one follicle approaching maturity and preparing to shed an ovum or yolk for passage down the oviduct.

The ovary
{: .right}

Some infections, such as salmonellosis, infect the ovary via the bloodstream so that the disease can in some cases pass into the fully developed egg and infect the embryo. This is one cause of dead-in-the-shell and weakly nestlings. In times of stress, excessive cold, food shortage or other forms of bad management, the ovary will not develop to the point of shedding yolks, even in the breeding season.

The ovary is sometimes the site of tumours (see Chapter 24).

The ovum is normally shed directly into the funnel-shaped opening of the oviduct which surrounds part of the ovary. Sometimes, however, the ova fall into the body cavity, from which there is no escape and no possibility of re-entering the oviduct. This may be due to two eggs entering the duct almost simultaneously resulting in one being returned and dropped into the abdominal cavity. At other times, spasm or obstructions of the oviduct may result in a partly formed egg being propelled back up the oviduct and into the body cavity. The displaced yolk or egg acts like a foreign body and irritates the peritoneal lining of the body cavity, eventually causing peritonitis (Plate 1/16).

Egg Peritonitis
{: .right}

The egg yolk, made up of a high proportion of protein, is slowly absorbed by the peritoneum. Once in the bloodstream this unaccustomed substance seems to produce a type of allergic reaction as it is now regarded by the body as a foreign protein. This is manifested by outward signs of illness, including depression. An outflow of inflammatory fluid or peritoneal exudate results in the abdominal cavity being filled with discoloured stringy exudate and remains of unabsorbed yolk material. The peritonitis may cause distension of the abdomen and result in respiratory distress. The peritoneal exudate is usually sterile, but if the yolk material becomes infected by bacteria such as *Escherichia coli*, the bird dies

270

rapidly. The peritoneal fluid may be yellow, cloudy grey, greenish, reddish-brown or black, according to the length of time that the peritonitis has been present.

In egg peritonitis gut action may be initially speeded up, causing diarrhoea, but later inactivity on the part of the gut produces little or no faecal droppings. In non-infected cases a bird with peritonitis can live days or even weeks in indifferent health, gradually losing weight, until eventually death occurs. In severe cases of abdominal distension caused by yolk material and exudates, rupture of the abdominal wall may occur. In such cases diagnosis can be difficult unless a small sample of abdominal contents can be obtained by puncturing or opening the abdomen in the midline. It is sometimes possible for a veterinarian to operate, flush and pick out all abnormal fluid and solid material, lubricate the abdominal organs with an antibiotic or saline solution and then suture the abdominal wall. Recurrence, however, may occur. If the bird is valuable and a non-breeder or pet, the oviduct and ovary can be surgically removed. No bird keeper should attempt such an operation himself, especially as even in the most skilled veterinary hands the recovery rate is poor. The alternative, however, is euthanasia or a slow death.

The Oviduct Although cage birds are not induced to lay daily like poultry, some species such as budgerigars or zebra finches are encouraged to lay, hatch and rear several clutches in each season, and this can be more than the hen's constitution can tolerate. Chilling caused by drafty or damp nesting quarters or poor nutrition may also affect the normal functioning of the oviduct. Spasm or cramp of the organ is one such result. The normal progress of the ovum down the oviduct, which is slow and intermittent, can be checked and even reversed at any stage of development. This may result in excessive amounts of albumen being deposited, and sometimes a double shell may be laid down. Such an abnormally large egg may be passed with difficulty or it may be impossible to pass. On occasion the egg can cause a rupture in the oviduct wall and then pass into the abdominal cavity. Another effect of spasm is for the developing egg to be halted in its passage down the oviduct long enough for water to be extracted from it, thus leaving a hard ball of egg material. Spasms with or without bacterial infection cause inflammation of the oviduct wall and result in thickening and increased production of mucus as well as albumen and calcium salts, thus leading to a total obstruction. In spite of these developments, ripe ova may continue to be produced by the ovary, enter the top of the oviduct and result in further impaction.

Atony or paralysis of the oviduct is another closely related

271

condition (Plate 2/16). When this occurs, a normal fully or partially developed egg may be held up in the oviduct owing to insufficient muscular activity for its expulsion.

Egg-binding is usually attributable to spasm or atony of the oviduct mentioned above. Excessively large, mis-shapen eggs are other causes, these being commonest at the beginning or the end of a laying period. In species kept in isolation as pets, especially budgerigars, an unmated hen may start to produce eggs, even sometimes late in life, and subsequently develop difficulty in laying which leads to egg-binding. Although the absence of a place suitable to lay may be a contributory factor, the cause of egg-binding in older birds is probably lack of tone in the muscles of the oviduct and abdominal wall rather than muscular spasm. Exhaustion due to over-breeding and out-of-season breeding is an important point in aviary birds. Dietary deficiences are probably only of importance in so far as they affect general health and condition: Obesity for example, is very important in this connection. Severe deficiencies are much more liable to result in failure to ovulate or failure of the ovum to develop fully into an egg, than to cause egg-binding.

Egg-binding

Inflammation of the oviduct—salpingitis—is generally accepted as a common cause of egg-binding and associated defects in the process of egg production.

Chilling disturbances, especially in the night while roosting, or damp nesting quarters, all tend to cause egg-binding. Although muscular contractions occur, they are not smooth and co-ordinated and a constriction develops in front and behind the egg. This results in straining and exhaustion, and sometimes prolapse of the cloaca or even the lower part of the oviduct. (Plate 3/16).

Time honoured remedies consist of holding the bird over a jug of steaming water and anointing the hind quarters with olive oil or liquid paraffin. Although this treatment is claimed to be successful by some breeders, in the author's experience more than half of the birds treated in this way, fail to produce an egg. The handling and further delay merely weakens the bird. Any muscular spasm present is liable to be prolonged or increased by the handling and steam. The sticky oil on the feathers reduces their insulating powers and makes the bird more prone to chilling and infection. Manual manipulation is the only method of treatment likely to be successful (see Chapter 28).

Sometimes a cystic distension of the oviduct occurs. This causes general malaise, the inability to lay eggs and a gradual soft enlargement of the abdomen. If the abdominal wall

Cystic Oviducts

272

is cut an enlarged oviduct is noticed. The enlargement may occur throughout its length or be only a localized swelling, which is sometimes like a pouch on one side of the duct. The oviduct is usually a creamy colour covered by a few small blood vessels. Occasionally it is grey in colour and the swelling more angular, with clear watery contents containing solid, cheesy masses or particles. Both types probably represent a chronic inflammatory process with outpouring of mucus and abnormal albumen which contains broken-down yolk material. Bacteria are seldom found in this material. Bulges in the oviduct wall probably indicate where an egg or yolk had previously been retained. No medical or surgical treatment can restore normal function to oviducts affected in this way.

Clinical signs may be vague. Straining does not necessarily mean that there is some form of obstruction. It is important not to confuse egg-binding and dilated oviducts with other causes of abdominal distension. However, to decide whether the genital or alimentary tracts are affected or if a tumour is present in the abdominal cavity can be very difficult.

Egg Abnormalities

Double-yolked eggs may be the result of two simultaneous ovulations, or the division of one completed ovum in the ovary or oviduct. The frequent laying of double-yolked eggs, however, suggests that there is often irregular passage of an ovum down the oviduct resulting in it being caught up by a succeeding yolk so that the two become enclosed in one membrane and shell. Not all abnormally large eggs are double-yolked. The extra bulk may be due to albumen which was added while a normal yolk was retained for an unusually long period in the area of the oviduct where albumen is laid down. This may happen when there is a mild inflammation present. Extra large yolks are only occasionally found and their significance is uncertain.

Small yolkless eggs are sterile. They do not usually cause any trouble and may be considered normal if passed occasionally at the beginning or end of a laying period. If they are produced frequently, they may indicate an inflamed oviduct; aberrant yolks shed into the peritoneal cavity; chronic, infectious condition of the ovary, or in aged birds a fibrous, cancerous or degenerative ovary.

Soft or shell-less eggs are most likely to result from calcium deficiency as the result of providing inadequate amounts of soluble grit. Even with adequate grit, however, overbreeding or the end of a normal season may be heralded by one or two unshelled or otherwise defective eggs. If a series of such eggs is passed, inflammatory changes may be suspected, affecting the shell-secreting glands of the oviduct and resulting in inhibited secretion. Conversely, although secretion may be

273

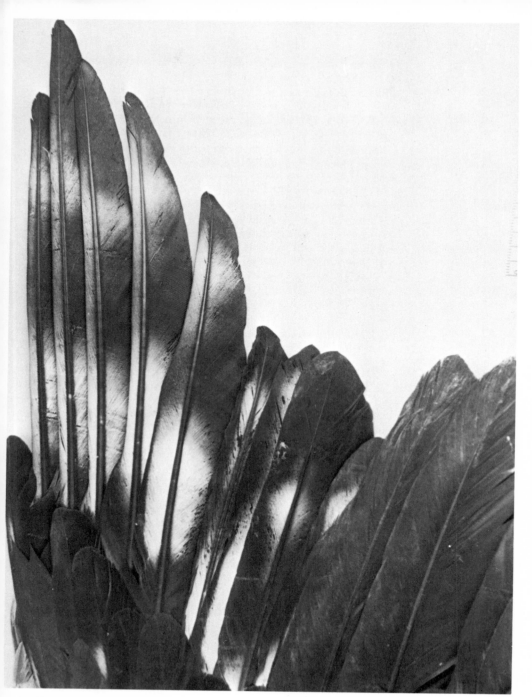

Bateleur eagle (*Terathopius ecaudatus*). Depigmentation of primary and some secondary wing feathers. Cause unknown, but possibly due to a deficiency of vitamins such as pantothenic acid: see Chapters 2, 3 and 23. (I.F. Keymer and T.C. Dennett, Z.S.L.)

normal, the egg may be passed through the oviduct too quickly for sufficient shell to be deposited. A soft-shelled egg remaining in the lower part of the oviduct does not appear to initiate the normal reflexes and the egg may therefore be deposited anywhere or even retained.

Eggs stained by blood and excreta are often of no significance. Excreta on the shell may indicate a mild urinary or alimentary upset or merely a poor state of hygiene in the nest. The contaminated eggs should be gently washed and dabbed dry with absorbent cotton wool. Excessive rubbing to remove stains should be avoided because it damages the pores and may even result in bacteria entering and infecting the egg. The usual cause of blood-stained eggs is a small tear of the cloacal mucosa or rupture of a minute blood vessel, perhaps as the result of passing an abnormally large egg. No treatment is possible and usually only one or two eggs are affected in this way.

Broken eggs may occur because the shells are too thin or they may be the result of accidents, such as a fright from a cat or other marauders while the hen is on the nest. Rodents or snakes may be responsible for broken eggs in outdoor aviaries, ground-nesting birds being commonly affected.

Soft-shelled or normal eggs laid accidentally on the floor can become a focus of curiosity for other birds, resulting in egg pecking, breakage and eventually egg-eating. It is uncommon for cage birds to eat their own eggs intentionally, but sometimes this may arise and the action becomes a vice.

Egg-eaters and careless egg-layers are best isolated lest the bad habits are copied by others. Special attention should be paid to diet. Freedom from boredom is also important. Attempted control of the habit in individuals by using such methods as de-beaking or fitting opaque "spectacles" as used in poultry, are not practicable for cage birds.

Sterility of the Female
An obvious cause of failure to breed is disinclination to accept the male. Early stages of courtship may be tolerated or even encouraged, but "treading" is strongly resisted. With newly imported or nervous species this may be partly due (as in the cock) to unsatisfactory surroundings and can sometimes be overcome with time and by keeping the birds in a spacious and natural aviary away from disturbance. Hormonal deficiencies or imbalances can also cause loss of libido. Alternatively, neoplasms involving the ovary, especially in budgerigars, can have a similar effect and can also produce homosexual tendencies.

Other Causes of Sterility
These include various inflammatory conditions of the oviduct, obstructions by degenerate egg material, and torsion or

twisting of the oviduct, especially in association with rupture of the abdominal wall. Any illness of sufficient severity will inhibit ovulation, this being more sensitive to such conditions than is the production of sperms in the male.

The interplay of birds' pituitary, thyroid, adrenocortical and gonadal hormones is extremely complex and imbalances are common. However, in budgerigars the changes in the colour of the cere do not necessarily reflect gonadal changes: they may merely relate to an altered state of health.

Sex reversal

Intersexes are rare. These birds are intermediate in appearance between male and female and usually show no sexual interest in other birds. A few show bisexual behaviour patterns, but all are sterile. Anatomically, the gonads may be undeveloped or contain both testicular and ovarian tissue.

True complete sex reversal occurs more frequently in the female than in the male. If the functional left ovary is destroyed by disease or surgically removed, the rudimentary right ovary may enlarge, but instead of becoming a normal ovary it develops testicular tissue, so that the hen gradually changes sex. It develops male plumage and in rare cases may even fertilize another hen. Sex reversal in the cock, with a change to female colouration, posture, fat distribution and behaviour is less common.

Medical treatment using hormones seldom has any permanent effect.

SELECTED BIBLIOGRAPHY

BLACKMORE, D. K. (1969). Diseases of the Reproductive System. In *Diseases of Cage and Aviary Birds,* p.321–329. Ed. Petrak, M. L., Philadelphia. Lea and Febiger.

HASHOLT, J. (1966). *Diseases of the female reproductive organs of pet birds.* J. Small Anim. Pract. 7, 313–320.

PECKHAM, M. C. (1965). Reproductive Disorders. In *Diseases of Poultry.* p.1201–1205. Eds. Biester, H. E. and Schwarte. H. L. 5th Ed. Ames, Iowa. State University Press.

THE CIRCULATORY SYSTEM

The diseases of this system of the body are usually only correctly diagnosed at *post-mortem* examination. The names given to a large number of diseases diagnosed purely on the clinical signs during life often represent in fact various disorders of the cardiovascular system. Examples include so-called pneumonia, cramps, enteritis, paralysis, fainting, vertigo, various suspected nervous disorders and sudden death.

The circulation of the blood has several important functions, which briefly are the supply of soluble food substances and oxygen, the removal of waste materials and gases and the transport of water, heat, hormones, antibodies and other necessities of life (see Chapter 2). Failure of that transport system, even when only partial or temporary, affects the body in several ways and in varying severity. All tissues and cells are dependent upon blood supply, but especially the more active, specialized cells. The brain is temporarily damaged in a matter of seconds and permanently affected in a minute or two, by any failure of the blood to bring it oxygen and remove carbon dioxide. Glandular tissue takes somewhat longer to be permanently damaged; the gut, lungs and muscles even longer; while skin, bone, the cornea of the eye, and ligaments and tendons are among the most resistant tissues. Developing feathers and skin will even continue to live some hours after heart failure, while muscles will twitch for several minutes in a dead bird.

When the heart ceases to beat, or severe loss of blood so lowers the blood pressure that the brain is deprived of blood, death of brain tissue and of the entire bird soon follows. In severe shock as the result of injury, fright, adrenal gland failure or exudation from severe burns, the blood pressure is lowered, partly and possibly by damage to the heart from toxic substances liberated from injured tissues, but mainly due to the reduction of blood volume which occurs. Under these circumstances the amount of oxygenated blood reaching the nerve cells is insufficient for their survival. Fainting or loss of consciousness then occurs, often leading to death. Short of this, the lowered arterial and the raised venous blood pressures lead to a failure of tissue fluid to be drained from the lungs and oedema or water-logging results. This oedema and subsequent congestion hamper the gaseous exchanges in the lungs, and again the oxygen supply to the brain falls off, preceded by panting and so-called asthmatic breathing. Infection and exudates in the lung and air sacs have a similar effect on the oxygen supply to the tissues.

Birds most likely to suffer from circulatory troubles are those which are inactive, nervous, obese, aged or inadequately fed. Inactive and fat birds store up fat, cholesterol and waste metabolites in their bodies. When only the normal fat depots aie utilized this is a relatively harmless process, but when excessive fat and cholesterol begins to be deposited elsewhere, such as in the heart, liver and kidneys it impairs their functions. When deposited in the layers lining the blood vessels themselves it leads to constriction of the lumen and the heart begins to show signs of strain. At first the heart enlarges and then its walls thicken in an attempt to make up for the additional work. The extra work, however, begins to have an adverse effect on the heart muscles, unless the obesity is corrected. The cardiac muscles stretch further in an attempt to contract more forcibly and therefore gradually become thin and weaker. The stretching also damages specialised cells in the heart muscle and the rhythm of the heart's beat is deranged. It is obvious that such a chain of events leads to a very inefficient circulation.

Outward signs of illness due to a failing circulation do not always show in the same order and include lack of energy, difficult or rapid breathing, unusual nervousness, fainting and many other signs of damage to nerve tissue. These signs will often continue in varying degrees of severity until death results. In other cases, especially where certain organs have already been left slightly damaged by a previous illness, digestive disorders such as a reduced appetite, vomiting and diarrhoea or toxemia from kidney failure may be the factors leading to eventual heart failure.

Just as the efficient transport of food, gases and waste products is hampered, so are the defence mechanisms of the bird. The production and maintenance of leucocytes and antibodies in this state of lowered vitality is severely hindered at a time when it is most needed. Microrganisms in the air pass into the congested and oedematous lungs during breathing and find this type of environment admirable for multiplication in the absence of efficient defences. The lungs are relatively susceptible to disease even in healthy birds, but in those with a poor circulation they are often the first organs to become infected.

Enlargement or Hypertrophy of the heart

In response to increased demands from the body the heart will become enlarged. An energetic bird will have a proportionately larger heart than a more sluggish one. Free flight in a large aviary permits better development of the heart muscle than confinement in a small cage. Sudden and violent bouts of energy in a caged bird—provoked perhaps by the entry of marauders—are liable to cause stretching of the heart muscle without any compensatory thickening. A fatty heart is more likely to dilate than a normal one. An enlarged and thick-walled heart is a powerful one. A stretched heart is weak and tends to beat more quickly and in a disorganized manner. In a large bird this can sometimes be detected by listening carefully with a stethoscope, when fluttering faint tapping sounds can be heard. At other times the heart sounds are unusually loud and sloppy, resembling a noise such as a small polythene bag being suddenly blown up and collapsed several times a second. Considerable experience, however, is necessary in order to recognize the significance of heart sounds.

Rupture of the Heart

This is occasionally found at necropsy, it usually being an auricle which ruptures, because during excessive dilation of the heart, the valves separating the auricles and ventricles cannot close properly, so that on ventricular contraction the backflow of blood is forced at high pressure into the thin-walled auricles. When inefficient valves are combined with degenerative disease such as atheroma affecting the large arteries (see below), it may be the vessels which rupture rather than the auricles. Disease of organs which require rich supplies of blood such as the liver or kidneys, may result in hardening or obstruction of the arteries due to back pressure of the blood and therefore impaired nutrition of the vessel walls themselves. In order to supply these demanding organs, the heart has to step up its output, again resulting in dilation which may lead to rupture.

Arteriosclerosis, Atherosclerosis, Calcification and Other Diseases of Blood Vessels

Arteriosclerosis is the name given to any thickening, hardening or calcification of the arteries. Atherosclerosis (Plate 1/17) is the deposition of fat, compound carbohydrates, blood and blood products, calcium and fibrous tissue in the walls of the arteries and is a form of arteriosclerosis. The damaged lining of the arterial wall encourages various constituents of the blood to cling to it and form a thrombus or clot. When such lesions are widespread, the inelastic wall of fibrous tissue developed in the arterial wall interferes with the normal flow of blood, and the consequent poor blood supply to the damaged vessels, leads to further degenerations.

Arteriosclerosis has been reported most often in birds from zoological gardens, especially in members of the parrot family and birds of prey which live to a great age in captivity.

Calcification of areas in the heart muscle, large arteries and certain soft tissues may be a feature of endocrine, kidney, or dietary disturbance as well as senility. It is often advanced before any obvious signs of illness appear and is rarely a major contributory cause of death. It is commonest in aged parrots.

Thrombosis, as stated, can develop as the result of an atheromatous area in an artery. It is more common, however, following a crushing type of injury, or in severe generalized and localized infectious diseases. When a thrombus is dislodged and moves into the blood's circulation, it eventually reaches a vessel through which it is too small to pass. There it stops, completely blocking the vessel: this blockage is known as an embolus. If no other branch of the arterial tree provides an alternative supply of blood, the tissues beyond the clot become damaged and die. Vital organs like the brain, liver and endocrine glands have two or more supplies, but nevertheless tissue degenerations, and even death are still possible if embolism occurs in these organs. A blood clot formed in an infected crushed foot, for example, may end up as an embolism in the lung, or even in an area so distant from the injury as the brain, with disastrous results.

Degenerations of the heart and blood vessels, although quite common in cage-bred and captive wild birds, are rarely diagnosed until the affected bird is approaching circulatory collapse. Indeed the end may follow quite mild exertion in an apparently normal bird. There are no effective treatments once these diseases are established, but they can be prevented to a large extent by always providing space for plenty of exercise, at least until old age approaches.

Embarrassment of the blood circulation

This is seldom due to a disease of the circulatory system, but is usually the result of disease in organs surrounding the heart or large blood vessels. The commonest cause is pressure from tumours or exudates, which prevents adequate filling of the heart or hinders its action by obstructing the outflow into blood vessels. Pressure in the body cavity, as produced by dropsy or by diffuse fat deposits, is tolerated better by the circulation than by the lungs. When such fluid or tumour formation is suddenly removed during an operation, the abrupt lowering of pressure in the abdomen allows the veins to fill more fully. But since the total volume of blood in the circulation, can only be increased by slow absorption of fluid from the tissues, this results in inadequate blood return to the heart and sometimes heart failure, thus accounting for the relatively poor survival from such operations. Tumours of the ovary and testes which cause only localized pressure can be removed more safely as their removal immediately allows improvement of the circulation. Fluid in the pericardial sac occurs in several infectious diseases and debilitated states and seriously hampers the inflow and outflow of the blood to the heart.

Apoplexy must be mentioned here since the cause lies in the circulation. Clinically it can be defined as sudden loss of sensation and motion, generally as the result of haemorrhage or thrombosis in the brain. Sudden congestion, thrombosis, or haemorrhage into a part of the body may result from an injury causing violent increase in local blood pressure; in generalized rise of blood pressure (for example as the result of panicky efforts to escape); injury; degenerations in the blood vessel walls or because of some abnormal effect of nerves on blood vessels in various organs. Signs associated with apoplexy almost always include loss of consciousness, derangement of bodily movements, general circulatory collapse, and often death, either immediately or after a recovery lasting anything from minutes to days.

Generally, treatment is of no avail because the site and nature of the lesion can seldom and only approximately be determined. Complete rest is essential in a darkened box or cage with all obstructions removed to lessen the likelihood of further damage. An equable temperature is important and vitamin, mineral, dextrose and soluble protein dissolved in the drinking water should be readily available. Handling, especially for the administration of medicaments or alcoholic stimulants such as brandy, should be avoided at all costs.

Dropsy or ascites are the names given to the collection of watery fluids in the peritoneal cavity which results from poor draining of the liquid released from the arterial capillaries of the abdominal tissues. Ascites is usually associated with kidney disease or abdominal tumours, cysts, or diseases of the reproductive system which cause pressure on the veins draining blood back to the heart. More rarely, it results directly from a general failing circulation of one of the types already discussed. It is thus a sign of a disease process, and since all its causes are serious, they should be found and if possible treated, whereupon the ascites may disappear.

Varicose veins, although well known in humans, are rarely encountered in animals. They are occasionally seen, however, in canaries (Plate 11/11). The cause is not always obvious, but in some cases it is probably due to injury or traumatic hindrance of the return flow of the blood at a point in advance of the affected area.

There is a great deal of overlapping of clinical signs in the various disorders of the cardiovascular system. Activity tends to decrease as the degenerative processes develop, and this may be incorrectly attributed to increasing age or even be unnoticed. In a few cases nervous activity increases, the bird becoming agitated, panicky and prone to bursts of flight, self-pecking or other unprovoked activity. The body weight in such cases usually falls rapidly. A temporarily increased rate of breathing sometimes occurs. The bird may fall off the perch at night while roosting or have bouts of fainting at varying frequencies. Leg or wing weaknesses, incoordination of leg, wing, head or other movements, crossing or trailing one or both wings, flaccid or spastic partial paralysis of the feet or entire legs may all be noted. Teetering on the feet, falling forwards onto the beak, throwing back the head and somersaulting are all late signs. Shivering, intermittent fluffing of feathers, temporary or permanent blindness and deafness are other signs which may appear. Most of these are evidence of nerve-cell damage in the brain or spinal cord, generally due to lack of oxygen from deficient blood supply or occasionally due to actual pressure on nervous tissue.

Prevention depends entirely upon maintaining correct standards of management and especially nutrition; ironically, however, many disorders of the cardiovascular system develop only in birds which have been well cared for and have therefore lived to an advanced age. Most free-living birds die young owing to the numerous hazards which they encounter in the wild, so that degenerative diseases are rarely seen, particularly of the cardiovascular system.

By the time most of the above-mentioned signs appear it is usually too late for any treatment to have effect.

Diseases of the Spleen

There are no diseases which are specific to the spleen, although it often shows lesions in such generalized diseases as tuberculosis, pseudotuberculosis, salmonellosis, pasteurellosis, ornithosis, lymphoid leucosis and some blood protozoan infections.

In pigeons, rupture of the spleen due to ornithosis occasionally occurs, leading to sudden death.

The spleen is not infrequently a site of tumour growth; this, however, is usually secondary, the primary focus being in another organ.

SELECTED BIBLIOGRAPHY

FIENNES, R. N. T-W., (1969). Diseases of the Cardiovascular System, Blood and Lymphatic System. In *Diseases of Cage and Aviary Birds,* p.291–302. Ed. Petrak, M. L., Philadelphia. Lea and Febiger.

PECKHAM, M. C. (1965). Diseases of the circulatory system. In *Diseases of Poultry,* p.1190–1198. Eds. Biester, H. E. and Schwarte, H. L. 5th Ed. Ames, Iowa. State University Press.

THE NERVOUS SYSTEM

A distinction must be drawn between diseases specifically affecting the nervous system, and those which affect the whole metabolism, and produce nervous signs.

Clinical Signs   Nervous signs indicating involvement of the functions of the nerve tissue, are extremely common in cage and aviary birds. At times they are so spectacular as to obscure the real reason for their appearance; the important lesions may often be in organs remote from the main centres of the nerves. Signs of nerve involvement can be divided into three main groups; those where normal function is lost or impaired, *e.g.,* paralysis, blindness; those where activity is increased, such as excitement and twitching; and those where function is obviously deranged or abnormal, such as convulsions, throwing back the head, and asymmetrical leg or wing movements. The paradox of such a grouping is that all three types can be outward manifestations of the same disorder.

The causes of nervous clinical signs can be listed as follows:
1. Pressure on the brain, spinal cord or a nerve—for example, by a tumour, inflamed tissue, blood clot or depressed fracture.
2. Inflammation or destruction of a portion of nerve tissue resulting from injury, infection or poison.
3. The loss of full nerve function involving brain and/or spinal cord and nerves. This can result from circulatory or respiratory disorders resulting in a lack of the oxygen vital to the health of nerve tissue, or from infectious diseases which cause a high body temperature or pyrexia and thus interfere with brain metabolism.
4. Abnormal development or functioning of nerve tissue due to a deficiency of vitamins or other nutriments.
5. Pain which causes reluctance to use a part of the body such as a limb or the neck, and is manifested as a type of paralysis.
6. Scarring or fibrosis and contraction around nerve tissue, resulting in the stretching or strangulating of a nerve.
7. Immobilization of a joint by fibrous tissue or bone proliferation, leading to degeneration of muscle then nerves, and finally nerve atrophy.

283

8. Abnormal levels of calcium or magnesium due to disorders of the parathyroid glands producing twitchings, or coma and death. Other endocrine disorders may also be involved, but are mostly unproven: thyroid deficiencies and excess have been shown to cause changes in nervous, as well as chemical activity.

Nervous signs can be divided into generalized (Plate 1/18) and local (*e.g.*, Plate 4/18); this is a practical approach, but by no means always a reliable distinction. When a leg is partially or completely paralyzed the cause generally lies somewhere between the spinal cord and the affected part. Convulsions and incoordination (Plate 2/18 and 3/18), however, are generalized signs and suggest brain involvement, although paralysis may also be produced by quite a small lesion in the brain or brain stem.

This type of paralysis includes that of the toes and foot; "sliptoe"; clenched feet; "cage paralysis" and flaccid and spastic paralysis or paresis of the whole or part of a leg. **Paralysis of the Legs and Feet**

A painstaking examination is necessary, not only of the limb but also of the entire bird, before the causes of most of these clinical signs can be elucidated. On many occasions the cause cannot be found during life, and even a detailed necropsy using laboratory aids seldom provides the reason for the symptoms. Nevertheless these disorders are extremely common in cage birds.

Firstly, such external factors as cold, draughty or wet quarters, predisposing chills or inflammation of nerves, muscles or joints (neuritis, myositis or arthritis) must be ruled out. A viral infection, such as Newcastle disease or Marek's disease, or a dietary imbalance may sometimes be implicated. It must be realized that quite often a diet which contains the bare minimum of vitamins or amino acids, just adequate for the growth of young stock, can be made deficient in vitamins by adding a high protein food supplement. Conversely, adding high-energy foods such as oil-rich seeds, can adversely affect the enzyme systems of the body and increase the deficit of amino acids and vitamins in the diet. Some of these induced deficiencies may be recognizable in chicks and growing stock; but they are also believed to occur in adults, although little critical experimental work has been carried out on mature birds. Deficiencies are most likely to appear in growing chicks, breeding females and ailing or ageing birds.

Specific lesions involving the spinal cord or nerves to the legs are difficult to pinpoint unless they are very large, and therefore they can usually only be suspected on circumstantial evidence. They include tumours of these structures (rare even in budgerigars); bony protuberances of the vertebrae which pinch the spinal cord, sciatic or other large nerves as they emerge from the spaces between the vertebrae; Marek's disease; injury; local infections and other inflammations of the nerve trunks or spinal cord.

In addition, there are conditions which appear at first sight to be paralysis of some kind, when in fact the lameness is due to interference with the functioning of bones, muscles, joints, ligaments or tendons. In this category can be included fractures, bony or other growths involving the muscles or the tendons passing over bones or joints, arthritis, sprains, perosis, cut or torn tendons or muscles, scar contractions, "bumble foot" and severe "scaly leg".

In order to try and diagnose these disorders it is necessary to examine the posture, general health and mode of walking and flying. The hand should also be passed gently over the entire bird, particularly the loins and hip region. In the case of so-called "cage paralysis", "clubbed foot" (Plate 4/18) and "sliptoe", which are sometimes different degrees of the same processes, nothing may be found by such examinations. The next step is to supply a vitamin supplement, either as an elixir or preferably by injection. It should contain riboflavin, nicotinic acid, thiamine, biotin, choline, vitamin B_{12}, vitamin E and the amino acids, lysine, cysteine and methionine. If the cause of the paralysis is a dietary deficiency or imbalance, the bird will generally recover in from one to three weeks or sometimes in a few days after such treatment.

If in spite of combined medical treatment and supporting dressings the use of the limb does not return, it is likely that the paralysis has not only worsened, but that there is a spinal swelling or other deformity present, such as a tumour or bony masses (exostoses), causing pressure. With disuse, muscles will atrophy and they may even be partly replaced by scar tissue, so that the tendons will contract causing the limb to hang in a flexed position. A useful indication of true nerve involvement is when only one group of muscles, such as the flexors or the extensors of the knee, hock or toe joints is affected. Usually the muscles supplied by the damaged nerves are soft and flaccid, but sometimes they are tense, contracted fully or spastic. In complete, flaccid paralysis (Plate 5/18) the leg will stay more or less in whatever position it is placed. In the spastic type (Plate 4/18), on bending or flexing the joint or limb and releasing it, the leg springs back to the straight or extended position. With a knowledge of anatomy of the nervous system, it is possible to determine which bundles of spinal nerves are involved and sometimes pinpoint the trouble. Unfortunately however, this does not indicate the type of treatment required, although it does tend to limit the cause to a local lesion rather than a dietary deficiency or other generalized disorder.

Paralysis of both legs (Plate 5/18) is serious, since birds are unable to take off without the use of their legs. However, unless the condition also involves the wings, a bird with paralyzed legs can fly quite strongly once launched.

Paralysis of the Wings

The procedure for diagnosing the causes of paralysis of the wings is similar to that for the legs, but wing paralysis is much less common. Frequently one wing tip or wrist joint is seen to be held higher than the other, and the wing tips are often crossed. When the bird is held by its legs in an upright position and lowered sharply, the weaker wing spreads less fully and may beat at a slower rate than the normal wing. This may be due to nervous incoordination (Plates 2/18 and 3/18) or ataxia of the wing, but it may also be because of muscle injury, pain, fracture, sprain or dislocation of the shoulder or elbow joints, bone tumours or arthritis. Paralysis or weakness of both wings, strongly denotes a spinal or hind-brain lesion, or occasionally viral infections such as Newcastle and Marek's diseases. Damage to one side only of the brain or spinal cord, will produce effects in only one wing. Most unilateral wing disabilities are due to lesions of the wing, and in budgerigars the various types of tumour associated with the elbow region come high on the list. In most other species, bone and joint injuries are the commonest causes.

In true paralysis involving some nerve tissue damage, medical treatment is generally useless. Provided the limb is rested, injuries will often heal without treatment. Tumours involving the brain or spinal cord are untreatable. When the brain lesion is a haemorrhage from cranial damage, or a disorder of the cardiovascular system, some arrest of the process may be possible through changes in diet, exercise or management. Usually, however, it is only a matter of time before the trouble is seen to be incurable and sudden death may follow at any time after the onset of signs. If breeding stock is involved, it is probably best to destroy affected birds unless the cause is dietary.

Paralysis of the Neck

This is relatively uncommon in birds. The so-called "limber-neck" of chickens and waterfowl due to botulism, and the type of neck paralysis seen in turkeys due to deficiency of folic acid are rarely if ever met with in cage and aviary birds. Most cases are due to severe injury to the head or neck; concussion or hind-brain damage, general weakness or brain tumours. When brain tumours are present, however, twisting or torticollis (Plates 6/18 and 7/18), "star-gazing" (Plate 8/18) or other grotesque attitudes are more common than a lowering of the head. Generally treatment is useless.

286

Tremors, Shivering and Twitching

These signs may indicate a highly nervous temperament, chilling, low blood magnesium as the result of parathyroid disease, other metabolic disorders or deficiencies in the diet. They may also occur in the early stages of infectious diseases; as the result of heat stroke, certain poisonings, particularly by insecticides containing phosphorus; carbolic acid poisoning, overdoses of some drugs and also when there is loss of body fluids caused by haemorrhage, exudations, diarrhoea or vomiting.

In order to ascertain the possible cause of these signs it is necessary to investigate all aspects of management, especially in relation to other birds kept on the same diet or with the sufferer. When there is a flock problem which has arisen over a short period, poisoning or dietary deficiencies such as calcium and/or magnesium, should be suspected.

Slow rhythmic twitches of a part of the body, such as a wing (Plate 9/18) are rare, but occasionally met with in parrots and budgerigars. The cause is unknown and treatment usually ineffective, although vitamin supplements and sedatives will sometimes produce some relief from the violent twitchings.

Fits, Convulsions and "Epilepsy"

Convulsions of various types are quite common in cage birds and are sometimes a prelude to death. Birds may have short-lived but recurrent attacks, which subside after a week or two but recur months later. Some birds completely recover either with or without treatment. Usually, however, the convulsions become progressively more severe or frequent and the bird eventually dies.

Epilepsy, or epilepsy-like convulsions are named after the well known but still incompletely understood disease of human beings. In cage birds only some of the characteristics of epilepsy occur. The bird may be sitting quietly on its perch when it suddenly cocks its head as if looking or listening for something: the eyes remain open and the muscles become rigid. This is followed by rapid vibration of the wings, these being raised a little from the body. In some cases the feathers are erected, the whole body becomes involved in the violent movements, the legs stretch out and the bird thrown off its perch, to lie unconscious and still convulsing. After several seconds the vibrations lessen, the wings slowly return to the closed position, the bird moves its head, and then struggles with difficulty to its feet. It usually sits on its breast somewhat dazed for a matter of hours before returning to its former activity and alertness. Additional signs which are sometimes seen, include throwing back of the head (so-called "star-gazing"), deviation of the tail sharply upward or to one side, a croaking sound as if the thoracic muscles are forcing air out of the partially closed throat and temporary paralysis. Involuntary excretion of faeces or urine is uncommon; the salivation which occurs in man is unknown in avian "epilepsy".

Fits or convulsions of this kind can be caused in several ways. In young stock, deficiencies of riboflavin, thiamine, nicotinic acid, other vitamins and amino acids may be responsible. In older birds, hormonal imbalances may be at least contributory causes, or more rarely, tumours or other lesions of the pituitary gland. When birds of all ages and especially several species are affected, toxic seed dressings such as organophosphorus pesticide poisoning should be suspected. If a more limited number of birds appear sick and die after a series of convulsions, then an acute bacterial infection may be suspected. Toxaemia from massive liver or kidney destruction—whether by infectious, metabolic or poisonous agents—is also a relatively frequent cause of convulsions prior to death. In the isolated bird, fed on a reasonably satisfactory diet, changes in the circulation, or more probably brain disorders resulting from an inefficient blood supply to the brain, are more likely causes. Inactive, middle-aged and obese birds, especially if pampered and fed on unnatural tit-bits, are most prone to convulsions. Even moderate exertion, such as a panicky flight around the cage brought about by the presence of a cat or strangers, may be sufficient to start a series of fits. Sometimes, however, they start spontaneously or when the bird is handled and can be immediately fatal. The cause may be oxygen starvation to the brain or even rupture of its blood vessels due to a sudden increase of blood pressure.

Convulsions may result from poor nutrition, poor oxygenation or local pressure on nerve cells. It is probable that, in addition to a weakened heart or blood vessel walls due to fatty infiltration, the adrenal cortical tissues of affected birds are incapable of adequate hormone production.

Convulsions and other evidence of brain or nerve damage may sometimes be due to concussion. Flying into an object, or even tight wire netting, can cause severe haemorrhage inside the cranium and produce nervous signs, often only a short while before death.

In all cases, a full clinical examination is necessary before the cause of any type of fit can be found and treated. It is essential to provide affected birds with complete quiet, a dim light and a concentrated, balanced and easily digested diet. An adequate supply of fruit, green stuffs, yeast, egg, liver, and wheat germ is advisable, with meat or gentles in some cases. Perches should be placed across the floor of the cage. The temperature should be kept constant between 60° and 70°F (15° and 21°C). If recurrences of the fits are expected a mild sedative such as metoserpate hydrochloride or metomidate hydrochloride, an anticonvulsant drug or a tranquillizer, such as acetyl promazine or chlorpromazine, may be used under the supervision of a veterinarian. When an infectious disease or other organic disease is suspected antibiotic or other treatment may be necessary. In most cases, except those of dietary origin or as the result of a minor injury, the prognosis is poor.

Fainting and Vertigo

Loss of consciousness without convulsions, is not infrequent. It may follow staggering or other types of incoordination, such as circling or rolling. It probably arises from causes similar to those which produce the epileptic type of convulsions. Vascular or cardiac diseases causing anaemia or anoxia of the brain cells are among the reasons. Overdosing with certain drugs and affections of the balancing mechanism in the middle ear are occasionally responsible, hence the name "labyrinthine vertigo". Signs of dizziness or fainting should always be considered potentially dangerous. Although hereditary tendency to these conditions has been noted in canaries and some other birds, this has not yet been fully studied and the composition of the diet and general health should always be checked first.

Apoplexy

Apoplexy has already been discussed in the previous chapter, because although the clinical signs may denote a nervous disorder, they are in fact due to disease of the cardiovascular system.

"Hysteria" and excessive Nervousness

Some individuals as well as certain species are notorious for their excessive excitability in response even to quite normal sounds or visual stimuli. Hyperexcitability is liable to be hereditary in nature, although a placid bird can be rendered excitable by subjecting it to irregular hours of artificial light, incorrect handling or frightening situations.

Hyperexcitability is often associated with gasping and panting respirations and many birds affected in this way are incurable. Others slowly recover after a period of repeated sedation or tranquillization. Hysteria is essentially a functional disorder and *post-mortem* examinations often fail to reveal the cause.

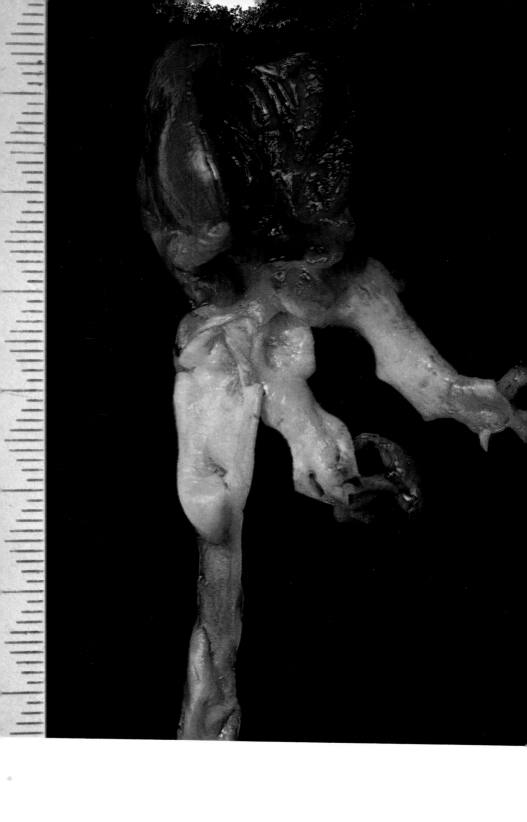

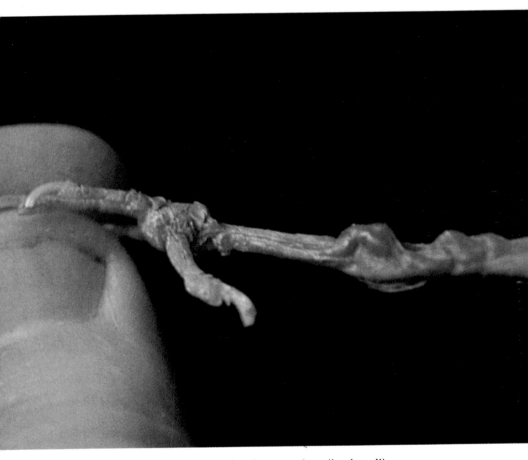

Plate 2/17. Severe varicose veins in a canary. (L. Arnall)

Plate 1/17. Heart, with associated arteries, from a red-billed toucan showing severe atherosclerosis. The arteries have been partly opened to show the yellowish coloured deposits lining the thickened arterial wall. In normal arteries the lining (intima) is white and smooth. (I.F. Keymer and T.C. Dennett, Z.S.L.)

SELECTED BIBLIOGRAPHY

HASHOLT, J. (1969). Diseases of the Nervous System. In *Diseases of Cage and Aviary Birds,* p.331–338. Ed. Petrak, M. L., Philadelphia. Lea and Febiger.

THE ENDOCRINE SYSTEM

Very little is known about the diseases of the endocrine system in birds; most available information deals with the budgerigar.

The Pituitary Gland

This gland lies on the underside of the brain, roughly in the centre of the floor of the cranium. It is given its common name of "master gland" because it largely controls all the other ductless glands. It may be damaged by infection, overstimulation or the growth of tumours. It is so complex and so inaccessible surgically that any derangement will almost inevitably prove fatal. A diseased pituitary gland causes abnormal development in a young chick. Growth may be either slowed or quickened and parts of the body may grow at different rates, producing monstrosities. In the grown bird anatomical proportions are unlikely to alter greatly, but metabolism is either stimulated or retarded. Tumour formation involving overgrowth of true glandular tissue will stimulate, while non-glandular tumours will tend to replace the gland and lessen pituitary hormone output. Because of the complex nature of the chemical products produced by the pituitary, and because of the fact that most of these chemicals act indirectly on body tissue by stimulating or suppressing the output of other glands, the ensuing diseases are numerous and variable.

The result of a diseased pituitary gland for example may be a stunted, nervous bird, or a sluggish, obese balding one. Interference with water and mineral metabolism may result in increased thirst. Resistance to shock or infections may be lowered in some cases and some birds may show abnormal sexual behaviour or sex reversal. In Britain, tumours of the pituitary gland have so far figured among the rare avian tumours, but in North America some surveys have shown them to be among the commonest types in budgerigars. Some pituitary affections of birds are possibly manifested by a proportion of the dead-in-the-shell and newly hatched monsters, so commonly met by budgerigar breeders.

The Thyroid Gland

This gland is situated astride the syrinx at the lower end of the windpipe or trachea and lies at varying distances inside the

293

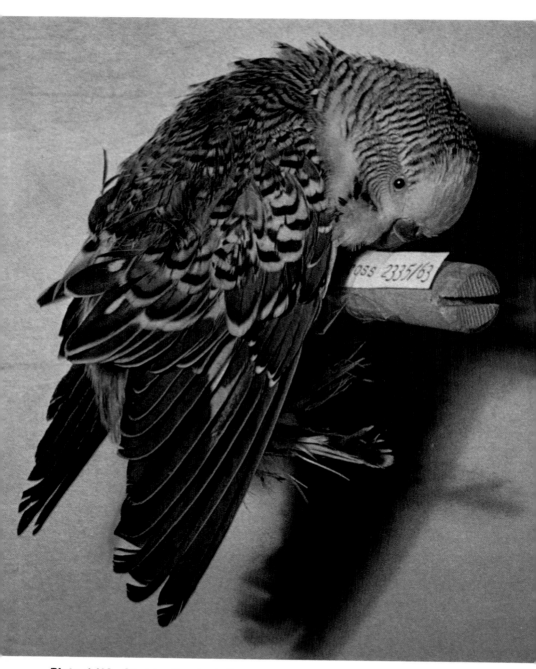

Plate 1/18. Severe disorientation and depression. Inability to grip perch with claws. Budgerigar has unkempt and debilitated appearance. Cause unknown. (L. Arnall)

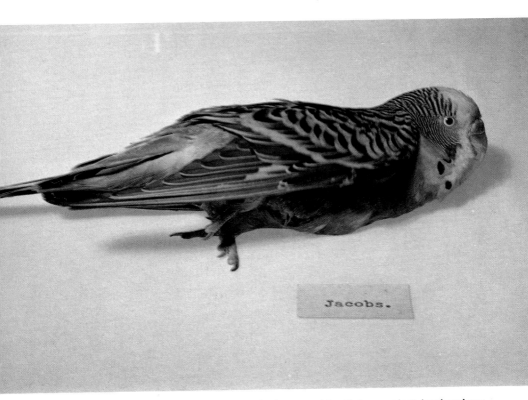

Plate 2/18. Incoordination with ataxia (crossed feet) in an alert budgerigar. (L. Arnall)

thorax according to species. In most it is only a short way behind the clavicles. Its main function in the young is to influence the growth rate. In the adult, after growth is completed, the gland "goes into low gear" but continues to control the metabolic rate.

When the thyroid gland is overactive, development is rapid, but since bodily activity is also overstimulated, weight increase is less than normal. Precocity results, including sexual precocity and premature ageing. When the gland is underactive, development is slow and a weak, retarded bird results. In severe cases, the bird cannot fend for itself; it is even unable to find food and usually starves to death at an early age. If the thyroid becomes underactive in an adult, the main changes are increase of weight due to deposition of fat, loss of activity and a partial moult with poor feathering and lethargy. The slowing of many bodily functions may also be apparent, together with the excretion of small, constipated droppings, a fall in body temperature and slower heart and respiratory rates.

Not all fat birds show clear-cut thyroid changes and thyroid enlargements and tumours are not confined to obese birds. The proportion of birds with both abnormalities, however, is too great merely to be ascribed to coincidence.

Overweight almost always decreases with progressive thyroid enlargement; consequently by the time obvious swellings and digestive and respiratory embarrassments are apparent, the bird is generally normal in weight or thin, weak and lifeless. Sometimes such birds may give the impression of being fat due to fluffing-up of the feathers. One indication of a previously obese bird is the coarseness and pinkish-yellow colouration of the skin, especially of the undersurface where it hangs in limp folds below the lower throat, breast and abdomen.

When overactivity of the thyroid develops in an adult, a common sign is nervousness shown by darting movements and tremors. The plumage remains in good condition but has a washed-out appearance due to loss of pigment. This is mostly seen in canaries and budgerigars which, when treated with thyroid, moult and rapidly grow a new, though paler plumage.

The manifestations of thyroid dysfunction described in young birds arise spontaneously, from an upset of the physiological control of metabolism. Microscopic examinations of thyroids from both adults and young at necropsy, may fail to show more than moderate evidence of overactivity or enlargement. Several species and budgerigars in particular, however, may develop excess growth of certain cells in the thyroid gland. This growth can be huge (Plate 1/19), without obviously affecting glandular function or conversely small, yet with the far-reaching results. An enlarged thyroid gland is called a "goitre" whether the output of thyroid hormone is normal, increased or decreased. Although most types of goitre found in man have occasionally been seen in birds, they are mainly rare.

Some enlargements of the gland are the result of a lack of the raw materials it needs to produce thyroxine, the active hormone. Such raw materials include iodine and the amino-acid tyrosine. Both these substances are relatively low in the diet of seed-eating birds in captivity and most reports of low thyroxine output or hypothyroidism occur in gallinaceous, psittacine and passerine birds, the groups favoured by aviculturalists. Fish- and insect-eating birds on the other hand usually obtain an adequate supply of iodine and tyrosine. Hyperthyroidism (high thyroxine output) has been diagnosed occasionally.

Early clinical signs of enlarged thyroids are bouts of continuous squeaking with each inspiration. On holding the bird near the ear expiration is heard as a low hiss. As the days pass, the squeak becomes incessant and quite beyond control. Breathing becomes increasingly difficult, weight is lost, the bird gasps for breath and sits huddled on its perch. Progressively less food is taken, because swallowing becomes difficult owing to constriction of the opening between the crop and proventriculus, due to pressure from the enlarged thyroids. Eating also interferes with the respiration. In this advanced stage the effort of trying to escape when approached or handled may be sufficient to cause heart failure. If the enlargement is mainly in a backward direction it presses on the veins entering the heart, or in very advanced cases on the heart itself and causes cardiac embarrassment. If the breast or back is auscultated at this stage, bubbling sounds may be heard which indicate that back pressure of blood in the great veins and lungs has caused congestion and oedema of the lungs. Such a bird is prone to chills and infections. Death, however, may occur before a swelling is detectable in the neck. In fact those birds with neck swellings (Plate 2/19) usually show relatively slight clinical signs because the thyroid enlargement in such cases is less confined and protrudes into the elastic tissues of the neck.

Removal of the thyroid is rarely possible or successful and is likely to be fatal. The demarcation between normal and abnormal tissue is seldom visible, therefore it is not practical to remove only the abnormal portions. The large numbers of blood vessels and nerves, and the closeness of the oesophagus and trachea also make surgery impracticable. In some cases, a reduction of the mass or an amelioration of the clinical signs have followed iodine, tyrosine or thyroid replacement therapy, in the form of diets containing these substances. In

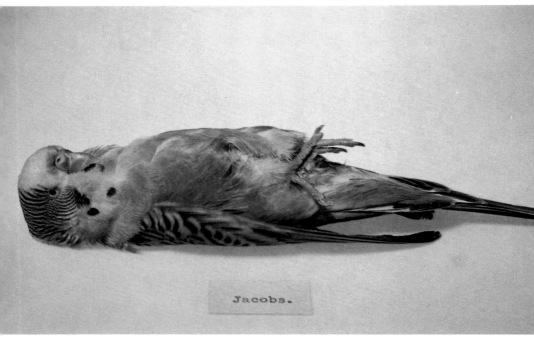

Plate 3/18. Same bird as Plate 2/18, unconcerned by being moved from prone to supine position. (L. Arnall)

Plate 4/18. Clenched or "clubbed" foot due to paralysis of extensor muscles of the toes. Budgerigar. (L. Arnall)

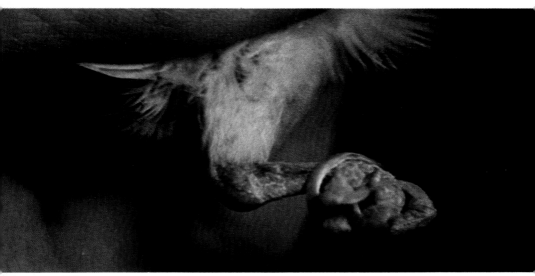

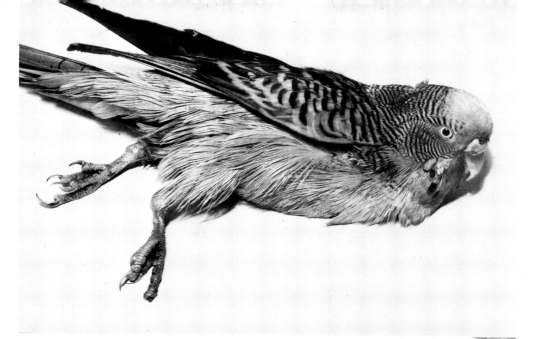

Plate 5/18. Budgerigar affected with bilateral paralysis of legs and respiratory distress. (L. Arnall)

Plate 6/18. Torticollis (twisted neck) and disorientation, but with the ability to stand when the feet feel contact with a flat surface. No pathological change found in brain on necropsy. Budgerigar. (L. Arnall)

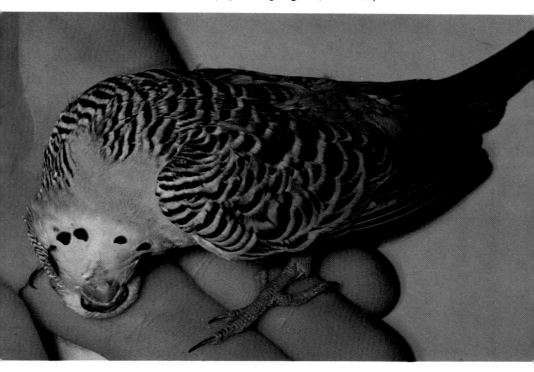

the main, however, the disease takes a relentless course leading to death. It is interesting to speculate how far breeding for size and weight or indeed any of the show characteristics of budgerigars may have contributed to the frequency of this unpleasant and common disease.

The Parathyroid Glands

The parathyroids are tiny structures lying just behind each lobe of the thyroid gland. As stated previously (Chapter 2) they are largely concerned with the utilization of calcium and phosphorus, influencing their level in the blood by varying absorption from the gut and mobilization from the bones. Calcium and phosphates are very important in the building and maintenance of bone—and in birds, egg-shell production —as well as for the conduction of impulses through the nervous system. In diseases affecting the parathyroids any of these activities may become deranged.

Direct proof is lacking, but experience with mammals and poultry provide considerable evidence that defects of parathyroid function also occur in cage birds. Although an outright lack of oyster shell grit in breeding females will result eventually in soft, non-shelled eggs, parathyroid hormone (parathormone) enables the birds to draw stores of calcium and phosphate from the bones for a time. The production of soft shells when an abundance of soluble grit is fed, denotes a possibly defective parathyroid gland. Fragile bones in adults and a tendency towards rickets in young parrots are probably related in many cases to abnormal functioning of this gland. A proportion of the vague, undiagnosable nervous disorders in adult birds of various species such as tremors, weakness, paralysis, convulsions and sudden blindness, have their parallel in mammals and have been related to parathyroid exhaustion or disease. Little research, however, has been done on the diagnosis and treatment of parathyroid disease in birds.

The Adrenal Glands

The two adrenal glands lie under the vertebral column just in front of the kidneys and are usually pinkish-cream in colour.

The adrenal gland is known as the stress gland. Whenever a bird is chilled, overheated, frightened, or if it is invaded by pathogenic organisms, this gland immediately stimulates whichever organ or mechanism is involved in the body's urgent defensive reaction.

The cortical tissue (covered in Chapter 2), also produces hormones which have a limiting effect on the body's inflammatory reactions. Any lack of this hormone will therefore allow repair processes to continue and pain to persist long after the cause of the trouble has ceased, producing such conditions as chronic arthritis and oedema. In an unsuitable

300

climate, on a deficient diet, after prolonged disease or after over-breeding, the gland can become exhausted beyond recuperation. This state of affairs probably occurs much more often than is realized, and quite likely accounts for many deaths attributed to shock.

Much research work is necessary before we can appreciate the full importance of this gland in birds. Some diseases in which a link-up with the adrenal cortex is suspected, include nephritis and gout, obesity, thyroid enlargement, French moult and other feathering disorders, as well as various diseases affecting the heart and circulation. Others include increased susceptibility to quite mild stresses such as being startled, quite brief or gentle handling, heat, cold, sudden exercise and the process of egg production and laying.

The Islets of Langerhans (Pancreas)

In mammals diabetes, which is a disorder of the Islets of Langerhans, is a well known disease, but there is virtually no evidence that it occurs in birds.

The Thymus Gland

There is virtually no information concerning diseases of this gland, although tumour formation has been reported in budgerigars.

The Gonads

Although the origins of both male and female gonads are similar, the secretions have diametrically opposite effects on secondary sex characteristics. The chemical structure of the male and female hormones, the androgens and oestrogens respectively, are similar not only to each other but also to vitamin D and a number of other body chemicals such as the cortisones and their derivatives.

The male hormones produce male characteristics and the female hormones produce female characteristics, but each sex gland or gonad also manufactures hormones which have a little of the effects of those of the opposite sex. Sometimes, however, hormonal disorders occur and give rise to varying degrees of sex reversal (see Chapter 16).

As birds have complicated patterns of territorial behaviour, peck orders and courtship display behaviour, it is not surprising that any bird departing even slightly from the norm is persecuted and often killed or driven away. Nature seems unable to tolerate a creature that is a little different from the crowd.

An imbalance of sex hormones can be manifested in several ways. For example, the bird will not mate or be mated, it will not sit on eggs or it becomes a bad parent and refuses to feed the young. Sometimes such a bird tries to mate a

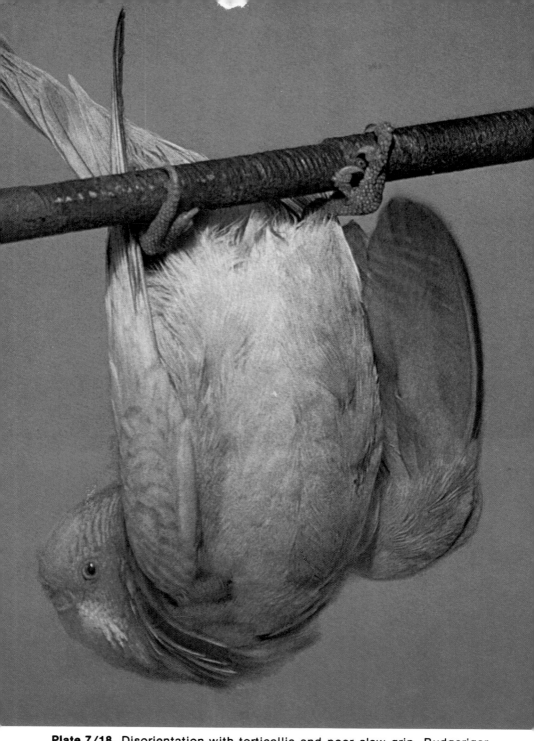

Plate 7/18. Disorientation with torticollis and poor claw grip. Budgerigar.
(L. Arnall)

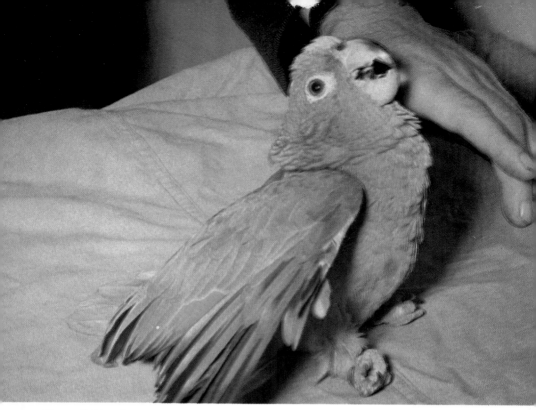

Plate 8/18. Opisthotonus (backward deviation of neck), lordosis and clenched feet in incoordinated yellow-fronted Amazon parrot. (L. Arnall)

Plate 9/18. Chorea or "St. Vitus Dance". A rhythmical twitch caused this bird to gyrate clockwise in jerks—a sign of brain damage. (L. Arnall)

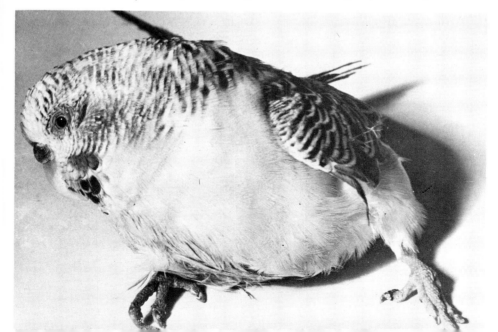

member of its own sex. From time to time, a bird may even show signs of being a nymphomaniac. Some of these states are of temporary or seasonal occurrence only; others are permanent.

Some of the abnormalities described above are accompanied by other physical changes, duller or brighter plumage, and development or atrophy of one or another of the combs or fleshy appendages. It is rare for a cock which has once fertilized a hen, later to lay fertile eggs or vice versa, but it is not unknown. In less advanced cases, a previously fertile hen may begin to mount females or a once virile cock will become less aggressive and begin to behave more like a hen.

These developments may represent either temporary exhaustion of the gland or excessive seasonal variation in its activity. Sometimes a pituitary lesion is responsible or possibly an adrenal degeneration or tumour. Abnormalities have on rare occasions derived from a dual or partially dual set of gonads, male and female, in the same bird, in which the pituitary or other glands allow one set to develop to maturity at puberty and the other some time in middle life. Malnutrition can halt sexual functions but it is unlikely to allow characteristics of the opposite sex to develop.

Both testes and ovaries are fairly prone to tumours, particularly in budgerigars. These tumours may or may not result in alteration of hormone secretion because they are formed of different types of gonad cell, only some of which secrete sex hormone. Those birds in which the tumour produces no hormones will show loss of sexual powers and characteristics only when the tumour cells have replaced the normal ones. Ovarian and testicular tumours in birds are significant mainly for the pressure which they exert in the confined body cavity by pressing on organs such as the kidneys, adrenals, liver and various parts of the intestinal tract (see Chapters 16 and 24).

In female budgerigars there is evidence that certain disturbances in oestrogen production can cause skeletal deformities. The disease is characterised by numerous bony deposits especially affecting the spine, sternum and skull, and is known as polyostotic hyperostosis (Plate 3/19). It has been produced experimentally by implanting the female hormone stilboestrol beneath the skin.

SELECTED BIBLIOGRAPHY

BLACKMORE, D. K. (1963). *The incidence and aetiology of thyroid dysplasia in budgerigars* (Melopsittacus undulatus). Vet. Rec. 75, 1068–1072.

THE ORGANS OF SPECIAL SENSE

Diseases of the eyes and ears are nearly always secondary to some other disease or infection. These diseases having already been covered in the relevant sections, the information is not duplicated below.

The Eye

As diseases of the eye are almost invariably consequent on such infections as pox, ornithosis, herpesvirus, *Mycoplasma* and erysipelas or vitamin A deficiency, it follows that symptomatic treatment of the eyes without consideration of other organs and tissues is unlikely to be effective. Inflammation of the eyelids (blepharitis) and conjunctivitis—inflammation of the conjunctival sac—are the commonest lesions of the eye. Conjunctivitis is a well known sign which leads to reddening around the eye. Keratitis, which is inflammation of the cornea, is often a sequel to conjunctivitis. It is frequently mistaken by laymen for a cataract, but this is deeper-seated in the eye, being an opacity of the lens.

Cataracts may involve one or both eyes. They are most commonly seen in old birds, particularly canaries, parrots and those birds of prey which live for many years in captivity. With increasing age, the opacities become denser so that the affected bird gradually becomes blind. A free-living bird would obviously be unable to survive for long with bilateral cataracts. In captivity, with food provided regularly and always placed in the same positions, a partially blind bird can remain in relatively good condition for many months. There is no satisfactory treatment for cataract in birds and the precise causes are unknown, although some cases may be hereditary (see Chapter 25).

The Ear

There is very little information available concerning diseases of the ears in birds. Like the eyes, however, they may be involved in generalized diseases, especially septicaemias.

Vertigo, which is discussed elsewhere (see Chapter 18) can be due to labyrinthitis or inflammation of the labyrinth of the ear.

Primary diseases of the ear are rare in birds, unlike mammals, probably because their ears are better protected.

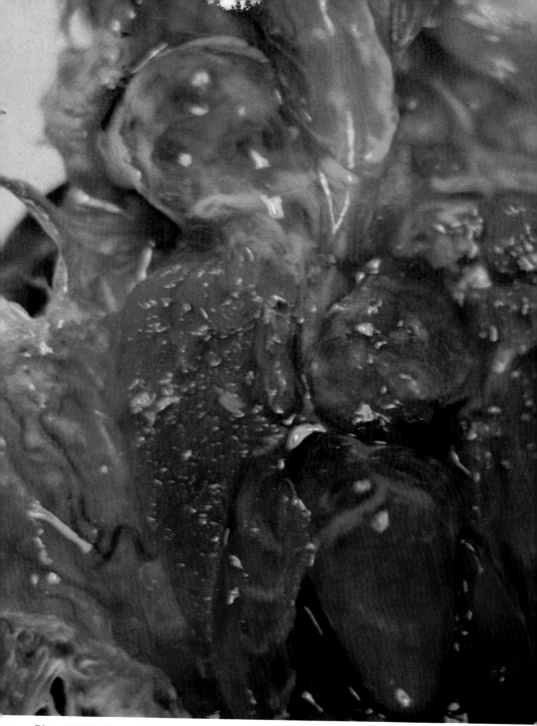

Plate 1/19. Thyroid dysplasia or goiter. The enlarged thyroid is the lobular spherical mass in the left hand corner of the picture. The heart can be seen on the right and the cut surfaces of the muscles in the middle. Budgerigar. (L. Arnall)

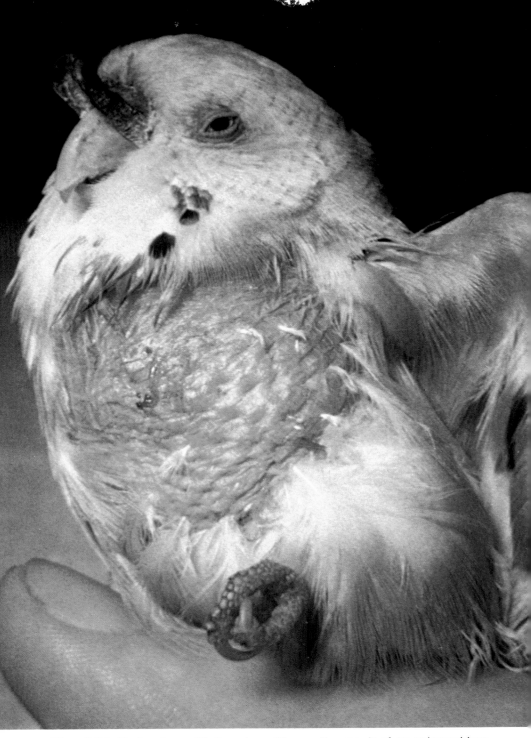

Plate 2/19. Budgerigar with throat swelling as the result of an enlarged hae-morrhagic thyroid gland. The cere shows marked "brown" hypertrophy. (L. Arnall)

SELECTED BIBLIOGRAPHY

SMALL, E. (1969). Diseases of the Organs of Special Sense. In *Diseases of Cage and Aviary Birds*, p.351–355. Ed. Petrak, M. L., Philadelphia. Lea and Febiger.

STARTUP, C. M. (1970). The Diseases of Cage and Aviary Birds, (excluding the specific diseases of the Budgerigar) p.46–58. In *Rutgers, A. & Norris, K. A., Eds. Encyclopedia of Aviculture, Vol. I.* London, Blandford Press.

INJURIES

The causes of injuries are numerous and usually unexpected; nevertheless, many mishaps can be prevented by common sense and good management. Luckily the great majority are trivial and many wounds heal rapidly in birds, whether or not they are treated. The majority are the result of flying into the boundaries of the cage and entangling a wing, foot or the head in wire netting or fittings. Night marauders, while not necessarily attacking the bird, usually cause panic and result in the bird knocking itself about. With pets which are given the freedom of a house or room, other hazards abound, such as open gas or electric fires, bowls or saucepans of hot water, light fittings, picture cords, etc. A fire may only singe feathers and burn off a few toes, but hot water and particularly fat have a penetrating heat which scalds the body as well. If death from shock does not occur in minutes or hours, infection of the damaged skin or pneumonia following the shock will probably kill in a few days (See later). Accidents will always happen, but forethought can prevent many.

Marauding animals are always a problem, both inside the house and particularly in outside aviaries. Sometimes rats, stoats and weasels, or even snakes may enter an aviary through a small hole in the netting which has developed unnoticed.

Special injuries occur under certain circumstances. Leg bands or rings, for example, may cause injury to the legs if they are the wrong size for the birds (see Chapter 29). Minor injuries may be manifested by ruffled plumage, patchy loss of feathers, small points of bleeding or simply dejection.

Wounds, especially due to fighting are common and vary in seriousness, sometimes resulting in the loss of eyes, limbs or even evisceration. It is surprising, however, how even free-living birds can survive quite severe injuries, including amputation of a leg or feet (Plate 1/21).

Feather pecking is common in intensively raised poultry (see Plate 2/21) and also occurs in other species (Plate 3/21). In an aviary of various species the larger birds are by no means always the culprits. Some, the cardinals and whydas for example, can be trusted with the smallest finches, weavers or waxbills, although less so with others of their own species. Cutthroat finches—especially in the breeding season—will

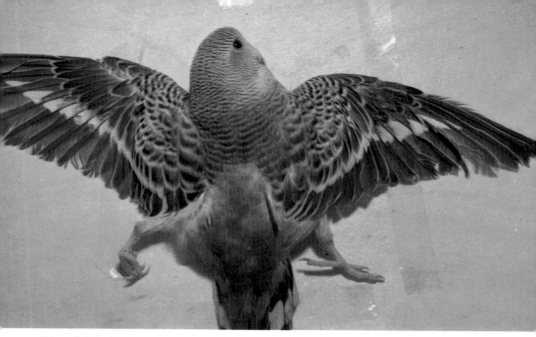

Plate 3/19. Hen budgerigar with hyperostosis of the spine, showing typical posture. (L. Arnall)

Plate 1/21. Feet amputated at tarsometatarsal level in a feral pigeon surviving adequately in the wild state. (L. Arnall)

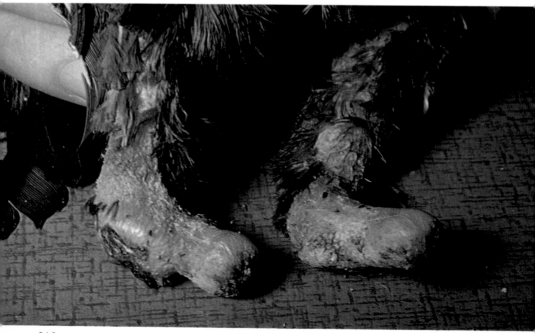

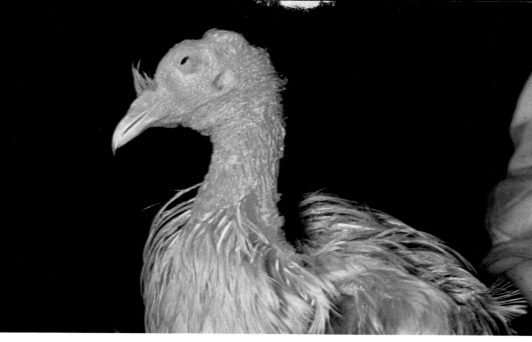

Plate 2/21. Alopecia of head and neck in the domestic fowl due to feather pecking by companion. (L. Arnall)

Plate 3/21. Granuloma due to repeated pecking on the elbow of a budgerigar. (L. Arnall)

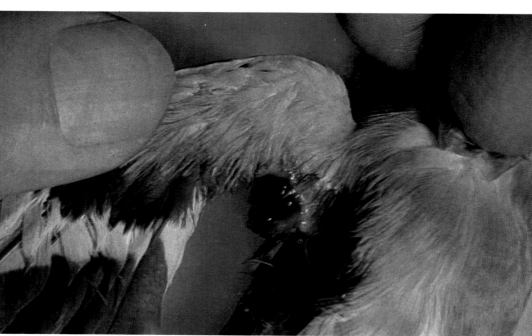

peck and bully most species and should never be kept with smaller or more peaceable varieties.

Under this heading are included scratches, cuts and bruises of the skin or deeper tissues. Where only a small area of skin is damaged, little more is necessary than bathing with a weak antiseptic solution or with salt water—approximately one teaspoonful of salt to the pint. If the wound is dirty, badly bruised or its extent is in doubt, it is wiser first to cut short or to pluck all the feathers around it. After cleansing the wound, an anti-bacterial cream or spray should be applied. Ointments must not be used because the body heat makes them soft and sticky; when this happens the bird becomes uncomfortable and bedraggled in appearance, whilst the heat-insulating property of the feathers is lost. As a result the bird is easily chilled and becomes susceptible to respiratory diseases. For similar reasons, oily creams must be used very sparingly: they should be gently rubbed into the wound until they disappear, and should have a base of "vanishing cream".

It is usually unnecessary to give antibiotics, except when wounds are extensive, of doubtful depth, or liable to involve an important structure like an air sac, the crop, the abdominal contents, the eye or ear.

Self-inflicted wounds sometimes appear to be the result of boredom, especially with a parrot kept alone in a small cage. Irritation due to ectoparasites, excessive moulting, skin inflammation, tumours, open wounds or sticky dressings may also be responsible. If such causes are removed or alleviated, then self-inflicted injuries will often heal in a few days. It may be necessary, however, to fit an Elizabethan collar, which is a lampshade-like ruff made of cardboard, polythene or thin aluminium to prevent the bird reaching the offending part. After two or three days this often breaks the habit. The bird usually resents the collar but it will do no harm providing that feeding is easy and the collar does not chafe its neck.

Covering wounds with bandages or other dressings is often liable to do more harm than good. In the feathered areas, such dressings may interfere with preening and with movement; they draw the bird's attention to the affected part, keep the wound excessively moist and usually retard healing. Not least, they are difficult to apply properly and unless tough and bulky, can be pecked into pieces; threads may then twine around a limb or the neck and interfere with movement and circulation, even to the extent of strangulation or amputation. But for some injuries as explained later, dressings may be necessary. If dressings are applied to legs, they must always be carried down to and include the toes. An even, gentle pressure must be maintained over all the area they cover, otherwise a part tighter than the rest may cut off the circulation and act like a tourniquet, especially if any inflammatory swelling develops under the dressing. Should this occur the entire lower leg may die and become gangrenous within a period as short as 24 hours. To prevent such a happening, sticking plaster should be folded around the limb in short pieces instead of being wound round and round. Where required with fractures, splints can be placed parallel to the shank and included in the fold of plaster.

Open wounds heal most quickly. They can be cleaned easily and drugs applied without difficulty.

Abscesses and Granulomas
Abscesses do not occur very commonly in birds when compared with mammals. Wounds sometimes become infected, but the infection is usually more likely to spread into the blood stream and internal organs causing a septicaemia and death, than to localize into areas of pus. Pus is a mixture of body fluids, living and dead white blood cells, and bacteria or other pathogenic organisms. Most of the organisms are engulfed by the specialized white blood cells known as phagocytes, which help to give pus its light colour. As stated previously, the blood and the lymphatic tissues and systems of birds are different from mammals and more like those of reptiles. Birds, for example, produce lymphatic cells in small specks of lymphoid tissue scattered throughout the body These and other differences probably account for the different response by birds, compared with mammals, to bacteria which usually form pus. Pus is nevertheless sometimes produced, but the localized response to infection tends to give rise to the production of diseased tissue in the form of chronic abscesses and so-called granulation tissue (Plate 4/21). The latter tissue is of the connective type and made up of fibre-producing cells and minute blood vessels. Sometimes it appears as quite large swellings or thickenings—called granulomas (Plate 3/21) because of their similarity to tumours, the suffix "oma" meaning tumour.

Abscesses can occur anywhere on the body; they arise from infected wounds, damaged feather follicles, blocked sebaceous glands, pressure and friction points, or beneath damaged skin. Abscesses can also form in internal organs as well as in the skin, occurring most frequently in the liver and spleen. They are often fatal and not diagnosed before examination, because their clinical signs are usually vague and typical of any sick bird affected with general malaise. On the scaled parts of the leg, abscesses can easily be confused with gouty swellings. Both appear as ivory-coloured bead-like pimples which when cut open yield creamy or sometimes crumbly contents: gouty deposits, however, are mainly around or near the joints.

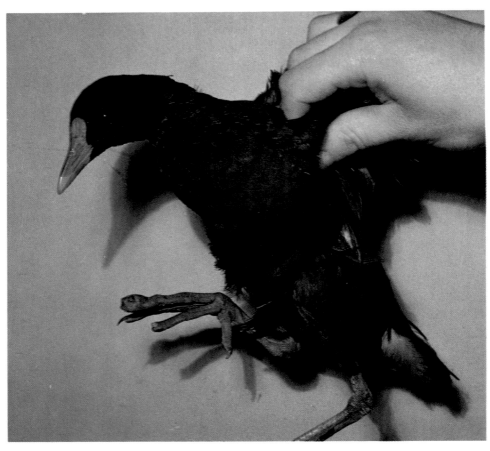

Plate 4/21. Granulating toe-tip and loss of 3 nails on right foot. Moorhen. (L. Arnall)

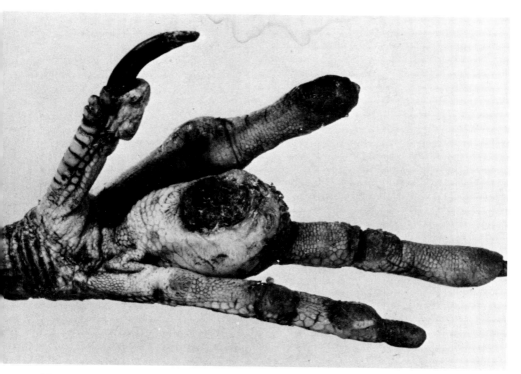

Plate 5/21. Chronic infective synovitis and arthritis or "bumblefoot" affecting a little egret. Note the marked swelling of the foot pad which also involves the plantar surface of the base of the middle toe. The extremities of the other anterior digits are necrosed and the nails have been lost possibly due to frost bite. The centre of the bumblefoot swelling is also necrosed (dark in appearance) due to pressure. (I.F. Keymer and T.C. Dennett, Z.S.L.)

The type of abscess commonly found on the toes and ball of the feet of birds is referred to by poultry keepers as "bumble-foot" and usually represents a chronically infected corn (Plate 5/21). It is essentially a normal abscess or granuloma, but owing to its position and continual pressure from beneath during perching and walking, the tissues are constantly irritated. The horny skin becomes undermined with infected granulation tissue, often becoming partly or completely surrounded by a thick fibrous capsule. Very little resolution occurs and normal healing is prevented. Dirty conditions favour the development of bumble-foot, which is caused originally by bacteria entering small scratches or wounds in the skin. It is particularly common in birds of prey

315

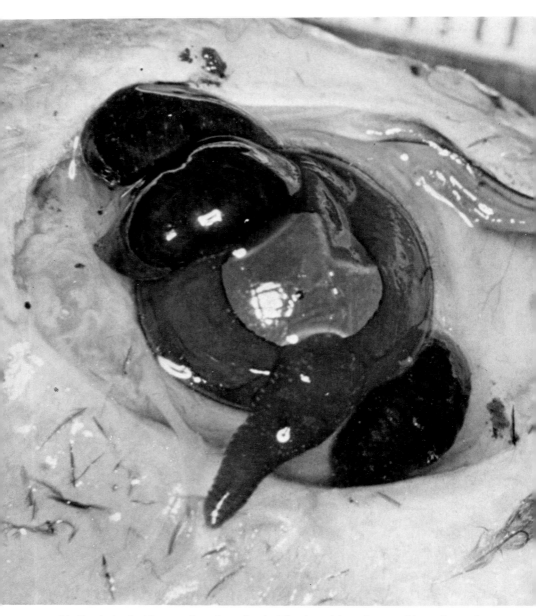

Mallard duck (*Anas platyrhynchos*). The head has been skinned to show four blood-sucking leeches (*Theromyzon tessulatum*) which are attacking the eye and conjuctival sac. The bird became infested when it was weakened by botulism (Chapter 22). The parasites are not helminths, but related to earthworms, i.e. Annelida. (I.F. Keymer and T.C. Dennett, Z.S.L.)

used in falconry and probably commences from infection of punctures in the ball of the foot produced by the bird's own sharp talons. This is most likely to occur when perches are too narrow and the toes insufficiently extended. Drastic cutting away of the tumour-like mass is usually necessary so that no raised rim remains. Haemorrhage is a danger here, but a powdered antibiotic or sulphonamide helps to sterilize the cavity, aids clotting of the blood and keeps out dirt and infection. In some cases it may be necessary to plaster over the toe or foot.

Granulation tissue is not confined to the skin. A ruptured abdominal muscle wall, the cere, a split beak (Plate 6/21) and pendulous, fat-covered breast in continuous contact with the perch, are all common sites. The avoidance of predisposing causes and removal of the affected tissue are the first steps in treatment. The fresh wound thus created is treated in the usual fashion.

Ulcers and Non-healing Wounds

An ulcer is an open, infected area on the skin or a mucous membrane which exposes the underlying tissues. It is usually a slow or non-healing area, a stalemate between the disease process and the body's defences.

As time passes, the edges of an ulcer often thicken into a rim. Bacteria or other organisms, especially those disliking a free supply of oxygen, flourish in the crater produced, but they are not necessarily the primary cause. Injuries, burns, penetrating foreign bodies or infections with such organisms as pox viruses or *Mycobacterium* (the cause of tuberculosis) may start the disease process. Dietary or other debilities may prepare the way for formation of an ulcer or help its progress. Tissues poorly supplied with blood, are common sites, such as the cornea of the eyeball or the surface of large growths over which the skin is tightly stretched. Typical internal sites are the lining of the crop in budgerigars, birds of prey and many other species, and the intestines in coccidiosis of gallinaceous birds.

It is important to understand before attempting treatment the many factors which favour the formation of ulcers. Careful observation of the bird in its cage and examination in the hand can help in finding the cause. The healing of many ulcers is slowed up by movement of the adjacent tissues, so prevention of such irritation is the first step in treatment. Many of the diseases associated with ulcers are discussed elsewhere. Assuming that the causes are eliminated, an external ulcer overlying normal tissue should be scraped until it bleeds, the lips of the ulcer trimmed off with scissors and their undersides also scraped. Caustics such as silver nitrate, ferric chloride, or a copper sulphate crystal may be rubbed into

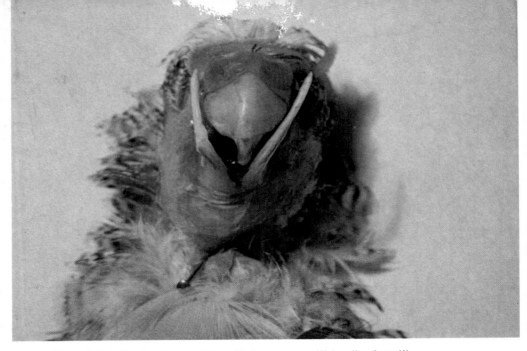

Plate 6/21. Budgerigar with split lower mandible. (L. Arnall)

Plate 7/21. Subcutaneous emphysema affecting the neck of a sulphur-crested cockatoo. (I.F. Keymer and T.C. Dennett, Z.S.L.)

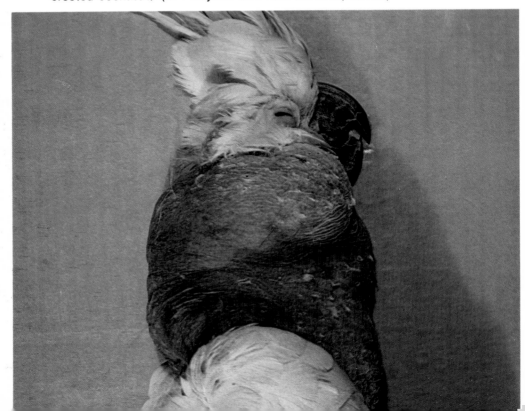

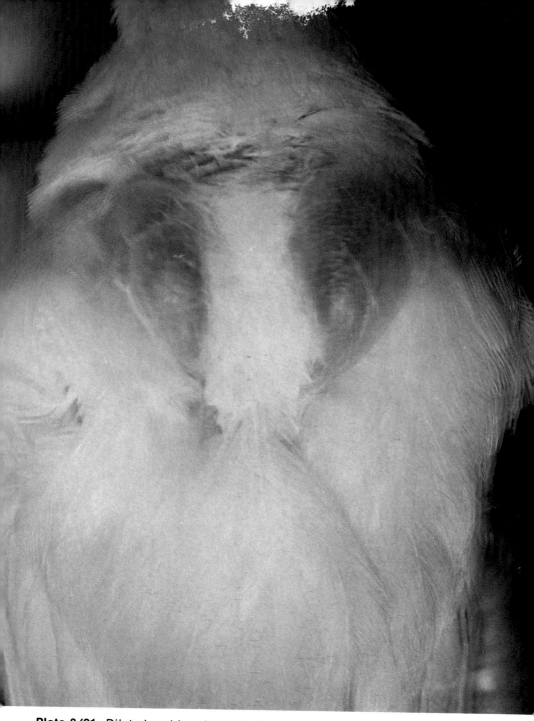

Plate 8/21. Dilated and herniated clavicular air sacs in the canary, visible from the back of the neck in the shoulder region. The bird has its head down presenting its back to the observer. (L. Arnall)

the wound to destroy the remaining infected granulation tissue and to check bleeding. A suitable anti-bacterial drug should then be applied. Chlortetracycline in powder form in a urea base is desirable to begin with, since it draws out infected fluids. Later, an oily antibiotic cream will help to maintain a clean wound both by killing bacteria already in it and preventing the entry of others. The application of a plaster bandage may be indicated for a short period or an Elizabethan collar can be used, depending upon the site of the ulcer. This should ensure quick, unhindered healing in birds which are used to being handled and tolerate a collar without undue distress.

Puncture Wounds

Lesions inflicted by teeth or claws, projecting pieces of wire, air-gun pellets or lead shot produce deep wounds, often severe internal injury and considerable haemorrhage. Such damage to the heart, lungs or intestines frequently causes sudden death and without careful examination of the carcase such deaths may variously be dismissed as "heart failure", "fright" or "chilling". In birds which survive, wounds of this type soon produce severe bruising and sometimes slow haemorrhage. Bacteria capable of causing disease are often deposited in the depths of the wound by the agent and become sealed in by congealed serum or blood. Although pus is relatively infrequently produced in birds, the usual pus-forming bacteria can still infect wounds and produce death of the local tissues. If virulent, the bacteria can spread and multiply in the blood, causing death by septicaemia and result in damage to any or all of the vital organs. Infection of deep penetrating wounds can often be avoided by the timely use of anti-bacterial drugs. Administration by mouth may be the safest route in some cases if the patient will drink and the breathing is not impaired. Subcutaneous injection is preferable to intramuscular, in birds which may be shocked. Antibiotics are indicated and suitable preparations are listed later.

Fractures

Fractured bones are a common feature in numerous types of serious injury. These are dealt with in Chapter 29 as the treatment is surgical.

Dislocations

Dislocations resulting from injury are much less common than fractures, although occasionally the two can occur together. The chief joints to suffer are the elbow, the stifle (knee), and the hock (heel), although the shoulder, the hip and the joints of the foot can also be displaced. In a dislocation, those

320

surfaces of the joint which normally slide over one another become displaced and stretch or tear the supporting tissues, that is the ligaments, tendons and muscles. As a result, the limb is deformed to a greater or lesser degree and may project stiffly at a bizarre angle, or become locked in an odd position. The muscles then cease to operate normally. Stretching or bending the limb, coupled with gentle squeezing across the joint between finger and thumb is often sufficient to replace the articular surfaces and produce an audible click, after which the joint resumes its normal movements. Reduction is more difficult, however, if ligaments are badly torn or fragments of joint surfaces have been broken off during the violence which produced the dislocation. In such cases, although replacement may still be possible, a further dislocation occurs when the bird is released. Under these circumstances, the limb should be fixed with adhesive dressings in such a position of rest that recurrence of dislocation is unlikely. Dislocations of the elbow and hock joints need for example, to be immobilized with the joint flexed to less than a right angle. In this position, the tendons which extend that joint tighten and assist in holding the articular surfaces together. Reasonably satisfactory repair usually occurs within six to fourteen days, depending on the bird's condition and size.

Congenital dislocations are not uncommon in budgerigars (see Chapter 25).

Subcutaneous Emphysema

This term merely means "gas under the skin". The gas is usually air which has penetrated the subcutaneous tissues through a skin wound or as the result of damage to part of the respiratory system. Some writers have described how air has been pumped into the surrounding tissues by the tongue and other muscular movements associated with swallowing, from a wound caused by something sharp in the pharynx or the throat. The accumulated air then diffuses down the neck and produces a puffiness of the overlying skin (Plate 7/21). The mechanism in all cases is similar. Puncture wounds and cuts involving layers of skin and muscles do not stay immediately opposite one another, since the layers slide over each other during movement. If the surface layer is concave and its elasticity allows it to lift, then air is drawn in. The air is then trapped and is pushed on the easiest course, which is along the planes between skin and muscle or between layers of muscles. After moving, the air becomes halted within the fat and connective tissues in the form of bubbles which crackle when the region is handled. Common sites of emphysema are the groin, the 'armpits', neck, entrance to the chest and over the shoulders (Plate 8/21). This type of emphysema is harmless but can be alarming to the owner, especially when the bird blows up into a grotesque shape within a few hours. Once access of air is stopped, however, the gases are slowly absorbed. Part of the air can usually be removed with a hypodermic needle and syringe, but the tissues will refill if the point of entry is not closed. A purse-string suture can be used to close a small external wound, but throat wounds or air sac ruptures without skin wounds, are impossible to repair surgically. Time will slowly heal most of them, but there is always the danger that air which carries dust and has not been filtered through the respiratory tract will result in inflammation and the formation of exudates which may block the air sacs and lead to pneumonia. Fungi, such as *Aspergillus*, and numerous bacteria flourish in these warm, moist and aerated wounds.

There is no effective cure for aspergillosis, but for bacterial infections the usual treatments for wounds should be used. Creams and ointments are useful for such lesions as they seal the wound; further protection can be applied by using a plastic skin in a solvent form as an aerosol sprayed on the affected parts.

Emphysema can also arise when certain gas-forming anaerobic bacteria related to those which cause the smell in gangrene, multiply in a deep and therefore airless wound. Such changes are preceded by obvious illness and loss of function of the part concerned, it showing reddish, green or black discolouration associated with coldness and insensitivity. This usually follows upon a very severe and probably painful inflammation. By the time the puffiness is apparent the bird is usually dying or dead. Although injections of penicillin, ampicillin or certain other broad-spectrum antibiotics are likely to be the most effective forms of treatment, they are usually administered too late for any hope of recovery.

Burns and Scalds

Burns are mainly caused by direct heat and chemicals. The most usual source is flames from open coal, gas or electric fires and cookers with hot metal surfaces or bars. Feathers provide considerable protection because they insulate the body for a moment, allowing the bird to escape or at any rate survive, if removed immediately from the heat. The areas which suffer most are the feet, the scaled parts of the legs and the eyes. Whole toes may be destroyed in the initial second on alighting, although they may not actually slough off for a few days. Immediate application of an antibiotic cream is the best treatment, preferably with an antihistamine or cortisone drug incorporated to reduce pain and shock. In an emergency, vaseline, olive or cod-liver oil are almost as useful. Oils

322

should if possible, be kept off the plumage, otherwise the already badly shocked bird is liable to further chilling from matting of its feathers. A humid environment of 70–75°F (21–24°C) is preferable to a higher temperature with low humidity. When toes are lost, the perches should be modified to provide a flat upper surface on which the bird can perch satisfactorily once the foot lesions are healed.

With chemical burns, the above treatment should follow after the corrosive has been removed as far as possible. Where acids are suspected, sodium bicarbonate (baking powder) solution will check further damage. With alkalis, such as caustic soda or potash which continue to penetrate the tissues deeply, dilute white vinegar is a useful antidote. Carbolic acid, coal tar products, and most other caustics can often be washed away with copious water, brine, bicarbonate or magnesia solutions. Antidotes for internal and external caustic burns will be found in the chapter on poisons.

Electricity is seldom the cause of burns because death usually occurs directly from electrocution.

Scalds directly affect only the outer layers of the body, but they have far-reaching effects on its functions. Hot water and especially hot fat, penetrate the plumage rapidly and cling for some time, thus scalding the skin further. As a result, although the feet and head may be damaged, it is the extensive skin damage over the body which produces most shock. The skin in this region quickly assumes a red, inflamed appearance, and the matted feathers allow rapid loss of body heat. When the body temperature is depressed, the lungs may become water-logged as a result of lowered blood pressure, shock and other factors. They are thus susceptible to invasion by infectious agents and pneumonia may occur within a few days. In severe cases it is the fall in blood pressure, loss of tissue fluids into the scalded area, and other aspects of shock which can kill the bird within a matter of hours. If the hot water or fat is inhaled in any quantity, death is virtually instantaneous.

Local applications of medicaments to the scalded area are not advised—except to the shanks and feet—unless it is of a non-sticky aqueous base, because they cause further matting of the plumage. Moderate warmth is advisable, as described for burns. Careful attention should be given to provide a diet which the bird will accept; milk may be given to drink and possibly an antibiotic and prednisolone supplement mixed with soaked seed or other food for a few days. It is impracticable to attempt to inject blood plasma substitutes or blood proteins into the veins in an effort to increase the circulating blood volume and draw fluids back from the tissues to the blood, except perhaps in large species. The usefulness of the method, however, is unproven in cage birds, and control of the technique is far too difficult except for an experienced veterinarian.

The provision of rest, quiet, reasonable warmth, fluids and easily digested foods will achieve more than drugs or complicated methods.

SELECTED BIBLIOGRAPHY

PECKHAM, M. C. (1965). Vices and Miscellaneous Conditions. In *Diseases of Poultry,* p.1162–1211. Eds. Biester, H. E. and Schwarte, L. H. 5th Ed. Ames, Iowa. State University Press.

TOTTENHAM, K. (1969). Wild Bird Casualties. In *Diseases of Cage and Aviary Birds,* p.500–501. Ed. Petrak, M. L., Philadelphia. Lea and Febiger.

POISONING

The study of poisons and their effect on the body is known as toxicology. It is a vast, difficult and fascinating subject. Toxin is the technical name for poison; but it is also used for harmful chemical substances produced by living organisms both animals or plants, including toxin-producing bacteria, fungi and other micro-organisms.

Substances poisonous to birds can be divided into a number of groups as outlined below.

Some plants contain substances which make them poisonous when eaten *e.g.* the fungus ergot (*Claviceps purpurea*) and green plants such as hemlock (*Conium maculatum*), nightshade (*Atropa belladonna*), corn cockle (*Agrostemma githago*) or yew (*Taxus baccata*), to mention only a few. A healthy well-fed bird will often reject some of these plants or seeds and it may even show resistance to the poisonous substances they contain.

Botulism   BOTULISM is a blood-poisoning caused by bacteria known as *Clostridium botulinum*. Ingestion of the toxin produced by the bacteria gives rise to the disease known as botulism. It is not an infection but a poisoning caused by the metabolic by-products of the bacteria. The toxin is possibly produced in living animals but normally in rotting food, carcases or other organic material and is often carried by maggots; it is primarily a disease of warmer climates where conditions are favourable for the organisms to multiply and produce the botulinal toxin. Man and probably all warm-blooded animals are susceptible to some degree. Certain species are more likely to suffer than others on account of their feeding habits. Some birds such as vultures which eat rotting carcases or its associated maggots appear to be relatively resistant. Water-fowl are most commonly affected, becoming poisoned in hot weather when the bacteria in the mud of stagnant ponds produce large quantities of the toxin.

It has been estimated that 25 ml. of botulinal toxin are sufficient to kill all the inhabitants of a city of two million people. In some countries the toxin has possibly been stock-piled for biological warfare, although this is now internationally outlawed.

325

Clinical Signs The toxin has its first effect on the central nervous system, producing muscular weakness usually within hours of being eaten. The neck, wings and legs of birds become paralysed, affected birds often drooping their heads to the ground with eyes half-closed, before becoming comatose and dying. Trembling, diarrhoea and shedding of feathers may also be seen. Mildly affected birds recover, although the toxin needs to be present in only minute amounts to be fatal to some small species. Cases in cage birds appear to be very rare.

Treatment and Prevention Control of the disease lies primarily in avoiding spoiled food. The organism can only multiply in an environment without oxygen; therefore gentles, fish, meat or egg food kept in screw-top jars and tins, or even carcases of dead nestlings or other birds, are potential sources of the toxin in hot countries or in cooler climates when they have been kept under warm conditions.

Once the source of poison has been removed it is essential to give a good laxative. This will void the offending material and increase the thirst. A purging, saline solution such as Epsom salts is preferable to an oil. Absorbent substances such as chalk, magnesium preparations or aluminium hydroxide can be given to take up any remaining toxin. After 8 to 24 hours, according to the species, light feeding can be resumed. In some countries, botulinal antitoxins are available for injection. These are available in various types, but for birds only Type C is effective.

PAINTS AND WOOD PRESERVATIVES include lead from fresh or flaking paint, also creosote and tar. Budgerigars may die from lead poisoning as a result of nibbling and eating the "leaded lights" of pseudo-tudor windows.

HERBICIDES, FUNGICIDES AND INSECTICIDES cover a wide range of chemicals which are mainly used as sprays on crops. They are liable to contaminate green food, seed or insects eaten by cage birds. Phenoxyacetic acid derivatives, paraquat and dinitro compounds, chlorates, chlorophenols, and T.M.T.D., D.D.T. and other chlorinated hydrocarbons, such as B.H.C., D.D.D., aldrin, endrin, dieldrin, chlordone and toxaphene are or have been widely used. Many of these compounds are stored in the fat-containing tissues of the body, and are thus cumulative in effect.

MOLLUSCICIDES such as copper sulphate and metaldehyde used for killing slugs and snails, are of importance only in water birds and other species which may eat quantities of poisoned molluscs.

RODENTICIDES are for killing rats and mice. The older and simpler substances, such as phosphorus, arsenic, zinc phosphide, cyanides and strychnine, have gone out of general use. But they are still obtainable in some countries and are a danger to animals if the poisoned bait is left in accessible places. Newer substances widely used as rodenticides, insecticides and acaricides, include the organic phosphorus compounds, such as parathion, malathion, schradan, dirnefox and dipterex, some of which contain sulphur, fluorine or nitrogen atom groupings and are developments of some of the most revolting poison gases created during the last war. They are frequently used in agriculture as crop sprays. The commercial ones now in favour are a little more toxic to mammals than D.D.T., but some, for example parathion, are much more toxic to birds than to mammals; some in fact are very dangerous merely on contact with the skin. Some accumulate in the liver from repeated small doses and if other organo-phosphorus compounds are taken as well, their toxicity is increased. They kill by so deranging the nervous system that increased excitability and uncontrollable convulsive movements lead to paralysis of the muscles. Some substances also cause massive liver or kidney destruction and contribute to the nervous effect by creating toxic by-products in the blood and tissues. The danger of these organic substances is their ability to spread easily through many tissues on account of their similarity to the normal chemicals of the body. Many are chemically stable and persist in soil, vegetation and animal tissues.

DISINFECTANTS AND DISINFESTANTS are numerous and valuable in the maintenance of hygiene, but they must be used sensibly. Some people when using disinfectants unfortunately work on the principle that "If one spoonful is good, five spoonfuls must be five times better!" This is exactly when trouble is likely to arise.

Removal of all birds from cages and aviaries is essential when noxious paints, aerosols or gases are used. Hydrocyanic acid is one of the most poisonous substances to man, mammals and birds, but phenol or cresols, carbon monoxide, sulphur dioxide and many others can be highly dangerous. Birds must not be replaced in disinfected quarters for some hours or days, depending on the persistence and toxicity of the chemical which has been used.

DRUGS in excessive quantities can virtually all be toxic— as can even foods in excessive amounts. The safety of a drug depends on its "therapeutic index", which is the ratio of a lethal dose to a useful or therapeutic one. With some drugs, for example vitamins, the safety margin is very wide, but some antibiotics and many of the newer drugs need to be used with care. Anaesthetics and some of the older worming or purgative medicines can be particularly dangerous and should never be used except under the guidance of a veterina-

327

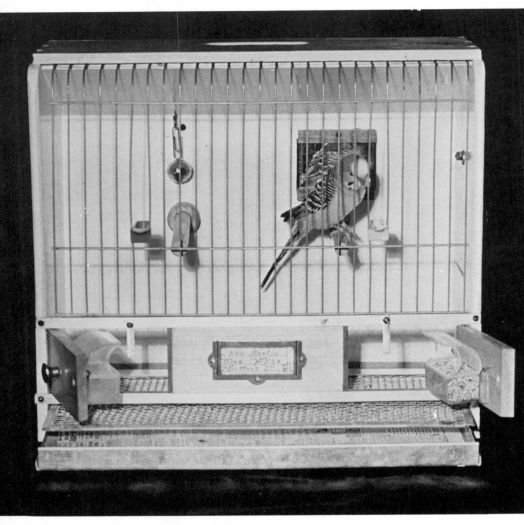

Example of a common, small and unsatisfactory type of cage. Cages of this construction should only be used for exhibition purposes, or for purposes during which birds are required to be housed for extremely short periods of time.

rian. As cage-bird species differ in their ability to deal with overdosages, care is always necessary.

GASES, such as carbon monoxide or anaesthetics in excessive amounts are lethal.

All except malicious poisoning is accidental and is usually due to thoughtlessness or simply ignorance. Untidiness, for example, after repairs to cage or aviary can lead to an inquisitive bird pecking at or eating toxic paints or other substances. Leaving the car running in a garage near to an enclosed aviary may result in carbon monoxide poisoning. Allowing labels to fall off packets or bottles which contain pesticides or dangerous drugs may result in poisoning if the contents are inadvertently used for the wrong purpose.

Intentional poisoning is rare in birds. With dogs and cats, where disturbance from noise or dug-up flowerbeds result in campaigns of neighbourly hate, for every case of deliberate poisoning confirmed there are many others where the owner is mistakenly obsessed with the idea that the sudden death of a pet has been caused by a machiavellian, pet-hating neighbour! Since cage birds are mainly harmless and unobjectionable, the proportion dying unexpectedly from deliberate poisoning is very small indeed.

As far as chlorinated hydrocarbon compounds such as D.D.T. and organo-phosphorous compounds are concerned, the minute amounts of the tasteless and odourless chemical necessary to cause illness or death can only be identified by a few specialized laboratories and often only by the company of manufacture. The testing procedure is extremely expensive and such poisoning must often remain only suspected. It is essential, however, in all cases of possible poisonings to be able to suspect certain specific substances, if poison tests are to be carried out; contrary to popular belief there is no single test which will demonstrate the presence of "a poison".

A further complication in diagnosing poisoning is that some poisons are cumulative, being stored in the liver, endocrine glands or fatty tissues. The clinical signs may thus start long after the bulk of the toxic dose has been eaten or absorbed. The fourth or fifth batch of contaminated seed for example, may coincide with the first signs of illness. Similarly, there may be a long delay after crops or garden plants near an outside aviary have been sprayed several times, before any of the birds show signs of poisoning.

A veterinarian should always be called in when poisoning of any type is suspected. When a specific substance is strongly suspected, a telephone call to the nearest chemist may reveal a specific antidote; this, however, should only be administered under veterinary supervision since the cure may prove more toxic than the suspected poison!

329

SELECTED BIBLIOGRAPHY

CLARKE, E. G. C. & CLARKE, M. L. (1967). *Garners' Veterinary Toxicology*. 3rd Ed. London, Baillière, Tindall & Cassell. 477pp.

HUNGERFORD, T. G. (1969). Poisoning. In *Diseases of Poultry including Cage Birds and Pigeons,* p.381–392. 4th Ed. Sydney, London, Melbourne. Angus and Robertson.

PECKHAM, M. C. (1965). Poisons and Toxins. In *Diseases of Poultry,* p.1212–1252. Eds. Biester. H. E. and Schwarte, L. H. 5th Ed. Ames, Iowa. State University Press.

ROSEN, M. N. (1971). Botulism. In *Infectious and Parasitic Diseases of Wild Birds,* p.100–117. Eds. Davis, J. W., Anderson, R. C., Karstad, L. and Trainer, D. O. Ames, Iowa. State University Press.

METABOLIC DISEASES

This group covers those diseases where the chemistry of the body has been disturbed. Sometimes we can explain how and where the mechanism has gone wrong, but we can rarely explain why. There is no obvious cause—such as an invasion by bacteria or other infectious agent. In a proportion of cases it is possible to trace the trouble back to a derangement of the hormone production of the ductless glands. As explained in Chapter 2, these hormones or so-called chemical messengers modify the rate and type of activity of many of the basic chemical reactions necessary for the life of each body cell and of the body as a whole. When hormones are produced in too small or excessive amounts, the body's complicated reactions cease to work properly.

Some of these disorders happen for no apparent reason, while others come about as the result of too much stress being placed on a particular system of the body. At first the organism takes the strain and gets along normally for a while. Eventually, however, illness in some form results. The stress may be starvation, unsuitable food, exhaustion, inactivity, fear or exposure to extremes of temperature. Sometimes a gland may be directly damaged by injury, or it may be replaced by tumour cells. The change of tissue cells from normal to those of a cancerous type could even be said to be a metabolic disorder; but since this tends to complicate an understanding of metabolic disorders, tumours are dealt with elsewhere (see Chapter 24).

Carbohydrates

The relationship of carbohydrates to disease is threefold. Carbohydrates (which include starches, sugars and cellulose) may be actually deficient in the diet: this is extremely rare in the average range of avian diets except when the bird is starved, fed grossly abnormal foods, or is completely off nourishment for some reason. Carbohydrates may be inadequately metabolized due to lack of certain vitamins, an excess of indigestible fibrous food, mechanical interference with digestion, or pancreatic disease affecting digestive processes. Thirdly, they may cause disease by virtue of their quantity being excessive in the diet in relation to other essential foods.

Defects in carbohydrate metabolism are common even when the proportion and types of these foods are correct. Normal utilization depends first on absorption from the gut. If gut movement or secretions are abnormal, including those in the stomach and from the pancreas, regurgitation or diarrhoea are liable to result. The causes are numerous and include vitamin deficiencies, infections, foreign bodies, exhaustion of the adrenal cortical tissue and some types of poisoning. In old age, spontaneous carbohydrate digestive disturbances arise especially when good quality protein is low in the diet. Excessive dietary intake of carbohydrates is not necessarily associated with overeating. Highly efficient digestion and absorption, with an impairment of the "overflow" mechanism of surplus food can lead to the accumulation of excessive amounts of body fat. Normally this is deposited in special fat depots designed for the purpose, under the skin, lining the body cavity, and so forth. In certain glandular dysfunctions and other disorders due to almost unknown causes, fat may be deposited practically anywhere in the body, such as in the connective tissues which hold the various organs together. This fatty infiltration is most noticeable in the highly active organs such as the liver, heart and kidneys, which it severely hampers.

Fats and oils

A lack of fats and especially oils tends to hinder the absorption of the fat-soluble vitamins A and E, and results in their deficiency even when they are present in the food. If fats in the diet are low, the carbohydrate and protein constituents also are not efficiently used. Although recognizable illness may not show itself, the bird tends to overeat, converting carbohydrate to body fat which has a damaging effect on tissues, particularly the arteries, and makes the bird sluggish. A high fat diet may upset the digestion, and tends to reduce the appetite; unless excessive, this produces a lean but active bird with a glossy plumage.

Mineral oils such as liquid paraffin are not absorbed and in lubricating the alimentary tract they also remove valuable fat-soluble vitamins, these becoming excreted in the faeces. Vitamins such as A and E are oxidized and damaged by substances in rancid oils. The oily seeds like linseed do not suffer from this rancidity, while still intact and fresh; but heat-treated pellets, dead stale gentles, and above all stale cod-liver oil are important causes of ill health from vitamin destruction. The chemicals which cause fat rancidity are themselves poisonous to birds.

Fats are a concentrated source of energy, but they are largely replaceable in this function by carbohydrates; some oils or unsaturated fats are, however, more chemically active and appear to be essential for growing chicks, if not for adult birds. Most seeds and nuts contain these "oily fats" and are therefore preferable to animal fats, except fish oils.

Proteins

Even when analysis of a foodstuff may show a reasonable proportion of protein, say 12–16 per cent, it does not necessarily mean that the protein it contains is of value to birds. Much vegetable protein is of poor quality because it contains insufficient of the essential amino-acids. In fact, seeds commonly fed to cage birds, such as the millets and maize, are low in total protein and are also deficient in methionine, cysteine, tyrosine, and certain other amino-acids. Turkish hemp, niger seed, teazle, and some other so-called "tonic foods" are better in this respect. When poor quality protein foods are fed, health suffers according to the tissue most starved of amino-acid nourishment. Since glandular tissues, muscle and skin have high requirements of those amino-acids which contain sulphur, prolonged periods on a diet deficient in this way lead to hepatic and renal disease, poor breeding, scurfy skins, faded plumage and muscle weakness.

Excessive protein in the diet of grain-eating birds increases the requirements of vitamin B12, which may produce signs of vitamin B deficiency, especially in nestlings. Scavenging and meat- or fish-eating birds normally flourish on a diet containing 25-30 per cent good quality protein. Not only does their diet contain considerable amounts of B12, but their constitution is adapted to this high protein diet. The protein requirements of birds in general appear to be higher than those of mammals. The high requirements of breeding hens and nestling chicks are met by the parent providing much animal protein in the form of invertebrates such as insects or in the case of pigeons the special fluid known as crop-milk and a similar proventricular secretion in budgerigars. In captivity, a common source is egg food.

A long-term result of both very high or very low amounts of protein in the diet is the deposition of gouty deposits through the body. This may be the result of stress and exhaustion of normal kidney tissue, toxicity of the amino-acid glycine, or damage to the kidneys by lack of the raw materials for their repair.

Vitamin Deficiencies

With one or two notable exceptions, there has been very little experimental work on vitamin deficiencies or imbalances in cage birds. Most of our knowledge is derived from information on the effects of deficiencies in the fowl, turkey, duck, or pigeon applied to similar symptoms in cage birds. This may not always lead to a clear understanding of such diseases,

333

especially as single deficiencies or excesses rarely occur naturally.

Deficiencies of this vitamin lead to lowered resistance to disease, especially by the skin and mucous membranes. Mucous membrane lines the mouth, nostrils, pharynx and the alimentary, respiratory, urinary and genital tracts. The tubular glands branching off from these tracts may become blocked by damaged cells and exudate, whilst the tubules of the kidney are also affected. It is not therefore surprising that lesions caused by vitamin A deficiency may be widespread. The clinical signs most commonly seen in young pigeons and some other birds, consist of rattling, respiratory sounds, and mucoid or purulent discharges from the eyes, nostrils, mouth, and even the vent. The discharges are partly made up of abnormally thickened, horny membrane and portions of dead cells thrown off the mucous membranes. If the inside of the mouth is examined, ulcers and cheesy, necrotic or diptheritic membranes can be seen, the latter occurring as soft, whitish, loose deposits which partially block the nostrils, throat or glottis. Beneath the eyelids and in the sinus below the eyes a thick, cheesy deposit sometimes builds up and causes a bulge in the overlying skin; these exudates are partly produced by bacteria which flourish in the damaged membranes. Other features of vitamin A deficiency are dullness of the plumage, weakness and poor appetite, and unsteadiness which suggests that even nerve function may be impaired. When a breeding female is deficient, the eggs she produces show a high incidence of dead-in-the-shell and weakly chicks.

Post-mortem findings include pale kidneys and sometimes gouty deposits on several organs.

Deficiency of vitamin A is most likely to be confused with trichomoniasis, candidiasis (moniliasis), pox, and possibly aspergillosis, since all these show similar exudates in the upper respiratory and alimentary tracts.

Treatment can be carried out by injections or oral dosing of vitamin A or by providing foods containing a high proportion of the vitamin. But since infections sometimes also play a part in severe deficiency, the use of broad-spectrum antibiotics may also be necessary. It is often preferable to destroy affected young birds because normal growth and development is seldom completed and they remain stunted and disease-prone.

A clinical hypervitaminosis A (excess of vitamin A), does not appear to occur as a problem in birds.

A deficiency of this vitamin (see also Calcium and Phosphorus deficiency), which gives rise to rickets in the young, should be suspected when chicks of any species develop a bow-legged appearance with swollen joints. Affected birds are also stunted, and limb fractures may occur without any marked violence or accident having taken place. Deficient adult hens lay thin or soft-shelled eggs and the clutch size may be reduced. Leg weakness in adult birds, softening of the beaks and claws, fractures or bending of the bones, including caved-in ribs, denote vitamin D deficiency which is called osteomalacia, or adult rickets. Small knob-like swellings can also sometimes be felt on the ribs at the junction of the vertebral and sternal parts.

Deficiencies of vitamin D_2 and especially D_3 in birds prevent absorption of calcium and phosphorus, both of which are essential in order to strengthen the bones and support the body.

A marked excess of vitamin D_3 which can be reproduced by repeated administration of the vitamin in large amounts, rarely occurs. When it does, however, it is liable to cause kidney damage. Calcium salts become deposited in the walls of the kidney tubules and in the walls of blood vessels, especially the major arteries as they leave the heart. This syndrome has been seen in aged parrots and cockatoos although it is not possible to relate its occurrence to excess vitamin D_3 in the diet.

Treatment by administration of vitamin D_3 in deficient birds is best carried out by injection, which is quicker than by giving it in the diet.

Vitamin E No reports of softening of the brain due to lack of this vitamin have been made in cage birds. It is also known as encephalomalacia and results in "crazy chick disease" in poultry.

In foodstuffs, vitamin E protects oils and vitamin A against destruction by oxidation or rancidity, but in doing so is itself destroyed. There is therefore a constant danger of a deficiency of this vitamin when foods are fortified with cod liver oil.

Deficiency of vitamin E seems to show itself differently in different species and includes wastage of muscle fibres, the encephalomalacia referred to above, exudation or dropsy of the tissues, and enlarged hocks. Adult birds do not often appear to suffer severe damage to the testes and reproductive powers as do some mammals, but this possibility should be borne in mind when confronted by problems of infertility and breeding. Although hens deficient in vitamin E continue to lay eggs, the embryonic development is impaired and embryos are liable to die early in the incubation period.

Crippling hock enlargements are quite commonly seen in some cage-bird chicks, but whether any of these cases are due

335

to deficiencies of vitamin E is uncertain. Provision of fresh natural foods, such as the germ of wheat and other grains and some green foods, is preferable to dosing with the vitamin when a deficiency is suspected.

The Vitamin B Complex

The vitamins in this group are so closely interdependent in their functions that it is customary to deal with them together. It is likely that if one is lacking, the others are also. Deficiencies of this complex can only be suspected with reasonable certainty when the symptoms are similar to those proved to be caused by deficiency in other birds and mammals, and when also the birds respond to treatment by restoring the suspected vitamin deficiency in the diet.

Leg and wing weakness, clenched feet, "slipped-toe", curled toes and other evidence of neuromuscular disorders suggest aneurine (thiamine) or possibly riboflavin deficiency, especially in chicks; although there are many more likely alternative causes, such as arthritis or injury, and in adult budgerigars pressure from a renal tumour on the sciatic nerve.

Other nervous signs (see Chapter 18), such as tilting back of the head, weakness of the neck, violent tremors, convulsions, inco-ordinated movements sometimes leading to coma and death, may signify a shortage of aneurine or pyridoxine or perhaps a folic acid deficiency. In adults, such signs are often attributable to circulatory or respiratory disease, head injuries and brain tumours, or the terminal stages of some infectious diseases.

Poor feathering, including stunted feather growth or loss of pigment in the feathers may be due to riboflavin, pantothenic acid, or folic acid deficiency; such causes, however, as French moult, protein deficiency, thyroid or pituitary disease must not be overlooked.

Dermatitis of the scaly parts of the legs and scabs on the head near the beak and on the eyelids are sometimes due to deficiencies of riboflavin, pantothenic acid, and biotin, as well as acute lack of vitamin A or oil.

Deformities of the skeleton, especially the long bones of the limbs and beaks, and swollen hocks, make investigation into the diets of affected chicks and breeding hens worthwhile. Possible deficiencies include pantothenic acid, nicotinic acid, biotin, folic acid, and choline as well as vitamin D_3 and minerals such as calcium and phosphorus.

Calcium and Phosphorus

These are so closely interdependent in their actions that they will be considered together. Both minerals are essential to the diet and need to be present in the correct ratio. The ideal ratio varies somewhat, not only according to the age of the

336

bird and whether or not eggs are being produced, but also possibly according to the species. Generally speaking, however, the proportions of phosphorus to calcium should be between 1.5:1 and 3:1, provided that sufficient vitamin D is also supplied to assure absorption of the minerals. Most of the calcium in avian foods is absorbed. No common food is rich in this mineral, but green foods, especially clover, and animal foods supply a proportion of the requirements. The remainder comes from the soluble or shell grit, which is eaten in noticeably greater amounts by breeding birds. Phosphorus is abundant in the common cereal foods fed to birds, but a large part is in an unavailable form. Animal foods such as gentles contain much less, although it is mostly absorbable.

Calcium is most likely to be deficient in the diet of young birds and provision of calcium in the form of soluble grit is essential. Certain disorders of the kidneys and gut, however, may lead to a deficiency owing to inadequate absorption.

Rickets and osteomalacia are the result of deficiencies or abnormal ratios of calcium to phosphorus in the diets of chicks and adults respectively. Brittle and easily fractured bones, result from these two diseases. The clinical and radiographic changes seen in the bones of young parrots and other young birds are sometimes similar to those reproduced in dogs on a diet containing normal amounts of calcium and very high phosphorus, with normal or high vitamin D_2 intake.

In breeding birds, shell-less or thin-shelled eggs are often laid and the embryos are stunted or chicks weakly on hatching. Although phosphorus comprises barely 1 per cent of the shell of eggs, it is nevertheless essential to its construction. It is also present in chemical combination in egg yolk. When birds are breeding, the extra phosphorus excreted is much greater than that used in the egg itself. Species which will eat manufactured crumbs or meals can be given a bone-meal additive to maintain a favourable calcium, phosphorus and magnesium intake.

Magnesium   This is seldom deficient in the diet because it is present in most avian foodstuffs, often in association with calcium and phosphorus. An excessive intake may lead to diarrhoea, possibly nervousness in poultry, and even deformed bones as a result of interference with the balance of calcium and phosphorus; but the latter minerals in adequate amounts and proportions will permit tolerance of a moderate excess. The mineral is essential for carbohydrate metabolism and in certain enzyme activities.

Sodium and salt   Neither deficiency nor excess of either are likely to occur in

337

cage birds owing to the high proportion of natural food usually fed and the unlikelihood of salted food being available or accepted by them. Extremes of both interfere with normal growth; excess produces severe thirst, weakness and possibly convulsions prior to death. Deficiencies are more likely to arise from an undue demand by the body for these elements when vomiting or serious exudation occur.

Potassium

This is so readily available in natural foodstuffs that a deficiency is improbable. The mineral is essential for the metabolic processes of the body and for the formation of all body tissues.

Iron and Copper

Iron deficiency can result from haemorrhage, from wounds for example, but more commonly from attacks by mites or ticks. Ulcers and other lesions that cause repeated small blood loss can also have a similar effect. Normal requirements are greatly raised when birds are laying and deficiencies may occur. Iron is closely linked with copper in the production and maintenance of blood and the constituents of eggs. Excessive iron supplied in the diet is not absorbed and is therefore harmless, but excessive copper is highly toxic, building up in and damaging the liver and other active organs. When copper is low in the diet, iron is absorbed and stored in the liver and is not used adequately in the manufacture of the blood pigment haemoglobin. Anaemia then results.

Sulphur

This is obtained in adequate amounts whenever the bird eats enough good quality protein, containing a high proportion of the amino-acids cysteine and methionine. Plant foods supply sulphur unconnected with organic substances in the simple inorganic forms such as ferrous sulphate. Egg contains a very high proportion of sulphur, and the characteristic smell of bad eggs is due to the production of hydrogen sulphide. A minute amount of sulphur is supplied by the vitamins aneurin and biotin. Even during laying, deficiency is unlikely to occur; but if it does, it will show itself largely as the thio-amino-acid deficiency (see protein deficiencies) which affects feathers, skin, heart, muscular and glandular tissues, as well as egg production.

Iodine

Iodine is liable to be deficient inland in areas where it is lacking in the soil and where birds eat nothing but local-grown food. Breeding increases the body's requirements for this element, so the young of parents on the borderline of insufficiency are most likely to show clinical signs of iodine deficiency such as thyroid disease or goitre. Fish-eating birds fed on sea fish derive adequate amounts of iodine from their diet and this type of goitre is hence unknown in seabirds. Even the oyster shell used as soluble grit contains an appreciable amount of iodine and so occurrences of goitre are comparatively rare except in budgerigars.

Enlargement of the thyroid gland in adult budgerigars is mostly the result of iodine deficiency; the affected gland contains inactive secretion, resulting in a lowered metabolism, sluggishness, ragged plumage with loss of pigmentation and a general slowing of bodily activities. In budgerigars, the most characteristic sign is laboured breathing associated with squeaking noises, this being due to pressure of the enlarged thyroids on the syrinx and lower trachea. In chicks and nestlings, the deficiency results in stunted growth and retarded mental and physical activities. Provision of an iodised supplement rapidly removes the clinical signs of disease except in far advanced cases. Many compounded cage-bird foods are nowadays impregnated with iodine. Certain foods can lessen the effect of the iodine available in the food; soya bean is an example.

Manganese Deficiency of manganese may play a part in the formation of enlarged hocks and slipped tendons sometimes found in growing cage birds, but this is not certain. Investigations into the rôle of the mineral in French moult of budgerigars have brought forth no definite evidence of this disease coming from manganese deficiency. The shortening and deformity of bones and spinal column in growing poultry when the diet is manganese-deficient, have not yet been reported in cagebirds but this is probably due to lack of research: this also applies to poor bone formation in the skeleton of the embryo and mortalities in the last third of the incubation period. Chemical analysis of bone and tissues would establish whether this or other deficiencies are responsible.

Other Trace Elements The rôles of molybdenum, selenium and zinc are incompletely known in cage birds. They probably assist in the development and maintenance of certain tissues.

Cobalt is important only inasmuch as it is part of the vitamin B12 molecule. If this vitamin is adequately synthesized by bacteria, no extra cobalt is required.

Water The intake of water, its utilization and excretion involve a very delicately balanced mechanism. Birds do not carry much useless water around with them in the form of urine. Nevertheless, their tissues contain almost 70 per cent water. Certain centres in the brain govern thirst and water intake; these are operated by changes in the chemical content of the blood, and this in turn is dependent on how much water is taken and excreted.

A bird has the normal stimuli to drink, but during some illnesses abnormal ones operate. These illnesses are salt or arsenic poisoning, when there is a high temperature associated with certain infections; heatstroke; loss of fluid by evaporation from panting in respiratory disease; loss of fluid in regurgitation, vomiting or diarrhoea; and when there is irritation to the kidneys. Excessive thirst is not always accompanied by loss of abnormal fluid. Even when it is, water intake cannot always keep up with water wastage. Soluble minerals and food substances are also lost when excessive vomiting, diarrhoea, or increased urine output occurs and these losses are not made up by drinking. Mineral deficiencies or imbalance will therefore result.

Water input, output, and reabsorption by the kidneys and gut are controlled by hormones from the pituitary and adrenal glands, which can influence the blood flow to the kidneys. Very many different diseases may interfere with some stage of these processes, which are designed to maintain a uniform balance of water in the bird. Some of the diseases are mentioned elsewhere in this book.

Roughage or Fibre

This important commodity if taken in an excessive amount, can be dangerous to health since it can cause impaction of the crop and gizzard where food normally stays for a time. This is especially true in debilitated birds. A diet high in fibre is often low in nutriments, and the functions of the gut are then impaired. A deficient bird is a weakened one and therefore the muscular power of the gut is also weakened. A laxative should be given followed by a more concentrated but easily digested diet: soaked or sprouted seed, egg, milk, cheese, liver, yeast or gentles, according to the species concerned. Treatment of impaction of the crop is dealt with elsewhere.

Insufficient fibre tends to produce a small amount of pasty, tenacious faeces which may matt the vent feathers or cause constipation. Under these circumstances the urinary excretion forms a relatively higher proportion of the droppings. When birds are fed concentrated diets lacking in fibre, there is a tendency for kidney disease and gout to occur.

Predominantly grain-eating birds, especially pigeons, are seldom affected with either excess or lack of fibre, although an unaccustomed bird allowed out into an aviary planted with grass and weeds may gorge itself on this roughage;

mineral deficiencies can make birds more prone to this habit. Crop and gizzard impactions are particularly common in large omnivores such as ostriches, emus, rheas and bustards. Members of the parrot and crow families, often given human food such as scraps and cake, are most likely to suffer from lack of roughage and it can lead to wasting or atrophy of the gizzard and gut muscles. Species such as fruit and nectar-eating birds with poorly developed gizzards do not appear to need fibre.

Obesity It is well known that some humans and animals, including birds, tend to become fat very readily. Others, however, remain slim, even though they may be eating far more. The differences lie in their metabolism, their rate of living.

Obesity can occur or be induced in many species of mammal or bird. It is often purely a result of overeating, coupled with inactivity in a protected environment. *Pâté de foie gras* is produced by force-feeding geese with starchy food until the liver is overladen with fat. This fatty infiltration of the liver is also seen in disease, during pregnancy in mammals, and in obesity in all species. At times, a normal volume of food intake, unbalanced or deficient in some way, results in obesity. The budgerigar is a common victim, although other birds are affected, including parrots, pigeons, quail and poultry. In budgerigars the incidence may be partly due to the fancier breeding for big, imposing birds. Prize winners in Britain are almost exclusively oversized and even a trifle obese; in their youth these birds are often quite active, but many become heavier and more sluggish after 18 to 24 months, the incidence of unhealthy or non-breeding birds being higher in the better show specimens. This fact is not readily admitted by breeders lest demand for their stock falls. Obesity in budgerigars and parrots may be a general weight increase or be confined to the breast (a major depôt of fat storage), thighs or other localized sites. In such birds there are generally degenerative changes in such vital internal organs as the liver and kidneys, and in the blood-vessel walls and heart muscle. These changes and the obesity result in an increased rate of breathing, especially after a short flight or other exercise. By placing an ear to the breast or back it is possible to detect rattling bronchial sounds together with rapid, faint heart beats or a very slow heart rate in later stages. The breathing sounds may suggest to the listener the presence of lung infection by viruses, bacteria or fungi, but their slow onset tends to rule out all but the fungal complication. Chilling and infections are a hazard for such sluggish birds and are quite common in those in which the respiration and blood circulation are hampered by the pressure of fat.

In a high proportion of obese budgerigars and those which

have previously been obese the thyroid gland has been found to be enlarged; this type of obesity is discussed in Chapter 19.

Medical treatment has proved quite effective in both slimming and rejuvenating budgerigars with "middle-aged spread". Firstly, however, the possibility of there being another simultaneous disease should be checked; the heart, kidney, digestive and respiratory systems should also be examined for natural functioning. In the absence of infections the obese bird should be transferred to a flight or aviary, either indoors or out depending on the circumstances of the weather. A slimming diet is best given to an isolated bird, although more exercise is possible where several birds share an aviary. If food is restricted, the stronger birds which are higher in the pecking order, will take the bulk of it. A daily ration of three to two level teaspoonfuls of high protein-content food, given at two or three evenly spaced times throughout the hours of daylight, is an adequate diet. No other seed is to be offered. A useful high protein diet is as follows:

Millet	2 parts
Spanish canary	2 parts
Hard rape	1 part
Niger	1 part
Turkish hemp	1 part
Teazle	1 part
Linseed	1 part
Egg crumbs	1 part

Other additions which may be made include finely minced meat and a range of fresh green stuffs and fruit—cabbage, Brussels sprouts, lettuce, spinach, groundsel, young lawn grass, carrot, turnip, apple, grape and orange.

Additional vitamins and minerals may be added in the form of fresh fish-liver oil and powdered supplement based on dried liver, yeast and wheat germ. Alternatively, a more accurately dosed multi-vitamin mixture can be dissolved in the drinking water. A more expensive but reliable method involves the use of the seed impregnated with vitamins supplied by several pet-food firms. But if only the husks are impregnated, such treated seed is of less value to birds like budgerigars which de-husk seed before eating it.

When a bird is being slimmed, its rationing should not be extended beyond 10 to 21 days (according to response) before a break is given. This is because budgerigars in particular have conservative eating habits and may select only certain seeds from the ration. Some birds will die of starvation rather than eat strange seeds. Ten days reduced diet followed by seven on normal food, repeated until the desired weight is reached, is a useful rule-of-thumb guide.

When localized breast (Plate 1/23) or belly fat deposits

(Plate 2/23) become so large as to ulcerate by friction against the perch, it is sometimes necessary to remove the mass surgically. The diseased skin is cut away and the fatty mass removed with a blunt instrument.

Ruptures of the abdominal wall are often a result of fat infiltrating and replacing much of the abdominal muscles (Plate 3/23). Fatty livers or other lesions causing an increase in the volume of abdominal contents exert an added strain on the abdominal wall. As this stretches, the damage stimulates a response towards attempted repair: fine blood vessels and cells which form scar-tissue appear in muscle remnants, producing a soft fleshy layer of so-called granulation tissue. This has very little tensile strength, and tension combined with gravity serve to make the distension more and more pendulous. As a consequence the oviduct, intestines or lobes of the enlarged liver protrude into the sac so formed and become tangled with strands of the abdominal muscle wall. The displaced organs can no longer function normally and retained eggs, cystic oviducts and bowel obstruction frequently result.

SELECTED BIBLIOGRAPHY

HUNGERFORD, T. G. (1969). Minerals and Mineral Deficiencies, p.44–55. Vitamin and Vitamin Deficiencies, p.55–97. In *Diseases of Poultry including Cage Birds and Pigeons*. 4th Ed. Sydney, London, Melbourne. Angus and Robertson.

MINSKY, L. (1969). Metabolic and Miscellaneous Conditions. In *Diseases of Cage and Aviary Birds,* p.491–497. Ed. Petrak, M. L., Philadelphia. Lea and Febiger.

TAYLOR, T. G. (1969). Nutritional Deficiencies. In *Diseases of Cage and Aviary Birds,* p.233–235. Ed. Petrak, M. L., Philadelphia. Lea and Febiger.

(See also references, Chapter 3)

TUMOURS, CYSTS AND SIMILAR STRUCTURES

A "tumour" simply means a swelling, and the use of the term is usually confined to swellings which are not directly caused by inflammation.

The term "neoplasm", has a roughly parallel meaning. It literally signifies a new growth, except that while it is initially developing it may not be recognizable as a swelling or tumour. The cells of a true neoplasm grow and multiply without the customary controls exerted by the body. The cells closely resemble the healthy cells from which they arise, but they are not arranged in any orderly fashion as they multiply and so far as is known they serve no useful function.

Tumours are occasionally found in most avian species, but neoplasms in budgerigars form a high proportion of that species' diseases, in which indeed they appear to be more common than in any other vertebrate animal.

Tumours can affect any area or tissue of the body (see Figures 1/24 and 2/24), including the blood, but a high proportion of tumours exist in, or just beneath the skin and produce a noticeable swelling. As time passes, more and more types are described and identified in cage birds, most bearing a close similarity in structure to those reported in man, mammals and especially poultry.

Types of neoplasms

Tumour pathologists or oncologists as they are known, have classified the diverse list of non-inflammatory tumours in several ways. Most tumours can be separated into those which are benign and relatively harmless and those which are malignant. Benign tumours are usually firm, enclosed in a fibrous coat, and fail to spread out of that capsule. Malignant tumours are generally softer, not encapsulated and tend to spread to other organs; they invade tissues by the easiest routes, such as between tissue masses and via the blood or lymph vessels, producing secondary tumours or so-called metastases. It is these malignant tumours which give rise to the disease known as cancer.

Oncologists classify tumours much further than this, however, depending on the origin of the cells from which they derive. It has been found that neoplasms correspond to almost

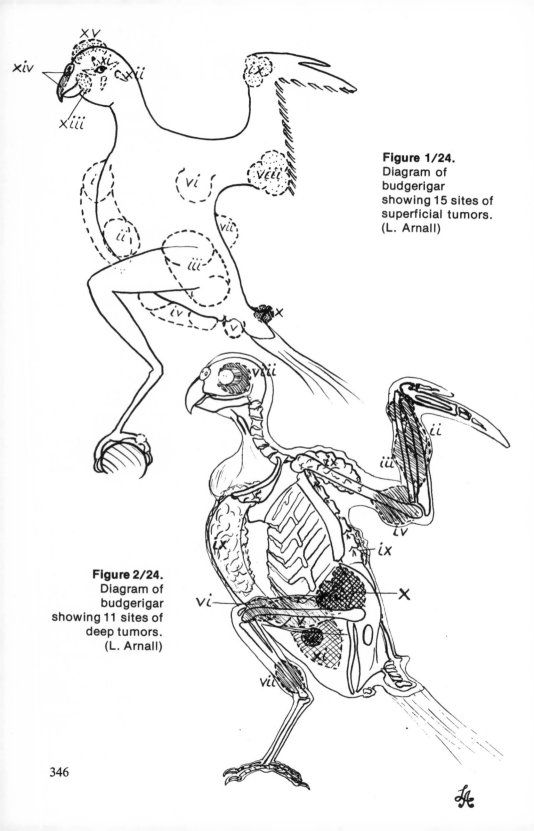

Figure 1/24.
Diagram of
budgerigar
showing 15 sites of
superficial tumors.
(L. Arnall)

Figure 2/24.
Diagram of
budgerigar
showing 11 sites of
deep tumors.
(L. Arnall)

every type of cell recognized in the body, but some come from cells occurring only at certain stages in embryonic development.

Benign tumours are usually named by adding "-oma" to the name of the tissue of origin. For example, a fibroma is a tumour of fibrous or connective tissue; a lipoma is a tumour of fat or adipose tissue; an adenoma is derived from glandular tissue, and an osteoma is a bone tumour. There are, however, some exceptions to this rule. If the tumours are malignant and resemble tissues which in the embryo were derived from so-called mesodermal tissues (see Chapter 2) they are known as sarcomas, those derived from ectodermal tissues being known as carcinomas. Thus a malignant tumour of fibrous or connective tissue is called a fibrosarcoma and a malignant, gland cell tumour is known as an adeno-carcinoma. Various odd terms such as papilloma are used for benign skin tumours or warts, this being an old name based on a fanciful likeness to a "little nipple". These names may sound a little confusing, but they are a neat way of describing the various neoplasms. Only a pathologist can pronounce the last word on the true nature of a growth, although a good guess can be made as to its type, from observing site, colour, consistency and speed of growth. A benign growth, if situated in a vital organ like the brain or the liver, can be as lethal as a malignant tumour owing to the vital space it fills and the mechanical pressure it exerts on surrounding tissues.

A tumour is not always a distinct sphere of tissue. Rapid growth in some neoplasms causes rupture of the capsule and exposure of the contents. Many tumours are multiple. They can start in several places at once, but sometimes fibrous tissue cuts a tumour into groups or clusters. Others, mainly the malignant types, allow groups of one or more cells to break off which are carried to different parts of the body by blood vessels or lymph and start growing wherever they are deposited. These metastases liberate chemicals into the system which rapidly lead to death. Birds, other than poultry, do not appear to be greatly afflicted by such metastasizing growths.

Normal Growths A number of structures are present on certain birds. These have functional or ornamental purposes. Some are present in one sex only and clearly play a part in courtship. The fleshy comb and wattles of poultry and the snood of turkeys both have a breeding and heat-regulating function. Some characteristics like the colours of the beak play a part in stimulating the response of nestlings to imminent food as soon as the parent appears near.

The cere of the budgerigar, the cere or wattle of the pigeon, the preen gland of numerous birds and the crest of the cardinal and cockatoo are all examples of specialized normal growths.

Some of these structures, for example the various feather variations and the distensible crop of the pouter pigeon, are man-made since they have been produced by selective breeding. Occasionally, as the result of breeding for an unusual type of feathering—the crested canaries for example—man has implanted in these birds the unwanted tendency to develop hereditary "lumps", which are feather cysts known as *"hypopteronosis cystica"* (see Chapter 25). The great majority of curious projections from the head and elsewhere in various breeds of canaries and pigeons are normal. Non-domesticated birds also show a wide range of feather variation. Although normal structures, these are by no means immune from disease, becoming injured or infected in the ordinary way and sometimes affected by neoplastic growths: seasonal variations in size and colour may also occur.

Some of the swellings found on the surface layers of birds are hard, hemispherical masses which make the skin bulge. They are painless and when the skin over them is cut, are seen to be lying free beneath the skin, apparently growing out of the underlying muscle, bone or other tissue. A deeper incision may reveal yellowish, cheesy contents which represent dead tissue. Lesions of this kind may be of several different origins. Some are abscesses which are relatively uncommon in birds, except for the chronic or so-called "cold" abscesses. The vast majority of such cheesy masses are devoid of any pathogenic bacteria. In racing pigeons, they are quite common in the breast and shoulder region; the contents are usually more fibrous and greasy than in other species, and sometimes contain a meshwork of fungal hyphae, usually *Aspergillus*. In such cases the swellings generally involve the interclavicular or subscapular parts of the airsac system. Sometimes a scar indicates where the exhausted bird has crash-landed into a wire or branch.

Pigeons, canaries and other species, especially budgerigars, sometimes develop skin swellings caused by fat tumours or lipomas. Usual sites are over the wings near the elbow or carpal joints, in the thigh (Plate 1/24) and less commonly on the neck and head. On the breast of budgerigars in particular, excessive fat deposits can sometimes assume tumour proportions. Skin lipomas are very prone to internal degeneration: the centre dies and may liquefy or become solid and granular, developing a greyish-pink or creamy colouration, which has little or no odour when opened. Some of these growths do not remain in the underlying tissues like a dome

Pathological Growths: Subcutaneous and Other Superficial Skin Growths

(the so-called sessile tumours), but separate and hang suspended in a fold of skin attached to the breast by small blood vessels, when they are known as pendulous or pedunculated tumours.

Sessile growths near joints are generally tumours of fibrous tissue or bone and are liable to be malignant. Fibromas can generally be removed by a veterinarian provided they are not too closely attached to muscle, bone or joints. Unfortunately it is seldom possible to be sure from external appearances whether such closely anchored masses are malignant or benign. Sarcomas and fibrosarcomas (malignant tumours) are almost as common as fibromas. Osteosarcomas, although less common than these, have been found affecting most bones of the limbs, the spinal column and also the skull. Perhaps the commonest bones involved are the femur, tibia, humerus, radius and ulna, especially near the joints.

When malignant tumours are suspected by a veterinarian, the only hope of saving the bird's life is amputation of the limb well above the growth. This would only be justified in a valuable bird needed for breeding, there being no evidence that such malignant tumours are hereditary. If a part only of any tumour is removed, especially a malignant one, it tends to speed the growth and spread of the remainder.

True skin tumours of birds papillomas (Plate 2/24), epitheliomas and carcinomas—are not common. Papillomas or warts seldom occur as frequently as they do in man and domesticated animals. A few sites which are prone to damage, such as the preen gland, the cere, the eyelids and the corners of the mouth, seem to develop a higher proportion of these tumours and related malignancies than other parts of the body.

Bizarre growths around the head are sometimes met with in budgerigars and less frequently in other birds. From their appearance they somewhat resemble horns (see Plate 3/24). In about half the cases, some evidence of knemidocoptic mange or "scaly face" is present, suggesting that the disease is basically an inflammatory response. In others not even pathogenic bacteria can be found. These horns generally grow out from the fleshy parts near the corners of the mouth, the eyelids and other parts of the face or mask as it is known in budgerigars. They are small knobs or pillar-shaped objects, beige or orange coloured, with a rough surface and are composed of a core of living tissue, well supplied with blood vessels, which is covered by scales of keratin and sebaceous material. They bleed profusely if incised, but can be pinched off, using ophthalmic-sized artery forceps. A little antibiotic dusting powder should be applied and an antiparasitic dressing may be necessary when *Knemidocoptes* mite infestation is suspected.

A number of non-neoplastic swellings may be confused with tumours. Near the joints, particularly those of the feet and to a lesser extent, the hock and tarsus (tarso-metatarsal region), shiny, creamy-yellow subcutaneous nodules which cause swelling, loss of joint movement and severe pain are generally signs of gout. Less frequently, the wing joints and cervical vertebrae are involved. Budgerigars are more frequently affected than other species.

Hard fibrous nodules on the soles of the feet, containing material like pus, sometimes covered with a strawberry-like swelling which has a tendency to bleed easily, usually represent infected corns. This type of lesion is called "bumble foot". It can be crippling, and prevent the bird from gripping its perch properly, as well as causing lameness.

Soft, fluctuating swellings anywhere on the body may be hematomas or blood blisters, cysts, or merely edematous areas. If they crackle on pressure, are translucent or give a soft hollow sound when lightly tapped, they probably contain air or gas and are emphysematous swellings (see Plates 2/11, 7/21 and 8/21).

Painful swellings of the limbs are liable to be fractures, or tumours of the bone-destroying type.

Feather cysts or so-called "lumps" in canaries, which are more correctly known as *hypopteronosis cystica* are hereditary and covered in Chapter 25.

Swellings affecting the Deeper layers of Muscle and Bone

In all species of vertebrates muscle is among those tissues least affected by tumours: cage birds are no exception. Tumours of other neighbouring tissues may spread between muscles or even infiltrate occasionally into muscle tissue itself, if malignant; but this is uncommon. Tumours of all three types of muscle—skeletal, smooth, and heart muscle—are extremely rare.

Bone is much more commonly affected than muscle, both by tumours (Plate 4/24) and affections of similar gross appearance. The benign slow-growing osteoma is rare, but chronic inflammatory bone thickenings are relatively common, and include periostitis, arthritis, gout, and certain other lesions of doubtful identity. Partially healed fractures can easily be confused with malignant bone tumours such as osteosarcomas (Plate 5/24). In such cases the affected limb is often swollen, hot and very painful; it is usually drawn up into an abnormal position. Manipulation will often show abnormal movement of the bone within the swelling. This is because the neoplastic cells invading the bone have caused it to fracture. This mostly occurs in long bones, such as the tibio-tarsus and tarso-metatarsus. When the bony orbit of the eye (Plate 6/24) or the spine is affected, a somewhat tender, hard or rubbery swelling is all that is obvious in the early stages. The faster the growth, the softer the swelling, because the most active tumour cells are incapable of depositing bone or calcium. Although not common, osteosarcomas are among the most unpleasant tumours of birds, being those most likely to metastasize.

The connective tissue is a common site of tumours. Fibrous, "fibro-fatty" (Plate 7/24), and fibro sarcomatous (Plate 8/24 and 9/24) tumours can occur anywhere in the body. Their consistency is the best guide to malignancy. A soft mass with little or no capsule is likely to be a cancerous or sarcomatous type.

Tumours of blood vessels rather than blood cells have rarely been reported.

Swellings of the Head, Brain and Spinal Cord In these areas, swellings are usually neoplastic in origin and the head, with its specialized, highly active parts, is quite a common site for tumours. Irritation of long duration such as is produced by a chronic infestation of the cere by Knemidocoptic mites or a deformed beak which hinders feeding, seem to favour the formation of malignant growths. Cancer, that is carcinomas (Plate 10/24) and sarcomas (Plate 11/24 and 12/24) of the beak, cere, forehead, eyelids and ear canal have been found both associated and unassociated with such irritations. Surgery is usually impossible, although cautery is successful in a few cases. Only a veterinarian, of course, should contemplate such drastic and potentially dangerous treatment. The mainly benign fatty and fibrous growths have already been dealt with.

Tumours of the brain and spinal cord are comparatively rare. Those confirmed on post-mortem examination in budgerigars usually affect the pituitary gland in the base of the brain. Clinical signs as the result of brain tumours vary enormously. With some tumours as the growth enlarges, the optic nerve may be compressed and result in blindness. General pressure on brain tissue results in abnormal behaviour, such as circling, staggering, inco-ordination of limbs and head, and metabolic disturbances. Local involvement of the area that controls feeding results in death within a few hours or a day or so, as the result of starvation. Diagnosis of the site, size and nature of brain growths on the basis of clinical signs is an unrewarding and virtually impossible exercise.

Swellings of the Internal Organs The diagnosis of a thoracic or abdominal neoplasm is often little more than an inspired guess. Circumstantial evidence may be present in abundance, but only in quite a small pro-

351

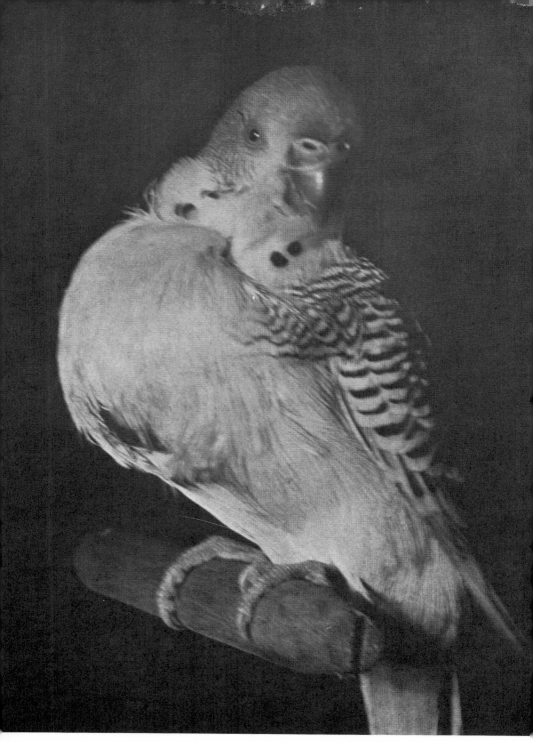

Plate 1/23. Budgerigar showing advanced lipomatosis of breast. (L. Arnall)

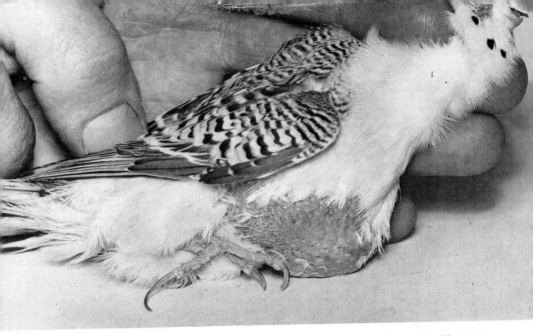

Plate 2/23. Abdominal swelling due to subcutaneous fat deposits (lipomatosis) in a budgerigar. (L. Arnall)

Plate 3/23. Pendulous, flaccid, abdominal rupture due to infiltration of the abdominal muscles with fat. Budgerigar. (L. Arnall)

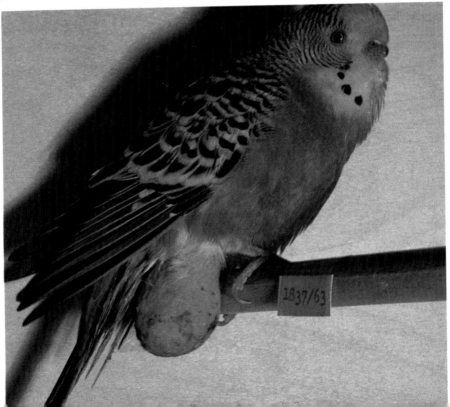

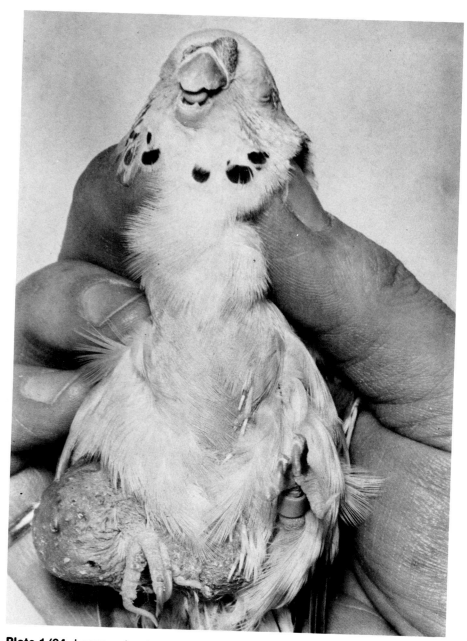

Plate 1/24. Large subcutaneous lipoma of the thigh of a budgerigar involving the right leg from hip to foot. Also note brown hypertrophy of the cere. (L. Arnall)

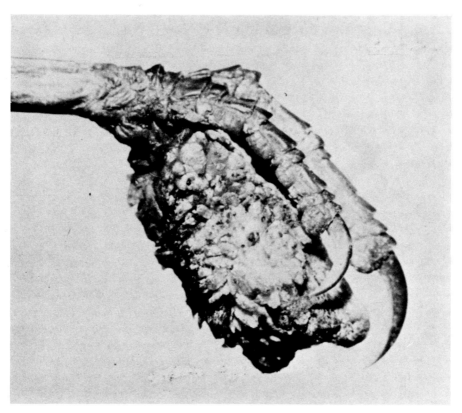

Plate 2/24. The foot of a wild chaffinch showing a tumour (papilloma) involving the hind digit; probably caused by a virus. (I.F. Keymer and T.C. Dennett, Z.S.L.)

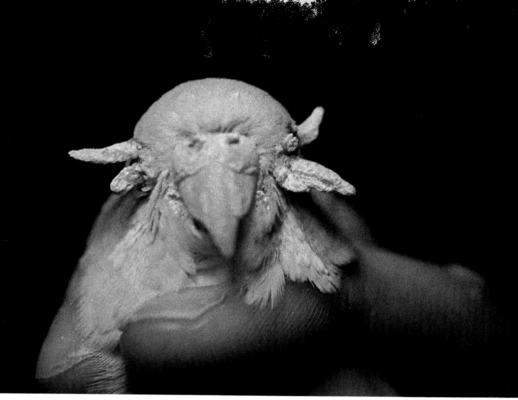

Plate 3/24. Horny structures around the eyes composed of keratin and sebaceous material, caused by *Knemidocoptes* infestation. Budgerigar. See also Plate 4/10. (L. Arnall)

Plate 4/24. Radiograph showing tumour involvement of humerus, ulna, radius and associated wing joint in a budgerigar. (L. Arnall)

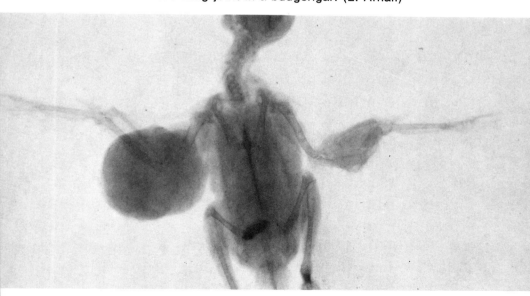

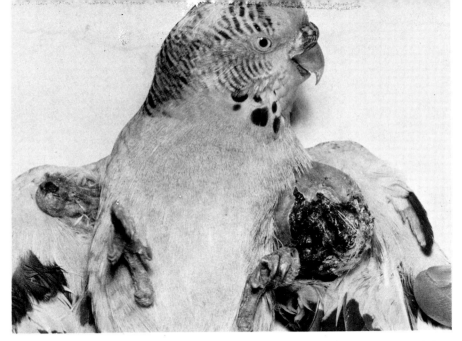

Plate 5/24. A 7-year-old budgerigar with tumours (osteosarcoma) involving ventral surface of the wing. (L. Arnall)

Plate 6/24. Sarcoma of the orbit of the eye with displacement of the eye and lids. Budgerigar. (L. Arnall)

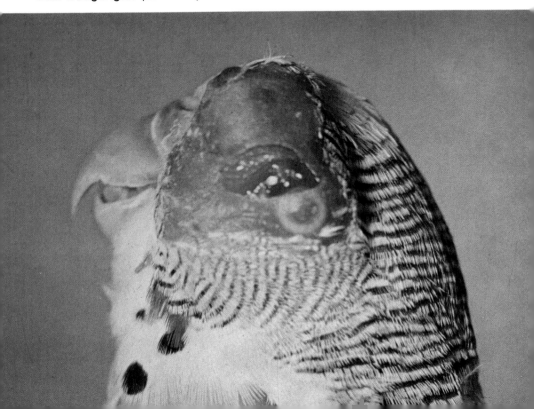

portion of cases can a swelling be felt in that limited area of the abdomen not enclosed by the bony skeleton.

Internal tumours cause illness in several ways:

1. By invading and destroying a vital organ, such as the liver or kidneys.
2. By liberating poisonous waste products into the tissue fluid and bloodstream.
3. By so enlarging and filling the limited space of the body cavity that neighbouring organs are squeezed and restricted in their action. Finally, they can no longer function adequately to support life.

The first two methods apply mainly to malignant tumours and the third to benign growths.

Organs which commonly become neoplastic are the testicles, ovaries (Plates 13/24 and 14/24), kidney (Plates 15/24 and 16/24), liver, spleen, thyroid gland, and lung; roughly in that order of frequency. Other organs are occasionally affected. Of those mentioned, all except the lung usually contain tumours composed of one or other of their own tissues, the lung being a frequent site of secondary tumours or metastases. More than one type of tumour can be present at the same time, the first to develop apparently having no suppressive effect on the development of another type in the same or another organ.

Because of their position, when any abdominal organs are affected by benign growths, the clinical signs produced as the result of pressure on adjacent organs are similar and indistinguishable from one another. The organs most sensitive to pressure are the lungs, heart and associated great vessels, and the gut. Pressure on the sciatic nerves caused by kidney tumours gives rise to leg paralysis.

Clinical signs denoting neoplasia of the internal organs include panting, gasping, tiring quickly, fainting attacks, fits of the epileptic type leading to inco-ordination and other nervous symptoms, constipation, diarrhoea, straining as if attempting to pass an egg, marked loss of weight, exhaustion and loss of consciousness. Swellings in the posterior part of the abdomen cause abdominal distension (Plate 17/24) which may even lead to rupture of the muscle layers of the abdominal wall.

Diffuse and malignant tumours invading the liver or kidney generally produce a wasting illness, with diarrhoea and watery, yellowish-white droppings and other evidence of indigestion which appear long before the abdomen shows enlargement.

Testicular and ovarian tumours, if they do not produce abnormal sexual behaviour patterns usually manifest clinical signs as the result of pressure on nearby organs, as well as abdominal swelling. They generally behave as benign growths and are among the few which are palpable through the

358

abdominal wall with gentle, intermittent probing of the fingers. Sometimes these tumours can be removed by a veterinarian under suitable anaesthesia.

Thyroid enlargements are not usually neoplastic but rather an overgrowth of the gland in an attempt to overcome the lack of such substances as iodine. Neoplastic growth, with or without excessive thyroxine production, is, like carcinoma of the thyroid gland, uncommon, although cases have been reported in budgerigars, parrots and pigeons. A description of clinical signs associated with thyroid enlargement is given elsewhere (see Chapter 19).

Leucosis   Leucosis is an abnormal multiplication of the cells which give rise to various types of white blood cells. All types of white cells, or rather their primitive formation stages, can multiply abnormally to form neoplastic tissue and give rise to forms of leucosis known as lymphatic, myeloid and erythroleucosis according to the types of cells mainly involved.

In spite of the excessive multiplication of blood elements in this way, only a small proportion of the circulating blood cells is altered, and so the term leukaemia or excess white cells in the blood is seldom appropriate. In poultry, lymphatic leucosis involving the nerves, liver and some other organs has a high incidence, and has been shown to be caused by a virus with an incubation period of several weeks or months.

In cage and aviary birds it is not yet certain whether leucosis occurs in the same forms in which it is seen in poultry, but pathologists have found similar diseases, especially in budgerigars (Plate 18/24) and less frequently in a few other species.

Clinical signs of leucosis include great loss of weight resulting in emaciation and death. Some birds show anaemia, and grey or yellowish diarrhoea often occurs when the disease is advanced. Appetite and activity are reduced, and handling or frightening the bird greatly increases its distress. When the bird is suffering from the nervous form of leucosis known as neurolymphomatosis or Marek's disease, partial paralysis of one or both legs occurs, or sometimes one or both wings. The leg weaknesses so commonly seen in caged birds, however, are much more likely to be due to other causes, there being many diseases which can produce similar clinical signs.

Except when more than one or two birds become affected in a single season, it is unlikely that the disease will be diagnosed except on post-mortem examination.

There is no treatment. Euthanasia is the only course when leucosis is suspected. It is inadvisable to continue to breed from stock which has bred affected birds. Birds which have been in contact with those affected or with parents of the diseased stock are liable to be infected as a virus is probably responsible for the disease.

Cysts

A cyst is a bag-like structure within a capsule of connective tissue and occasionally muscle. It is generally lined with a layer of secreting cells. Cysts normally contain fluid produced by this lining. Sometimes the contents are solid after water has been extracted from the secretion. Some authorities include under this heading hematomas, pockets of air in the tissues, and in fact all abnormal cavities.

True cysts can form almost anywhere in the body, but are particularly common in tissues containing gland cells, such as mucous and serous membranes, the liver, oviduct, kidney and the thyroid gland. Skin and subcutaneous cysts are fairly uncommon in cage birds, although the feather cysts of canaries are an exception. Degenerating fatty tumours with fluid centres, sometimes seen in budgerigars, can easily be mistaken for cysts. Experience helps to distinguish them, but only microscopic examination can reveal the true nature of these fluid-filled masses.

Plate 7/24. Large fibro-lipoma (benign tumour) involving the carpus. (L. Arnall)

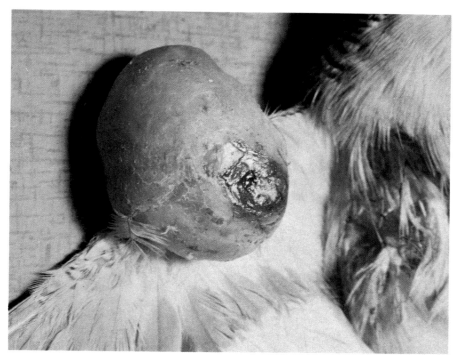

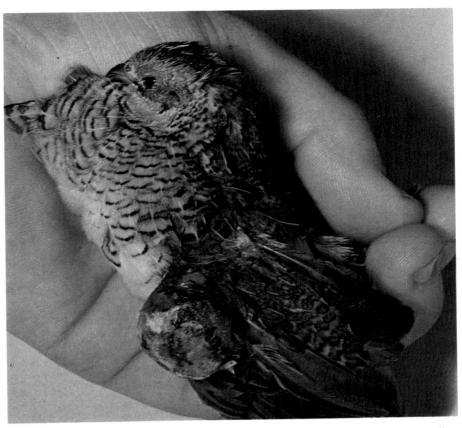

Plate 8/24. Chinese painted quail with fibrosarcoma of the elbow joint. (L. Arnall)

Cysts in the body cavity are even more difficult to diagnose than tumours. Most are found at necropsy or during an exploratory operation of the abdomen under anaesthesia. Cysts are not malignant, but sometimes they can cause severe illness and death as the result of their size. Cysts of the thyroid gland, sometimes encountered in budgerigars, are very well supplied with blood vessels and are easily ruptured if the bird is roughly handled. This can lead to death in a few minutes as the result of internal haemorrhage. Cysts or dilations of the oviduct are met with quite frequently in budgerigars and occasionally in other species and may simulate abdominal tumours or egg-binding. Peritonitis may ensue if retained egg material accumulates in these pockets of the wall of the oviduct. Painstaking removal of the entire oviduct through a midline abdominal wound may have to be undertaken by a veterinarian if the bird is to survive.

The remaining processes which may be confused with the tumours and similar swellings already dealt with in this chapter are almost entirely associated with injury or infection, and are therefore mainly inflammatory in nature.

Sudden or acute inflammations are accompanied by the classical signs of swelling, heat, pain and usually reddening and impaired function of the part which is inflamed. Long-term or chronic inflammations on the other hand are seldom very painful, are cool to the touch, often of the same colour or paler than the surrounding tissues, and although producing an obvious swelling do not usually interfere with the function of nearby organs, except sometimes mechanically, if near a joint or other mobile part of the body.

Chronically infected areas may be of the cold or dormant type, which are symptomless apart from the swellings they produce. Others which are exposed to scratching, pressure or other factors causing continuous irritation, develop into so-called granulomas (see also Chapter 21). These lesions caused by excessive production of repair or granulation tissue, contain scar-forming cells, numerous capillary blood vessels, and pockets of infection. The vitality of the area is so lowered by repeated minor injury and infection that complete healing becomes impossible. Common sites are the soles of the feet but also affected are the hocks, nostrils, third eyelid, angles of the beak, the fatty pad over the breastbone, the under side of the wing, the bastard wing, the tail and the preen gland. All these areas are prone to damage and most undergo repeated movement. Skin granulomas can be confused with tumours, the surface of which has undergone ulceration. This is often due to pecking or friction of some kind, almost invariably resulting in the destruction of the nerve endings and blood vessels in the skin. Necrosis or death of the over-lying skin inevitably follows the loss of blood and nerve supply. Granulomas and ulcerating tumours can usually only be differentiated with certainty from one another by examination under a microscope.

A special type of granulation tissue occurs in the remnants of the abdominal muscles, when these rupture after invasion by large quantities of fat or after enlargement of the abdominal contents by tumours or egg-binding. Granulomas in the abdomen are occasionally found to affect various organs, including the gut; in these sites they are potentially as dangerous as malignant tumours. Unlike true tumours, granulomas are sometimes associated with a degree of peritonitis.

Haematomas or blood blisters are really confined haemorrhages. When blood vessels are torn or otherwise damaged, and the blood cannot escape from the wound to the surface of the skin or into a large cavity such as the abdomen, it collects in spaces between layers of tissue where it is trapped and produces a local swelling. In view of the small amount of blood loss needed to kill a small bird, such lesions are best left alone in case the excitement caused by handling results in further haemorrhage. In confined spaces, back pressure of the blood slows down the haemorrhage and clotting soon occurs. Left alone, the blood clots in haematomas and contracts, squeezing out serum which is slowly absorbed back into the lymph and finally into the circulation. The clot is gradually replaced by granulation and finally scar tissue, leaving nothing but a tiny nodule to mark its position.

Other swellings

Organs can be enlarged by an increased inflow of blood or a decreased outflow. This occurs normally in the wattles and other fleshy structures of some birds and is a seasonal and hormonal variation.

Sometimes swellings may reach the size of a tumour when there is obstruction to blood flow due to tumour pressure or rupture of tissues. Congestion or engorgement of tissues with blood hinders tissue fluid flowing back into the bloodstream and its build-up in the congested organ leads to oedema. Oedema or dropsy is really the accumulation of lymphatic or tissue fluid in the tissues between cells. In a mild form it accompanies almost all inflammatory conditions and many others as well. In mammals it is commonly associated with a failing heart as well as several debilitating diseases. Ascites or abdominal dropsy is caused by the accumulation of fluid in the peritoneal cavity, when tissue fluid produced in the abdominal organs fails to drain into the lymphatic system. It is usually produced as the result of damage to the liver and kidneys and also when abdominal tumours interfere with the blood circulation. Ascites occurs in birds and should be suspected when a large, soft, fluctuating abdominal swelling develops.

Oedema of the limbs or extremities is probably most frequently seen in foot enlargements caused by identification rings on the legs which are too small, becoming tight and interfering with the circulation. Once the swelling of an injured leg fills the space within the ring, the circulation to that limb soon ceases and lymphatic vessels, veins, and even arteries may be progressively blocked off by the strangulating pressure. The thin walled veins become blocked first, but the arteries continue for a time to carry more blood into the foot, so that the limb below the ring swells greatly. This swelling, partly venous engorgement but mainly oedema, persists until the ring is removed or the foot dies. Such a swelling if squeezed for a few seconds and then released, shows an

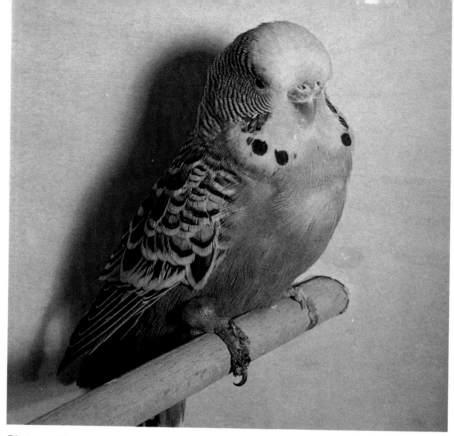

Plate 9/24. Fibrosarcoma of lower end of metatarsus and phalanges. Budgerigar. (L. Arnall)

Plate 11/24. Sarcoma involving the head of a Chinese painted quail. (L. Arnall)

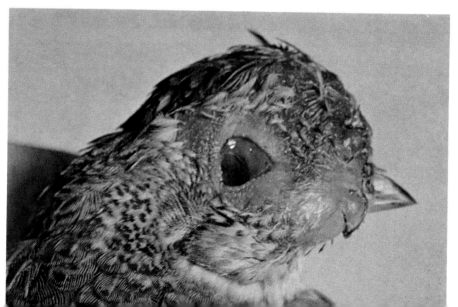

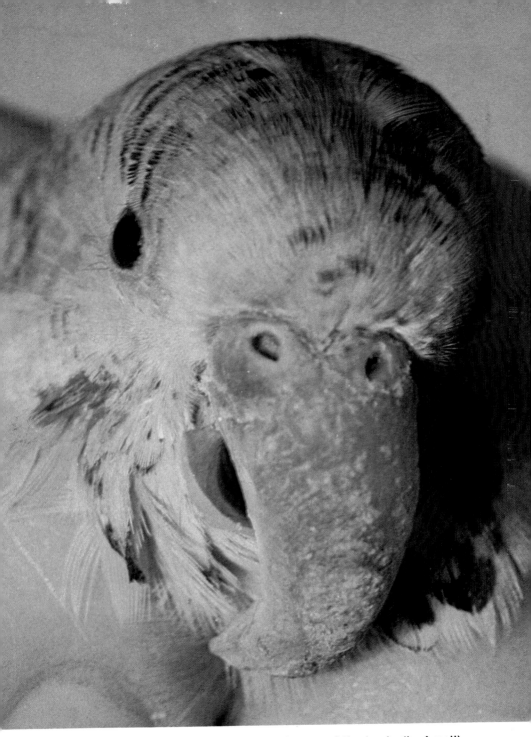

Plate 10/24. Budgerigar with carcinoma of the beak. (L. Arnall)

indentation for some seconds where pressed with the fingers —it "pits" under pressure. This pitting and blanching of the squeezed area, is a sure sign of oedema.

Treatment of oedema is related to removal of the cause when possible. In the case of pressure from a leg-ring the answer is obvious; often, however, no cause can be found.

In tissues which have been dropsical for long periods of time permanent changes will result, such as the deposition of fibrous material, especially around blood and lymph vessels. Thickened swellings of this kind can never revert to a normal state.

SELECTED BIBLIOGRAPHY

ARNALL, L. (1966). *The Clinical Approach to Tumours in Cage Birds. IV. Treatment of Cage Bird Tumours.* J. small anim. Pract. 7, 241–251.

BLACKMORE, D. K. (1966). *The pathology and incidence of neoplasia in cage birds.* J. small anim. Pract. 6, 217–223.

FELDMAN, W. H. & OLSON, C. (1965). Neoplastic Diseases of the Chicken. In *Diseases of Poultry*, p. 863–924. Eds. Biester, H. E. and Schwarte, L. H. 5th Ed. Ames, Iowa. State University Press.

PETRAK, M. L. & GILMORE, C. E. (1969). Neoplasms. In *Diseases of Cage and Aviary Birds*, p.459–489. Ed. Petrak, M. L., Philadelphia. Lea and Febiger.

SMITH, H. A., JONES, T. C. & HUNT, R. D. (1972). *Veterinary Pathology.* 4th Ed. Philadelphia. Lea and Febiger, 1521pp.

HEREDITARY AND CONGENITAL DISEASES

Hereditary diseases or tendencies are those carried by the genes of the bird's germ cells. They are therefore passed inexorably to the next or later generations, becoming inbred in the strain or family.

Non-hereditary, congenital abnormalities are characteristics of the individual which have been acquired at an early stage in its development.

A congenital disease is not transmissable; it is one which affects the bird from the time of hatching. "Congenital" literally means "born with". This includes infectious and nutritional diseases as well as abnormalities of development· The term congenital covers also the tendency to develop certain diseases in later life, these being "stamped" on the embryo during its development in the shell.

The terms congenital and hereditary are frequently misused, but because of the large gaps in our knowledge of avian disease this is not surprising. Unless proof of inheritance is present it is therefore safer to avoid the term "hereditary" and use "congenital" instead.

Infections and deficiencies in the parent may affect the health of the embryo and cause congenital abnormalities. The affected chick is weakened and the internal organs may be damaged and anatomically deformed if the damaging agent operates at the stage when primitive tissues are being organized to form limbs or other organs. In such cases the stunted or dead embryo may be suspected as suffering from an hereditary defect in development, when the responsible factor was really an acquired infectious agent or nutritional deficiency.

Accidental occurrences such as inadequately formed eggs; delay in fertilization, delayed egg laying or cooling of eggs in the nest may lead to imperfect development.

Important hereditary diseases are mostly due to anatomical, physiological, or biochemical disorders which affect the chromosomes of the germ cells. If a limb or eye for example does not develop properly it is almost certainly because of an unfavourable chemical environment in the developing embryo. A breakdown in the highly complicated chemical processes of the body has occurred and as these processes are necessary for most of the body cells, then there are liable to be far-reaching effects.

367

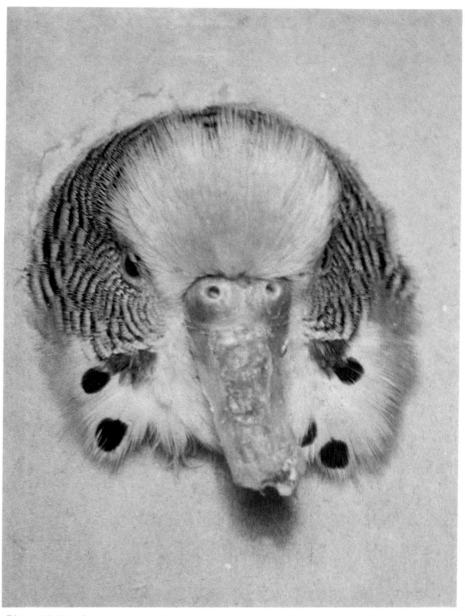

Plate 12/24. Carcinoma of the upper beak of a budgerigar resulting in lateral deviation of the beak, i.e. wrybeak. (L. Arnall)

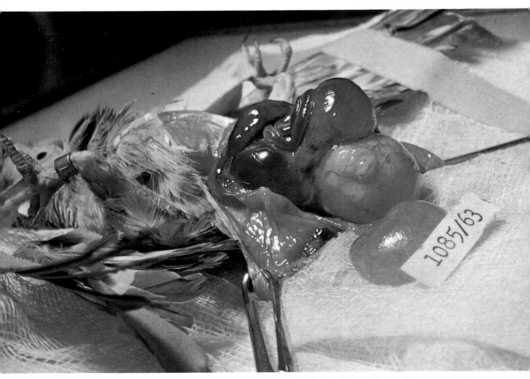

Plate 13/24. Huge ovarian tumour surrounded by large follicles or custs. The liver is congested and rounded. Budgerigar. (L. Arnall)

Plate 14/24. Ovarian tumour associated with egg peritonitis. Budgerigar. (L. Arnall)

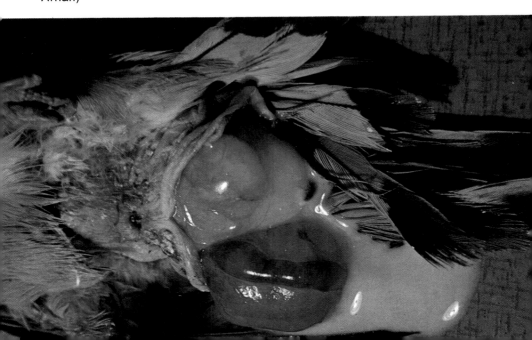

The importance of diseases that are really hereditary lies not only in the wastage of individually affected birds, but in the transmission of the defect within the strain or species, especially if it is linked genetically with characters such as colour, size, or other special features commonly selected by fanciers.

Examples of factors which are sometimes hereditary include the proneness of budgerigars to tumours, obesity and French Moult. But it must not be thought that these are diseases in which heredity is the only factor; environment, especially that of captivity, can greatly influence the incidence and degree of such undesirable traits. Although the extent to which tumour development can be controlled is probably negligible, exercise, less readily available and more varied foods, and restrained, seasonal breeding can considerably reduce obesity and its associated thyroid disorders, and perhaps even the incidence of French Moult.

Certain show points in birds such as carriage, size, colour and unusual types of feather may be associated with undesirable characteristics because some of the genes for these factors are situated closely together in the chromosomes. Some undesirable characters are merely incidental concentrations of bad qualities, intensified by in-breeding, (see Chapter 1). A successful free-living bird has to compete for food with others of its kind and it adapts to alternative foods or changes in environment. It is also able to flee or hide from its enemies. When man interferes by supplying a less challenging environment and by breeding for such factors as increased size, vitality is lowered and there is a tendency to disturb the metabolism of the strain. Small birds tend to be most active, whilst heavier birds tend to have relatively less tone or power in their muscles and other organs. Not only do they tend to be less fertile, but the hens are less able to expel their eggs. Curly, crested, or silky feathered birds usually have a plumage which insulates less efficiently and it also wears less satisfactorily than a normally feathered one. These birds are probably therefore more prone to chills and other diseases. Feather cysts are more likely to occur in unnaturally feathered varieties. Sometimes abnormal feathering is accompanied by constitutional weakness.

Lethal factors are abnormal genetic characteristics inherited by the offspring from one or both parents, which produce chemical or anatomical abnormalities that will not support life. Such factors intensified by in-breeding, produce embryonic deaths or monstrosities which cannot survive long after birth. Many monsters and dead-in-the-shell chicks occur in domesticated birds; and these are usually buried or incinerated by the owner. Among these specimens there are undoubtedly some examples of lethal factors, but so long as they are disposed of in this way statistical evidence of their hereditary nature will remain hidden. Only a few lethal characteristics in birds have so far proved to be hereditary. A skeletal stunting or achondroplasia in domestic pigeons is one example.

The Beak   Severely underdeveloped, abnormally long or shaped mandibles, as well as complete absence of a beak are encountered from time to time. The hereditary nature of such abnormalities is rarely tested by inbreeding, most examples being destroyed. A few are kept as curiosities, and provided such a bird can eat, the defects are of little disadvantage in captivity.

Beaks may be absent in one or both jaws, abnormally thin or thick, twisted, overshot or undershot, of a greater or lesser curvature than normal, make an abnormal angle with the head, be hooked in straight billed species or straight in curved-beaked ones. Some of these abnormalities are compatible with normal health, but others rapidly cause starvation.

The Eyes   Cataract (Plate 1/25), possibly of an hereditary nature, is fairly common in canaries. Eyelessness is a rarity, apparently reported only in budgerigars and pigeons. A milder form of microphthalmia or small eye may be hereditary, but it may also be related to vitamin A deficiency in the egg.

The Feet and Legs   Syndactylism (webbed feet) in land birds, and polydactylism (excessive numbers of toes) are occasionally encountered and of little detriment to the bird. Extra legs are more of an encumbrance and are likely to excite persecution or cannibalism in a flock or in the wild state. Often polydactylism is accompanied by other abnormalities—of the beak, wings or internal organs, for example—and specimens do not generally survive to adulthood.

The Hip and Pelvis   Skeletal deformities affecting mainly the hip and pelvis when the legs are spread horizontally are not uncommon, especially in six to 12 week old budgerigars. This results from a congenital pelvis and hip deformity in which the ball and socket is under-developed and sometimes dislocated. In such cases the bird is only able to climb in the corners of its cage where both feet can grip the wires simultaneously. On the floor of the cage, the bird behaves like a turtle on its back, paddling its legs, vainly searching for the ground. Spinal and other dislocations are also met with in nestlings and the stifle and

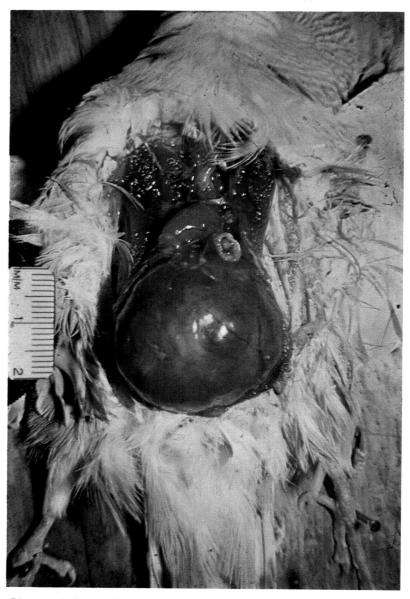

Plate 15/24. Cystic neoplasm of kidney occupying much of the abdominal cavity and displacing the heart. The alimentary tract has been removed. (D.K. Blackmore)

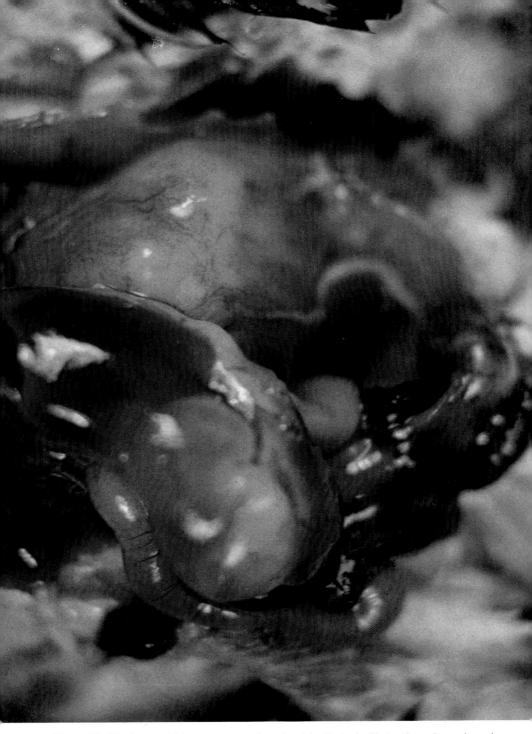

Plate 16/24. Large kidney tumour (nephroblastoma). Note the gizzard and intestine below part of the liver. Budgerigar. (L. Arnall)

hock joints are sometimes deformed. These defects may be truly congenital or they may be acquired as the result of a severe peck by one of the parent birds after hatching. When the deformities are seen in an otherwise normal bird which has not been injured they are almost certainly hereditary and must not be confused with severe rickets.

The Wings

Faults of the wing are rare. Various defects, however, have been reported such as: stunting of the bastard wing, ankylosed or fixed wing joints, and shortened wings (Plate 2/25) without a humerus or with stunted radius, ulna or metacarpals.

Other Abnormalities of the Skeleton

Apart from deformity of the spine, broad and flattened rib cages, and perhaps certain other deformities which are usually of dietetic, metabolic or traumatic origin, few abnormalities are hereditary in nature. A split sternum exposing the pericardial sac, and achondroplasia manifested by a grotesquely disproportionate stunting of the skeleton, have both been reported in pigeons.

The Plumage

Most unusual feather abnormalities are to be found in pigeons and poultry, which for centuries have been bred for amusement, curiosity, or decorative reasons. Many of the variations of plumage must have arisen accidentally as "sports". Examples are featherlessness, silkiness, crests, frills, "hoods" and "manes." It often takes many years and numerous generations of birds to fix such variations in a species, and sometimes losses are also incurred in the process of developing the desired new character. The crested canary, nowadays somewhat of a rarity, owes at least part of its fall in popularity to the discovery in the thirties that the desirable crest was a "dilute form" of feather cysts. These can be regarded as a characteristic which can be lethal because the ragged plumage they produce tends to cause irritation and thence self-pecking which may result in severe haemorrhage, possibly shock, and also encourage cannibalism. Feather cysts occur in the Norwich, crested and certain other cross-breeds of canaries and have been shown to be hereditary. The cysts are also called "lumps", dermal cysts and *hypopteronosis cystica* (Plate 3/25). In breeding for a soft, curled or tufted appearance of the feathers, an abnormal development has resulted. The young, growing feather becomes curled over in its follicle, so that the feather sheath fails to erupt. Several follicles behaving like this coalesce and produce a skin cavity or cyst containing abortive feathers and keratin, together with greasy material produced by the sebaceous glands of the skin. These cysts

374

rupture over the adjacent skin and present a beige, dry mass which swells similarly to the wax in a dog's ears and has an acrid, fatty smell. Such lumps can be single large masses or consist of numerous smaller ones. The feathers nearby are also disorganized, and give the bird a bedraggled appearance. When the lesions are extensive the bird appears depressed but can survive several seasons; the condition worsens, however, at each successive moult. Individual masses can be removed entirely or their contents scraped out, but new cysts tend to develop. The more diffuse type of cyst will sometimes respond to treatment with thyroid gland extract at the dosage rate of 1.5 mg./20 grammes body weight per day, either as a liquid by dropper or in the form of a powder mixed with the seed as a vitamin supplement, or preferably impregnated in the seed. A moult is thereby induced and once this has started the thyroid treatment can be stopped. The new plumage is generally paler than normal after such treatment. Affected birds should never be used for breeding purposes, whether or not the cysts have been cured by treatment.

It is often purely a matter of fashion whether an unusual feather colour, pattern or distribution is considered a rare and valuable show characteristic or a fault. What is introduced as an attribute in one breed may be considered detrimental to the health and quality of another.

The Central Nervous System This system is rarely affected by hereditary abnormalities. Ataxia or weakness due to under-development of the brain occasionally occurs in various species. The cerebellum is most often affected. Reduction of the brain tissue limits muscle power and control as well as coordination. An affected bird staggers about and is unable to maintain its balance or to fly. In pigeons the character is a recessive (see Chapter 1).

The Reproductive System Defects such as twinning (double-yolked eggs) and partial or complete division of single-yolked eggs may be hereditary in origin. Congenital abnormalities such as deformities of the skeleton and various organs have already been mentioned. On rare occasions two oviducts may be encountered (Plate 4/25).

It is undesirable to continue to breed from stock which produces occasional freaks. Though the abnormal young are destroyed, the apparently normal birds may still carry and transmit the undesirable characters even if mated to healthy strains.

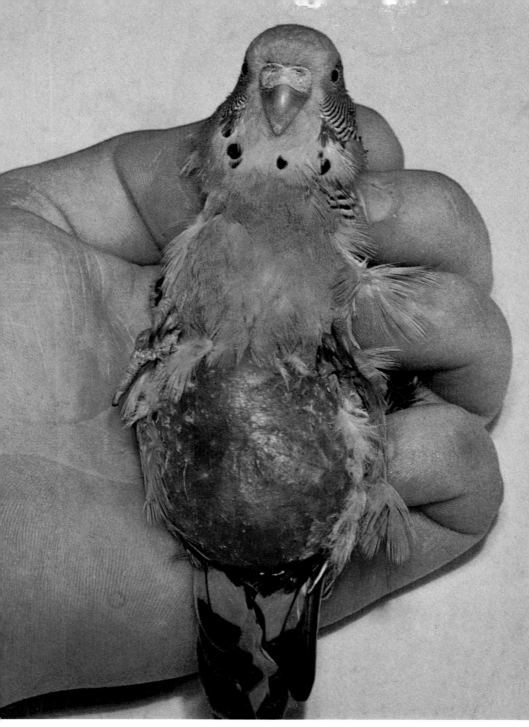

Plate 17/24. Discolouration of abdominal wall due to underlying pressure of the internal organs caused by ovarian tumour. Budgerigar. (L. Arnall)

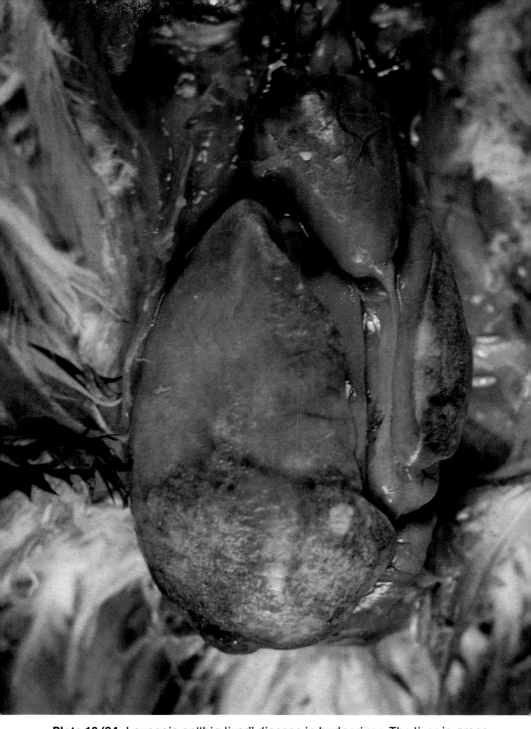

Plate 18/24. Leucosis or "big liver" disease in budgerigar. The liver is grossly enlarged and paler than normal. (L. Arnall)

SELECTED BIBLIOGRAPHY

BUCKLEY, P. A. (1969). Genetics. In *Diseases of Cage and Aviary Birds,* p.23–43. Ed. Petrak, M. L., Philadelphia. Lea and Febiger.

PECKHAM, M. C. (1965). Congenital and Inherited Conditions. In *Diseases of Poultry,* p.1205–1207. Eds. Biester, H. E. and Schwarte, L. H. 5th Ed. Ames, Iowa. State University Press.

SHOFFNER, R. N. (1965). Heredity and the Defective in Poultry. In *Diseases of Poultry.* p.77–99. Eds. Biester, H. E. and Schwarte, L. H. 5th Ed. Ames, Iowa. State University Press.

TAYLOR, T. G. & WARNER, C. (1961). *Genetics for Budgerigar Breeders.* London. Iliffe, 129pp.

GENERAL BREEDING AND REARING PROBLEMS

This chapter summarises only the factors which may be responsible for breeding difficulties, virtually all the points having been discussed in previous chapters. This information is of course most relevant to such common domestic birds as the budgerigar and the canary.

Breeding problems may be manifested at different stages:
1. Birds fail to mate.
2. Birds mate but no eggs are laid.
3. Only clear infertile eggs are laid.
4. Fertile eggs are laid, but they fail to hatch.
5. Eggs are laid, but are broken and/or eaten by the parents.
6. There is a high proportion of addled eggs.
7. There is a high proportion of dead-in-shell chicks.
8. Chicks have difficulty in hatching.
9. Weak nestlings are produced or deaths occur in the nest.

The causes of these problems are discussed below.

1. Failure to Mate The causes include:
(a) Immaturity of one or both birds.
(b) Senility affecting one or both birds.
(c) The birds are not a true pair, having been incorrectly sexed. This can easily happen with species in which the male and female plumage is similar.
(d) Fright and continuous or periodic disturbance.
(e) Dietary deficiencies, straightforward malnutrition or obesity. (See Chapters 3 and 23).
(f) Hormonal imbalance. (See Chapters 2 and 19).
(g) Infectious disease. (See Chapters 6, 7, 8, 9 and 10).
(h) Neoplasia of the gonads of either sex. This is mainly applicable to budgerigars. (See Chapters 16, 19 and 24).
(i) Congenital or hereditary disease. (See Chapter 25).
(j) Various disorders of the reproductive system. (See Chapter 16).
(k) Various disorders of the nervous system such as paralysis of the limbs. (See Chapter 18).

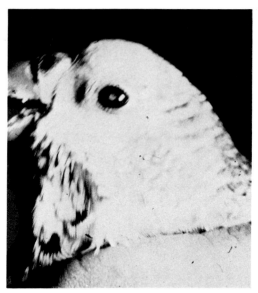

Plate 1/25. Opacity of the lens (cataract)in a budgerigar. (L. Arnall)

Plate 2/25. "Angel Wing" deformity—shoulder + elbow/carpal dysplasia. (L. Arnall)

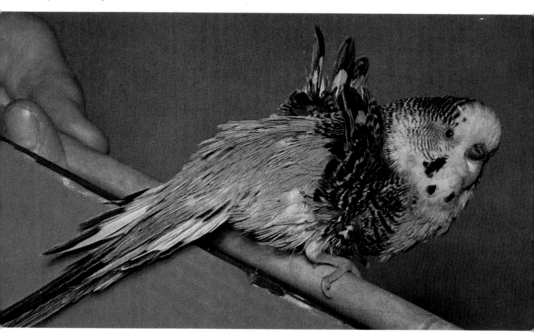

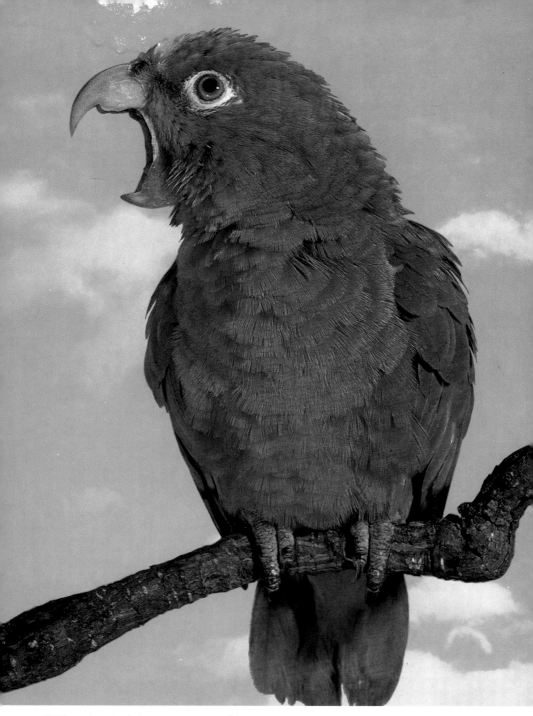

Yellow-fronted Amazon parrot (*Amazona ochrocephala*). There are several species of the predominantly green Amazon parrots. Another popular bird being the blue-fronted (*A. aestiva*) which has a pale blue instead of a yellow forehead. Recently imported Amazon parrots are a considerable hazard to health, because they frequently carry a virulent strain of psittacosis (Chapter 6).

(*l*) Unsuitable environment for breeding—not enough space, lack of proper nesting facilities, insufficient light, irregular use of artificial lighting, temperature too low, too high or too fluctuating.

(*m*) Excessive breeding.

(*n*) Incompatability: sometimes a pair of budgerigars, for example, will refuse to mate with each other, but will mate satisfactorily with other birds.

(*o*) Incorrect season; especially applicable if the pair are housed in an outside aviary.

2. Failure to Mate and no Eggs Laid

Causes:

(*a*) These factors listed above are applicable: *a, b, d-j* and *m*.

(*b*) Occasionally this is due to homosexuality. (See Chapter 16).

(*c*) Egg binding or other disorders of the female reproductive tract. (See Chapter 16).

3. Infertile Eggs

Causes:

(*a*) The following factors listed in paragraph 1, are particularly applicable: *b, c, e, g, i, j, m* and *n*, and less frequently some of the other factors listed may also occasionally apply.

(*b*) Absence of a cock: inexperienced bird keepers sometimes do not realize that a hen kept in isolation or inadvertently "paired" to another hen, may lay eggs.

(*c*) It is conceivable that prolonged or over-dosage of certain drugs may interfere with metabolic and especially hormonal processes and cause infertility of either sex.

4. Failure of Eggs to Hatch

Cause:

(*a*) Disturbance to the incubating bird by the owner, cats, mice or vermin, excessive noise, other birds or previous offspring, or even by its mate.

(*b*) Chilling of the eggs, due to disturbance (see above) or failure of the incubating bird to cover the clutch adequately, especially if fostering additional eggs.

(*c*) Accidental damage to an egg shell; for example, by handling or due to perforation of the shell by a very sharp or overgrown claw. Only a hairline crack in the shell may be sufficient to introduce faecal contamination and kill the embryo. Eggs may also be damaged when birds are disturbed.

(*d*) Certain infectious diseases may be transmitted from

the hen to the embryo and eventually kill it before hatching occurs. The organisms involved appear to include *Escherichia coli* and *Salmonella* spp. as well as perhaps certain viruses. (See also Chapters 6 and 7).

(*e*) Dietary deficiencies. (See Chapter 23).

(*f*) Hereditary disease affecting the development of the embryo. (See Chapter 25).

5. Eggs broken and/or eaten by the parents

Causes:

(*a*) Disturbance. (See 4*a* above).

(*b*) Poisoning by chlorinated hydrocarbons. This is unlikely to be encountered, unless the hen bird has recently been acquired from a heavily contaminated area of the wild. (See also Chapter 22).

6. Addled eggs

Addled eggs are those which after incubation are found to have decomposing contents. They may be infertile eggs which have decomposed due to the warmth of incubation or infection or from neglect and prolonged exposure by the sitting bird. Alternatively, they may be fertile eggs which have died due to infection, neglect, hereditary deformity or injury.

The causes will be found listed in sections 3 and 4 above.

7. Dead-in-Shell Chicks

There are a multitude of different possible reasons, and some are listed in sections 3, 4 and 6 above.

An additional cause is dehydration of the embryo; this may occur especially under conditions of artificial incubation when the humidity of the incubators is too low. Very little is known unfortunately about the humidity requirements of developing embryos of most birds except poultry. It is quite possible that some species such as aquatic birds may require a high humidity for satisfactory hatching.

8. Hatching Difficulties

The principles in section 7 above also apply to dead-in-shell chicks. In addition, a very low temperature will hinder hatching, as it will result in chilling and lowering of the metabolic rate of the chick.

A weakened embryo is unable to break through the egg shell with its egg tooth (see Figure 6/2) at the right time: indeed if the shell is specially hard or thick, even a healthy normal chick may be unable to break it. Disturbance by the owner will not help the chick; but if after several hours the egg remains "pipped", that is, the shell is broken in one place with the egg tooth visible, and the chick is obviously getting weaker, then the egg should be carefully opened and the chick released.

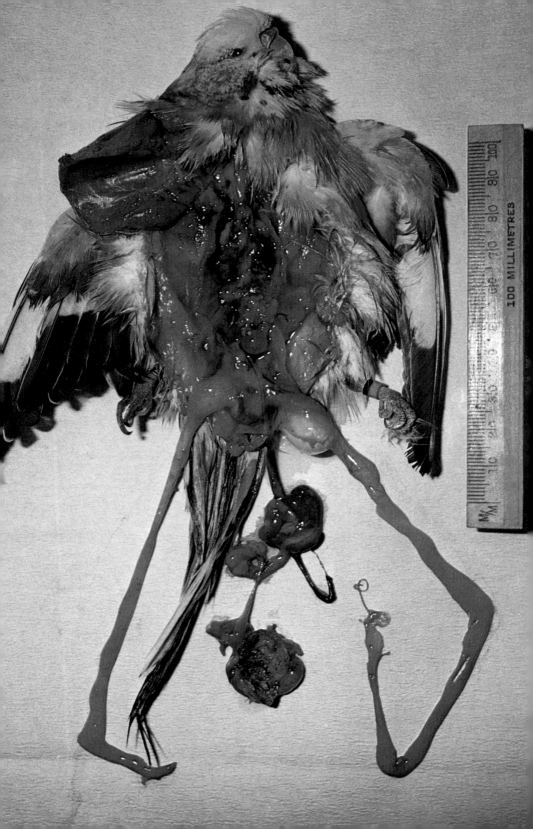

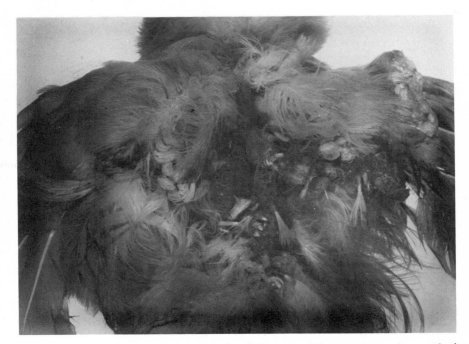

Plate 3/25. Norwich canary with feather cysts (*Hypopteronosis cystica*). Note the malformed and encysted feathers on the back and upper part of the right wing. (L. Arnall)

Plate 4/25. Congenital abnormality characterised by two fully formed oviducts in a budgerigar. No right ovary had developed and the left was normal and active. A fully formed but broken egg was causing impaction of the lower part of the left oviduct. (I.F. Keymer and T.C. Dennett, Z.S.L.)

The causes are again numerous and include:

  (a) Disturbance: deaths may occur if the young are neglected by the parents as the result of disturbance, (see section 4a above), or owing to illness or death of a parent. All result eventually in chilling and starvation of the young.

  (b) Dietary deficiencies. (See Chapter 23).

  (c) Infectious disease. (See Chapters 6, 7, 8, 9 and 10).

This short chapter cannot deal in depth with problems which often remain unsolved even by trained breeders with a lifetime of experience. It is the difficulties and the great challenge, with some species particularly, coupled with the moments of success, which makes bird breeding such an absorbing hobby.

SELECTED BIBLIOGRAPHY

General

BOOSEY, E. J. (1962). *Foreign Bird Keeping. A complete guide to breeding and management.* 2nd ed. London. Iliffe, pp. 384.

RISDON, D. H. S. (1953). *Foreign Birds for Beginners.* 8th Ed. London. Cage Birds. pp. 140.

RISDON, D. H. S. (1972). *Cage and Aviary Birds.* London. Faber & Faber. pp. 188.

RUTGERS, A. (1969). *The Handbook of Foreign Birds in Colour. Their Care in Cage and Aviary.* Vol 1, pp. 262. Vol. 2, pp. 230. Ed. Norris, K. A. London. Blandford Press.

RUTGERS, A. & NORRIS, K. A. (1970). *Encyclopaedia of Aviculture.* Vol I, pp. 350 and Vol. II, pp. 308. London. Blandford Press.

YEALLAND, J. J. (1958). *Cage Birds in Colour.* London. H. F. & G. Witherby Ltd. pp. 130.

Waterfowl

JOHNSON, A. A. & PAYN, W. H. (1968). *Ornamental Waterfowl. A Guide to their Care and Breeding.* 2nd Ed. London. H. F. & G. Witherby Ltd., pp. 110.

MARTIN, R. M. (1973). *Wildfowl in Captivity.* London. John Gifford. pp. 160.

Birds of Prey

WOODFORD, M. (1966). *A Manual of Falconry.* 2nd Ed. London. Black. pp. 194.

Gallinaceous Birds (except Poultry)

COOPER, D. M. (1972). *The Japanese Quail.* pp. 461–470. In U.F.A.W. Handbook on the Care and Management of Laboratory Animals. Edited by U.F.A.W. 4th Ed. Edinburgh and London. Churchill Livingstone.

DELACOUR, J. (1959). *Pheasant Breeding and Care.* 3rd Ed. Wisconsin. All Pets Books. pp. 108.

GERRITS, H. A. (1961). *Pheasants, including their Care in the Aviary.* London. Blandford Press. pp. 144.

TREVISICK, C. H. (1958). *Fancy Pheasants, Jungle Fowl and Peafowl for Beginners.* London. Cage Birds. pp. 104.

Pigeons

LEVI, W. M. (1974). *The Pigeon.* 2nd Ed. Revised with additions, Levi Publ. Co. Sumpter, S. C. pp. 667.

LEVI, W. M. (1965). *Encyclopaedia of Pigeon Breeds.* Jersey City. T.F.H. Publications, Inc., pp. 790.

MACRAE, R. R. (1969). *Management, Feeding, Breeding and Training of Racing Pigeons,* pp. 65–75. *In* Proceedings of the British Veterinary Zoological Society 1961–1970. Eds.

Keymer, I. F., Irvin, A. D. and Cooper, J. E. (Sept. 1972). Obtainable from the Hon. Sec., B.V.Z.S., C/o. B.V.A., 7 Mansfield Street, London W1M 0AT. England. Price £1.
WHITNEY, L. F. (1961). *Keep your pigeons flying*. London. Faber. pp. 240.

Psittacines

ARMOUR, M. D. S. (1956). *Exhibition Budgerigars*. 2nd Ed. London. Cage Birds. 159pp.
BEDFORD, Duke of. (1954). *Parrots and Parrot-like Birds*. Fond du Lac, Wis. All-Pets Books, Inc. 210pp.
BOOSEY, E. J. (1956). *Parrots, Cockatoos and Macaws*. London, Rockcliff. 162pp.
KEYMER, I. F. (1972). The Budgerigar. p.482–489. In *The U.F.A.W. Handbook on the Care and Management of Laboratory Animals*. Edited by U.F.A.W. 4th Ed. Edinburgh and London. Churchill Livingstone.
ROGERS, C. (1970). *Budgerigar Guide*. New York. The Pet Library Ltd. 250pp.
RUTGERS, A. (1967). *Budgerigars in colour: their care and breeding*. Ed. Rogers, C. London. Blandford Press. 256pp.
VANE, E. N. T. (1959). *A Guide to Lovebirds and Parrotlets*. London. Iliffe Books Ltd. 160pp.
WATMOUGH, W. (1960). *The Cult of the Budgerigar*. 5th Ed. London. Poultry World Ltd. 292pp.

Canaries and Other Passerine Birds

BATES, H. & BUSENBARK, R. (1963). *Finches and soft-billed birds*. New Jersey, T. F. H. Publications. 703pp.
KEYMER, I. F. (1972). The Canary, p.471–481. In *The U.F.A.W. Handbook on the Care and Management of Laboratory Animals*. Edited by U.F.A.W. 4th Ed. Edinburgh and London. Churchill Livingstone.
ROOTS, C. (1970). *Softbilled Birds*. London. John Gifford Ltd. 158pp.

MISCELLANEOUS DISORDERS

Heat-stroke   The excellent insulating properties of feathers and the almost complete absence of sweat glands in the skin limit the loss of heat. Insulation is essential for small birds and mammals when the temperature of the environment is well below that of their bodies, because the heat lost is proportional to the surface area of the bird: thus, the smaller the creature, the higher the ratio of the surface area to its body weight. Large birds lose much less heat by radiation.

When the surrounding temperature is high, the amount of heat transferred from the body to the outside air is less than when the temperature is low. If the air temperature approaches the bird's blood temperature, no heat is lost at all because there is no longer a difference in temperature between the bird and the outside air.

A bird can still lose heat even when the air temperature is higher than that of its body: this happens when the air is dry. The heat loss under these circumstances is purely by the cooling effect of evaporation. If the air is humid, however, evaporation is slower and it may be insufficient to keep the bird's temperature down to a safe level. If it rises too high, the bird suffers discomfort which can lead to collapse and death. In warm and humid climates it is therefore necessary to provide not only adequate shade, but to avoid stuffy buildings with high humidity. Moving air helps cooling, especially if the bird can wet itself in a bath. In addition to the heat lost by radiation, the bird also loses warmth in the air it breathes out, which has been previously warmed by passage through the lungs and air-sacs.

When the bird gets excessively hot, it pants and gapes. This uses up more energy and causes therefore an increased heat output. The bird also fluffs its feathers until they separate from one another, exposing the skin and facilitating heat loss by convection. The wings are held half-extended, drooping on the floor. If eventually the bird cannot lose sufficient heat, it becomes comatosed, sometimes with brief terminal convulsions. Its temperature may rise by 6°F (3°C) or more before death occurs.

Housing birds in hot weather in exposed wooden buildings without insulation and good ceiling space is liable to produce heatstroke unless there is a wide area of wire netting in front of the bird-house to permit a flow of air.

Immediate treatment consists of removing distressed birds to an air-conditioned room or spraying them periodically with cold water. Recovery is usually rapid, provided that body temperature has not risen too far. Birds which have been subjected to heatstroke may, however, be off-colour for a day or so and may afterwards be more prone to infections, particularly respiratory diseases.

The term "chilling" has been given to many undiagnosed illnesses in birds, mammals and man. True chilling is a stress syndrome in which the vitality of the tissues particularly that of the lungs is lowered, making them more susecptible to infections and other injurious agents. A severe fall in the temperature of the environment is one factor, but sudden starvation, shock, injury or exhaustion may affect the adrenal cortex and cause lessening of the body's resistance. **Chilling or Hypothermia**

Chilling from actual cold is liable to occur mainly in newly imported tropical birds or birds undergoing a heavy moult. The most extreme examples of the former type of chilling have been known to happen when birds are imported by air in crates in unheated compartments at 15–30,000 ft. from Asia, Africa or other tropical countries. Under these conditions the temperature in the freight hold drops well below freezing even in summer. The birds have no water, and the resulting stress on them is extreme. On arrival at their destination, such birds are usually comatose, with a body temperature often registering below the scale of the thermometer. Placing the birds in an environment of 90–95°F (30–33°C) quickly enlivens the majority, but a proportion will slowly die. Those which recover show for a time an almost obsessional thirst. During the subsequent days or weeks a steady number of survivors will continue to develop signs of various affections, it being essential to watch them closely so that appropriate treatment may be given without delay.

Hypothermia can also occur in acclimatised birds in temperate and cooler countries when their body heat is lowered as the result of insufficient or unsuitable feeding, extensive injury or major surgery, sudden heavy moult, oil contamination causing matting of the feathers, and wetting of the skin after the plumage has been washed with detergents. The mechanisms involved can only be reconstructed approximately by analogy with similar processes in mammals, but it is believed that a breakdown occurs in the control of blood sugar, liver and muscle glycogen levels as well as the levels of sodium, potassium, calcium, magnesium, phosphates, chlorides and other mineral ions in the blood and tissue fluids. The

390

effect on pancreatic (insulin), adrenalin and histamine production is not known accurately.

Shock

Shock is a process which is little understood, but of which everyone is aware. Research on it is constantly being carried out both in man and animals, although to only a limited extent in poultry and other birds. Knowledge of the complex mechanisms involved and even the definition of shock are constantly having to be revised.

Shock can be briefly defined as a depressive response to various stresses. Various types of shock are catalogued according to the cause, the system, the part of the body affected, the degree, the appearance, and the timing. Examples include the following:

Cause: Crushing, compressive, decompressive, haemorrhagic, electric, toxic, anaphylactic and surgical factors.

System or region: Neurological shock, causing pain due to marked nervous involvement.

Degree: Mild, severe.

Appearance of main clinical signs: Depressive or torpid, excitable or erethismic.

Timing: Primary, secondary, delayed or recurring shock.

Haemorrhagic shock is of particular importance and usually comes as a sequel to accidental or surgical injury. In old parrots and other species which live to a great age in captivity, haemorrhagic shock may occur spontaneously during a burst of activity after injury, being usually associated with degenerative vascular or heart disease. After stemming the visible external haemorrhage, subcutaneous injections of small quantities of hypo or isotonic saline should be made at various sites in quantities of up to 20 ml. per kg. of the bird's weight. The bird must not be made too warm unless its temperature is obviously low to the touch: 70–85°F—approximately 20–40°C—is recommended according to response.

Idiosyncracy and other Sensitivities

The part played by the phenomena described below, especially allergy, has been shown in recent years to be more far-reaching than was previously believed. The study of the nature, the production, and the action of antibodies and the antigens, or allergens which stimulate the reaction is known as immunology. Whether pathogenic microorganisms succeed in entering the body is largely controlled by the degree of immunity it has built up. Antibodies assist in the resistance to disease, and in the tolerance or rejection of grafts of tissues and whole organs to replace the diseased ones. The violent responses shown by the skin of some individuals or their internal organs to eating, inhaling or merely touching certain substances, and the occasional illness produced by blood transfusions or serum injections are all due to the production of antibodies. A study of immunology explains how disease is produced and why an agent can cause illness in one individual but not in another.

This is the exaggerated response shown by certain individuals, **Idiosyncracy** strains, or even species to contact, or entry into the body of a small quantity of certain foreign substances. From the first occasion on which the body cells meet this substance the response is there: the individual possesses this peculiar reaction from birth. An example of idiosyncrasy in many species of birds is the violent shock reaction and death which follows an injection of even low doses of streptomycin, when other species like mammals of equal size, would show no undesirable effects. An idiosyncratic tolerance or intolerance to barbiturate anaesthetic has been noted in individual men and certain other mammals. A dose which safely anaesthetises the vast majority of dogs or cats may kill one individual and yet leave another fully conscious. Idiosyncrasy is probably therefore the result of a congenital or hereditary peculiarity of metabolism, which only shows itself on the first challenge by the rejected substance.

Allergy is a much over-used word. People are heard to say that **Allergy** someone is allergic to certain people, when what is meant is merely that he dislikes them. Allergy is really a local response by tissues to the presence of a foreign substance at the second or a subsequent challenge. Allergic responses are virtually unrecorded in birds. To be allergic a bird must meet and be sensitized by the allergen or allergy-creating substance— usually a protein. When it meets the same substance, whether it be two weeks or even two years later, its tissues react violently with an allergic response. It is therefore an acquired response and is in fact a protective mechanism designed to repel invaders by building up a defensive armament. Unfortunately, the tissue reaction is not always beneficial to the health of the individual in question, and may result in local oedema, pain, shock or even cell death. The challenging foreign substances, which are usually large molecules like proteins and groups of sugars (polysaccharides), may be encountered by being swallowed, inhaled or merely through contact with the skin. Especially in man, such responses as dizziness, asthma, hay-fever, capillary haemorrhage of the skin, nettle rash, diarrhoea or vomiting may result when the second and later challenge occur. The amount of allergen required to produce these local effects need only be very small. When damaged by allergen-antibody reactions certain cells liberate

392

a substance called histamine, which produces pain, swelling and some signs of shock.

Allergic skin, gut or respiratory reactions must not be confused with the response to irritant and poisonous substances. These have a specific chemical reaction of their own and produce similar skin or mucous membrane damage in most species of birds or mammals. Only the degree of reaction may differ a little. True allergic reactions usually affect only a few individuals within a species. Allergies to milk, egg, horse meat, various fish, carpet dyes, grass or other vegetation, wool and very many other substances, have been found in mammals. Information regarding avian allergies, however, is almost non-existent, although oedema of the glottis and marked swelling of the fleshy head structures of pigeons and poultry have been observed following mosquito bites. In the absence of obvious causes, such lesions have been assumed to be an allergic response to inhalation or ingestion of various allergens. Antihistamine or cortisone-like drugs are most likely to be helpful in the treatment of rare cases.

Anaphylaxis More profound reactions by tissues of the body leading to severe shock and death are called "anaphylaxis" or anaphylactic shock. This is a violent and sudden response of an allergic type which is not limited only to those cells and tissues in contact with the allergen entering the body. The whole defence mechanism, geared for action by the first challenge, is let loose in the second or later challenges. In man and animals the second injection of serum (for example, an anti-tetanus inoculation) has caused some violent anaphylactic reactions.

Sera containing antibodies to specific infectious diseases have been little used in cage birds, and even then this has been mainly experimental. It is probable that with increasing knowledge of avian disease this practice will increase and anaphylactic responses to serum will become more important.

Corticosteroid drugs and antihistamines are most useful for lessening anaphylactic sohck.

Hypersensitivity Many so-called allergies are not allergies at all but hypersensitivities. For instance, many avian species react violently when injected with low therapeutic doses of streptomycin, dihydrostreptomycin, chloramphenicol and numerous other drugs they have never previously encountered. Signs of violent shock, collapse, coma and death usually result. The skin in such an instance is unaffected, though it may just be detectable that it has become paler than usual.

Hypersensitivity is merely an exaggerated response in an

393

individual to a dose of foreign substance which produces in the majority a normal or therapeutic response or even no response at all. It is a useful term for a state which includes idiosyncracy, allergy and anaphylaxis, until the precise cause of the reaction and its mechanism can be elucidated and named. Fleas and other ectoparasites produce such responses in both mammals and birds, and it is safest to refer to the abnormal response elicited as a "hypersensitive reaction".

Although experimental proof is lacking, it is quite possible that the bird which is constantly pecking at its skin or plucking feathers, wheezing, having loose droppings or showing necrosis of the feet, or other complaints, may be suffering from the result of allergic or other hypersensitive reactions to food or materials found in its cage. This is partly why radical changes in diet, environment and management are advocated in this book for several diseases where the cause is unknown. The reasons for any improvement can then be found by replacing the changed circumstances one by one until the same clinical signs of disease return.

Relief of oedematous swellings, laboured, wheezy breathing and other signs can be temporarily relieved by corticosteroid drugs and to some extent by antihistamines.

Photosensitisation

Photosensitivity is an exaggerated response to light, especially to sun or ultraviolet light. The response is a reddening of the skin which may progress to severe sunburn. White-haired mammals and possibly white-feathered birds appear to be most prone.

Such birds should be removed to an environment of subdued light and exposed only gradually again to sunlight.

Photosensitivity

This is an induced tendency to light sensitivity, which occurs as the result of eating certain plants or the administering of certain drugs. In cattle for example, the plants St. John's Wort (*Hypericum* spp.), kale and rape (*Brassica* spp.), as well as some sulphonamides and tetracyclines derange the metabolism to such an extent that the normal tolerance of the skin to certain wavelengths of light is lost and burns result. No proven cases, however, have yet been reported in cage birds.

SELECTED BIBLIOGRAPHY

BIESTER, H. E. & SCHWARTE, L. H. (1966). *Diseases of Poultry*. 5th Ed. Ames, Iowa. State University Press. 1,382pp.

HUNGERFORD, T. G. (1969). *Diseases of Poultry including Cage Birds and Pigeons*. 4th Ed. Sydney, London, Melbourne. Angus and Robertson. 672pp.

ANAESTHESIA

This part of the book is not intended to be a manual on "do-it-yourself surgery".

A veterinarian will not receive an amateur surgeon very warmly if he is presented with the failures and asked to put them right. A further consideration is that by virtue of his training the veterinarian knows far better than the layman what constitutes cruelty and what surgical procedures are justified. Nevertheless, there are occasions when veterinary attention may not be available within a reasonable time, especially in distant parts of the world. Medical doctors, nurses, zoologists, animal technicians or similar people may have to be called upon in an emergency. To the great majority of readers therefore, this section of the book is intended merely to outline what can be done.

Means of producing insensibility or suppressing sensation were sought for thousands of years before relatively harmless methods were found. At first, man was the subject of the experiments and the motives were not necessarily humane or in the cause of medicine: The reasons were indeed, often religious or recreational. Giving alcohol or some form of hypnosis were used increasingly until the last century as methods of lessening pain or fear. Although alcohol is normally no longer used, more and more sophisticated methods of hypnosis continue to be practised.

In testing various substances for effect and safety it was inevitable that mammals and birds would be used and in this way veterinary anaesthesia soon developed as a useful by-product of medical anaesthesia. From virtually nothing, these branches of medicine have progressed enormously since the beginning of this century. Doctors soon realized the convenience to the surgeon and veterinarian, and that it was also humane to develop drugs which depressed the activity of the central or peripheral nervous systems. These drugs have since proved their value in veterinary surgery by ensuring that little or no pain is felt by the animals involved.

Birds and also reptiles appear—unlike mammals—to be relatively insensitive to pain stimuli, except in the more specialized areas of the body such as the beak, nares, eyes, ears and cloaca. Methods of anaesthesia for birds, have therefore been developed only recently.

Anaesthesia may be general and produce loss of consciousness, or local, causing loss of sensation confined to certain areas by affecting the sensory nerve endings. The peripheral nerves of the skin, mucous membranes or muscles are most commonly affected by local anaesthetics.

Many species of non-domesticated birds, particularly those which have only recently been brought into captivity, become apprehensive and struggle when handled. The use of a tranquillizer is therefore often desirable before a bird is handled for clinical examination. If anaesthesia is to be attempted involving the use of a face mask, then a sedative called a premedicament is necessary in such cases.

Some anaesthetic drugs have sedative or analgesic properties when they are given in doses below those required for full anaesthesia. Although this means that they can sometimes be used intentionally as sedatives, it can make their use hazardous even in experienced hands if full anaesthesia is required. This is the case particularly with birds where accurate dosage rates have not been determined.

The various degrees of loss of sensation, through the stages of **Stages of** sedation, narcosis, and light, medium or deep anaesthesia are **Anaesthesia** gradual and indistinct and may not be recognized easily even by the expert veterinarian. The stage of anaesthesia is determined not only by direct observation, but by response to various stimuli. The responses or reflex actions to these stimuli vary considerably and depend upon such factors as the type of anaesthetic drug being used and the size, age, species and general health of the bird. In many cases, apparently similar individuals vary considerably in their reactions.

The stages of loss of consciousness can be classified on the basis of diminishing responses. They may, however, become apparent slightly differently from the customary order set out below. Indeed some stages may disappear simultaneously rather than consecutively.

Tranquillization: This is the onset of calmness. The bird is not nervous when approached and tends not to struggle when handled.

Sedation: This stage is marked by sleepiness. The eyelids droop; the head is held low and may be shaken; the bird is unsteady on its perch and may fall off. Although psittacines are unable to use the wings they are able to climb.

Narcosis: At this stage the bird sleeps and lies on the floor with the head and tail down. The wings are partly spread out; wing and leg movements are inco-ordinated. The bird will still flutter when handled and struggles briefly if subjected to a mildly painful stimulus, such as pinching the toe or touching the eyelid with a blunt pointed instrument: in budgerigars, a similar stimulus to the cere will produce the same reaction. Response to loud sounds is almost negligible and the bird can be placed carefully on its back without any struggling.

Light Anaesthesia: Although the bird is unconscious at this stage, there are still brisk reflexes when the toes are pinched. Feet and wing movements occur if the skin around the eyes or ears and the angles of the beak is pricked with a pin. There is no response to sound or vibrations and the respirations become deep and regular. At this stage minor skin surgery can be performed on most parts of the body and neck, thigh and basal parts of the wings.

Medium Anaesthesia: Responses to toe pinching and eyelid stimuli are sluggish, delayed or intermittent. The respirations continue to be moderately deep and regular and not appreciably slower than the previous stage. Loss of body heat is now quite marked and it is essential therefore to keep the bird warm.

Most operations can be performed at this stage, but some struggling may occur if the body cavity is opened or if the head and feet are the site of surgical interference.

Deep Anaesthesia: The toe-pinching and eyelid reflexes are absent, very delayed or intermittent. The respirations become slightly shallower and slower and may cease without warning. The heart may stop a few seconds after respirations have ceased or simultaneously. Immediate administration of oxygen or artificial respiration is necessary in such cases. If alphaxalone and alphadalone acetate injected, then intra-muscular injection of "Millophylline" (Dales Pharms) or "Bemegride" (I.C.I.) should lighten the depth of anaesthesia, stimulate respiration and avert a calamity. Obviously in an ideal state of general anaesthesia no cessation of respirations should occur.

Premedicants, Tranquillizers, Sedatives and Other Central Nervous System Depressants

Premedication is seldom necessary with inhalation anaesthesia unless to allay fear; but it will reduce the dose of injected anaesthetics by 20-50 per cent.

Phenothiazine derivatives, such as chlorpromazine and acetyl promazine, are tranquillizers when used in higher doses. Used judiciously, they can allay fear in wild or nervous individuals and allow safer handling for examination and the administration of anaesthetics.

Diethyl thiambutene hydrochloride acts as a sedative on the smaller psittacines within a few minutes when given sub-cutaneously, but it often makes the patient hypersensitive to sound. Although it may be approached or touched, high-pitched sounds may stimulate the bird and result in a few

397

seconds of vigorous, incoordinated movement. The drug is technically a narcotic: it is on the Dangerous Drug List in the U.K. and not available to unqualified persons.

CT 1341, a steroid anaesthetic, is a useful tranquillizer or sedative for nervous birds when used in small doses and given subcutaneously.

Ether (Diethyl ether)

Volatile Anaesthetics

Only anaesthetic ether should be used, never industrial ether, which contains acetone and other impurities. Ether is one of the most readily available of the volatile anaesthetic liquids and is probably the safest, even without special apparatus. It is best administered by pouring about 4 or 5 ml. onto a piece of cotton wool or gauze pressed into a narrow pot or similar receptacle. The bird's head is inserted into the container until surrounded by, but not in contact with, the soaked pad. When the bird becomes limp, the head should be withdrawn an inch or two from the pad and replaced only if the bird starts to make movements or noises. The quicker the emergency operation can be performed, the better the chance of recovery from the anaesthetic and the operation.

The bird must not be allowed to inhale the liquid ether. Most emergency operations are best performed under anaesthesia. The bird may be held gently by the head, feet, the wing and tail feathers; great care should be taken not to restrict the breathing with any pressure on the throat or thorax. Cautery by heat, for example for checking haemorrhage, must *never* be used with ether anaesthesia because of the danger of fire or explosion.

Chloroform

This *must not* be used on birds because it kills most smaller species in a matter of seconds from heart damage and cardiac failure. If the bird actually survives the anaesthesia, it usually dies later from liver damage.

Halothane and Methoxyfluorane

These are somewhat safer than chloroform but variable in effect and difficult to control without special apparatus.

Halothane is a highly potent anaesthetic which requires an oxygen supply and a special vaporizer to make it a safe anaesthetic for birds.

Methoxyfluorane is much safer than halothane, but it is less potent and may not produce full surgical anaesthesia.

Nitrous Oxide and Cyclopropane

These gaseous anaesthetics can be used only with complicated apparatus. The former is very safe but ineffective by itself. Cyclopropane is excellent for use in a fully equipped animal hospital, being a safe anaesthetic but inflammable and explosive even in low concentrations.

Local Anaesthetics for Injection

These are dangerous even in skilled hands and varyingly effective because of rapid absorption, dispersion and general systemic effects.

Surface Anaesthetics

Substances such as proxymetacaine hydrochloride, which is absorbed by raw surfaces, may be fairly safely used for spraying on extensive wounds before suturing.

Injected or Parenteral Anaesthetics

Pentobarbitone is a moderately long-acting barbiturate in mammals, in small birds it produces variable results, especially if given subcutaneously or intramuscularly. In the larger birds the depth of anaesthesia can be controlled more safely if it is given intravenously in diluted form, but the duration is unpredictably short unless a competent anaesthetist gives small additional quantities to maintain the depth of anaesthesia.

A substance called "Equithesin" (a mixture of pentobarbitone, magnesium sulphate and chloral hydrate) is somewhat more reliable and a little safer than pentobarbitone used alone.

Alphaxalone and alphadalone hydrochlorides by injection are not entirely safe. The effects and recovery take several minutes therefore great care must be taken to conserve body heat. The respiration rate is not a reliable guide to the depth of anaesthesia: sluggish toe-pinch reflex and eyelid touch reflexes persist almost to the point of death.

Recently metomidate has been used successfully as a general anaesthetic in various species including pigeons, pheasants, psittacines and birds of prey. It is given by intramuscular injection and is very safe. The anaesthesia can be supplemented with Halothane if desired.

SELECTED BIBLIOGRAPHY

ARNALL, L. (1961). *Anaesthesia and surgery in cage and aviary birds.* Vet. Rec. Part I, *73,* 139–142. Part II, *73,* 173–178. Part III, *73,* 188–192. Part IV, *73,* 237–241.

ARNALL, L. (1964). Aspects of Anaesthesia in Cage Birds, p.137–146. In *Small Animal Anaesthesia Symposium.* Ed. Jones, O. Graham. London. Pergamon Press.

GANDAL, C. P. (1969). Surgical Techniques and Anaesthesia. In *Diseases of Cage and Aviary Birds.* p.217–231. Ed. Petrak, M. L., Philadelphia. Lea and Febiger.

HUNGERFORD, T. G. (1969). Anaesthesia. In *Diseases of Poultry including Cage Birds and Pigeons.* p.582–585. 4th Ed. Sydney, London, Melbourne. Angus and Robertson.

SURGERY

Surgery is an art which cannot be outlined in a few paragraphs, nor can it be taught by reading—no matter how comprehensively. The competent surgeon is a craftsman with the skills of a dressmaker, carpenter, plumber, sculptor and engineer. He has to deal with an adaptive plastic material, living tissues, and although certain general rules and principles apply, he quite often has to change his techniques in the middle of an operation to cope with an unexpected emergency.

The Properties of Tissues: Normal and Damaged
Tissues differ in many respects—their strength, elasticity, blood supply, speed of healing, resistance to disease and degree of importance to the animal. Surgery is inevitably a destructive process and the removal of diseased parts, if it is to be adequate, means removing also some more or less healthy tissue. Surgical interference always produces some degree of shock. Even the closure of a clean, fresh wound by suturing causes further damage through holding the edges with forceps, washing with antiseptics, puncturing with needles and impeding blood supply to the tissues enclosed by the sutures themselves. There is always the risk of introducing pathogenic organisms. Damaged tissues swell, and after surgery the ligatures become miniature tourniquets, and are subject to extra tension. It is necessary unless the suture material is cat-gut and absorbable, to remove the stitches at the right time; this needs experience.

A bird's skin is much looser and less elastic than that of mammals and when suturing it is rather more difficult to ensure an air and water-tight closure of the wounds. On the other hand, it is easier to replace a torn flap of skin to its correct position since it does not contract so easily.

In small birds, all the tissues are very fragile and even the most sensitive pressures with forceps or needles may tear them. Even the lightest forceps must never be left hanging from a bird during an operation or they will tear away the tissues and may cause a fatal haemorrhage.

Haemorrhage is one of the great hazards in avian surgery. In large animals, vessels which are bleeding can be tied with

401

cat-gut, but in most cage-birds the blood vessels are so minute and friable that the ligature will cut through them. This is particularly applicable to those vessels in the subcutaneous fat. Pressure with a very light and springy pair of ophthalmic type artery forceps for one to two minutes will often stem the flow of blood. A touch with a low-current diathermy electrode is excellent, except when ether or cyclopropane is being used as an anaesthetic. Capillary haemorrhage can be checked with a light dusting of sulphonamide or antibiotic powder, since it absorbs water readily, does not dissolve and by partially solidifying helps to form a foundation for the blood to clot. Boracic powder or even chalk or flour may be used in an emergency when life is in danger. Because of the bird's loose and poorly elastic skin, pressure bandages do not prevent haemorrhage since blood from the cut surface seeps under the skin. This unhindered blood flow prevents clotting which is further inhibited by the lack of exposure to air.

Cleanliness is essential in all surgical procedures. All instruments must be sterilized before use and the hands must be thoroughly washed. Surgical instruments are best sterilized in a domestic pressure cooker for 20 minutes at 15 pounds pressure, or by boiling for 45 minutes in a covered saucepan. Chemical sterilization is suitable for items which are damaged by heat.   **Hygiene**

The site of the operation must also be cleansed. Accidental wounds are always contaminated to some degree and further contamination must be avoided if at all possible. Surgical wounds should theoretically be sterile: in practice the best that can be done is to pluck the feathers from around the site, wash the skin with soap or detergent antiseptic and finally wipe with a swab of surgical spirit, quarternary ammonium compound, mercuric chloride or preferably an antiseptic containing iodine. Contaminated wounds should first be washed thoroughly in 5 per cent sterilized salt solution. The bird is then held or, if anaesthetized, strapped on a cork mat using sellotape. The bird should be covered with a light sterile cloth or gauze with an adequate hole cut for the site of the operation. The surgeon then scrubs his hands and arms thoroughly for 10 minutes in medicated soap and water, finally applying a penetrating detergent or iodine-containing antiseptic before rinsing in clean water. He does not dry his hands unless a sterile towel or gauze swab is available and does not touch any unsterile object whatever. A freshly laundered white coat or other protective garment should be worn; the room chosen must be free from dust, food and animal residues.

Dressings, Strappings and Other Devices

As a general rule the fewer ointments, lotions, paints, adhesive tapes, collars, hoods, plasters or splints that are applied, the less uncomfortable the bird will be and therefore the less it will interfere with the operation site. Nevertheless, these devices may be necessary at times. Loose ends of dressings which can be pulled are to be particularly avoided, similarly overtight dressings which interfere with breathing or circulation and greasy preparations which mat the plumage and thus cause discomfort or chilling. Because it is difficult to maintain an active bird in one position and at the same time keep a slight tension on bandages or tapes when applying them, tissues which are distorted by dressing are a common cause of discomfort and interference by the bird.

An Elizabethan collar, which may be flat, cylindrical or cone-shaped protects the front parts of the body from pecking or the head from scratching with the feet; but it may chafe the neck and cause dermatitis if it is not carefully fitted. Birds with powerful beaks such as parrots, owls (Plate 1/29) and other birds of prey can tear adhesive tape, fibre-glass or Plaster of Paris dressings, and this may result in further fractures. It is essential that dressings should be comfortably fitted especially on these birds.

Surgical and Anaesthetic Equipment

1 Swann-Morton scalpel, No. 3 handle and blades Nos. 10, 12 and 15.

1 pair of fine scissors with sharp/sharp or sharp/probe points.

2 ophthalmic pattern artery forceps.

2 dissecting forceps, 1 with and 1 without teeth (transversely grooved).

4 suture needles—1 straight, round bodied, 1 straight, cutting (javelin pointed), 1 curved, round bodied and 1 curved cutting. Sizes 10-18 as appropriate.

1 reel of black cotton No. 40 and one reel of button thread nylon.

1 small pair of nail clippers.

1 cautery pin or radio soldering iron, 12 volt. *This must not be used with wet hands or when ether is employed.*

1 curette/probe for scraping out dead tissue and estimating the depth and directions of wounds.

2 gauze or cotton, operating cloths.

12 small, gauze swabs.

1 roll of cotton wool.

1 cork mat and pins.

1 reel each of $\frac{1}{2}$ and 1 inch zinc oxide, adhesive tape.

1 hypodermic syringe (1 ml. graduated in 1/100ths).

2 hypodermic needles, approx. 0.5×10 mm. for most injections, approx. 0.9×10 mm. for thick fluids and suspensions for injection or aspiration.

403

1 anaesthetic mask.

1 bottle anaesthetic ether—*not* the industrial type, which contains toxic impurities.

Surface absorbable or local anaesthetic.

1 eye dropper.

Hairpins or similar clamps of looped, springy, stainless, steel wire.

Drugs such as antibiotics, non-irritant antiseptic dressings, small, sterile tubes or bottles for specimens, may also be useful. A stronger pair of scissors may be included to be used for post-mortem examination if necessary.

There are many types of suture material available. Some of these can be absorbed rapidly by the tissues, others are slowly or never absorbed. Most absorbable, suture materials are expensive, especially in the sizes required for cage birds. Chromic, sterile cat-gut "00" and "000" gauge, with or without needle attached, is excellent for all tissues and dissolves in about 3 weeks. Number 40 cotton or button thread is satisfactory for suturing all tissues in larger birds and for ligatures in smaller ones; it is also ideal for suturing the skin wounds of most species. The Figure 1/29 shows the basic suturing or stitching methods which are most useful. **Types of Sutures**

The simple, interrupted suture can be used for almost all purposes including closing small wounds or larger ones where speed is not essential. It can also be used for tying tightly around the bleeding end of an artery in order to act as a ligature.

The mattress suture encloses a rectangular piece of tissue and serves to turn the edges of the wound outwards. It produces a better seal than other sutures in large wounds, and helps to control haemorrhage.

The continuous, mattress suture is a rapid means of closing a large wound and promotes healing if not drawn so tightly as to produce a sharp ridge of tissue.

The simple, continuous suture is easy to insert but produces an ugly wound. The main advantage is its ease and speed of use.

The purse string suture, as its name suggests, closes an irregular wound to a puckered purse or duffle-bag appearance. It is used for such procedures as correction of a prolapse of the cloaca; if the thread is drawn gently onto an object such as a thermometer in the cloaca, a small hole remains on its withdrawal for the passage of droppings.

It is essential to realize that sutures must draw tissue only into light contact with one another. If sutures are pulled too **Some Surgical Procedures**

tightly they cause loss of blood supply; the death of the enclosed tissue will almost certainly result unless the sutures
are removed or slackened after a few hours.

It is advisable for most purposes, to use round-bodied
needles of the milliner's type whether straight, half curved or
fully curved. Triangular, javelin pointed or cutting type
needles are likely to cut blood vessels and their use is indicated only for larger birds with a tough skin, when there is a
danger of tugging tissues with round-bodied needles.

Birds tolerate skin suturing without any form of local or
general anaesthesia and seldom indicate pain by movement
or voice except in the following areas: the head, especially
near the nostrils, eyes or beak; the scaled parts of the legs
including the toes, and the wings to a lesser extent; the cloaca,
and any area where the skin is stretched or pulled away from
underlying tissues in order to obtain a free edge for suturing,
or to clean out dirty or damaged tissues.

Most of the procedures discussed below are relatively
minor interferences and some of them can be carried out by
experienced breeders. But the more complicated should be
attempted by laymen only in exceptional circumstances, such
as when a veterinarian is unobtainable or when delay is likely
to cause severe illness or death of the bird. The methods of
diagnosing the various afflictions mentioned in this chapter
have been dealt with previously.

Treatment of   Skin wounds occur frequently and healing is most rapid
Simple Wounds   when they are repaired immediately. It is inadvisable to
attempt to repair wounds which are more than about 24
hours old because the edges become distorted and contracted
and adhere to the underlying tissues, making closure of the
wound difficult. Such wounds will not heal satisfactorily. If
left open, they tend to heal with the edges apart instead of
together and the exposed subcutaneous tissues will fill with
granulation tissue (see Chapter 21, Abscesses and Granulomas), unless the wound is freshened by trimming away the
edges and curetting the depth of the wound. The Figure
2/29 shows typical fresh wounds and the process of closure
on flat or convex surfaces.

When suturing a fresh wound, the most mobile part of the
edge of the wound—usually the middle—should be grasped
with the forceps and drawn to the most relaxed portion of the
opposite lip to fill the gap as neatly as possible without strain
on edges of the skin. A skin wound in a concave part of
the body such as the base of the neck, axilla or groin is
liable to draw in air if it is not adequately closed, which will
result in subcutaneous emphysema (see Chapter 21). Torn
strips of skin more than $1\frac{1}{2}$ to twice as long as the width of

405

Figure 1/29. SUTURE TYPES

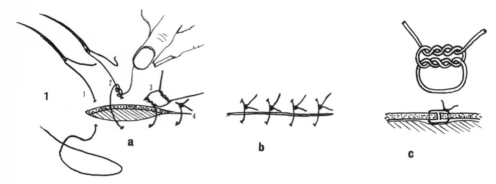

1. *Simple, Interrupted Suture* with double throw, nylon knot.

a) Stage (1) Surface view—insertion of needle and suture material; (2) Tying, loosely the first double knot; (3) Tightening first, double throw and loosely tying second reversed or "mirror image," double throw, knot, tight enough to draw wound edges into snug contact; (4) Tightening second throw making a double, reef knot.

b) Completed 4 double reef knots in surface view.

c) Transverse section of sutured wound parallel to first completed knot with oblique or perspective view of wound.

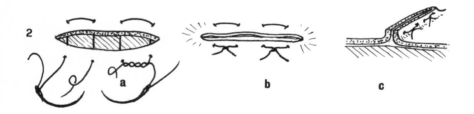

2. *Interrupted Mattress Suture* also using double, reef knot.

a) Surface view—insertion of two mattress sutures and tying of first, double, throw knot in 2nd suture.

b) Surface view—stages of tying first, double throw and tightening this; tying second, reversed, double throw and finished double, reef knot, tight enough to evert edges of the wound and gently oppose the underlying surfaces.

c) Transverse section through wound in front of first knot with a schematic perspective of the bulk of the wound after closure. Note the eversion of the lips of the wound and the opposed under surfaces of the skin. Also note the tent-like ridge this form of suture creates giving a larger opposed area of vascular (*i.e.*, well supplied with blood) dermis for stronger and more rapid healing.

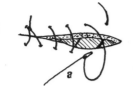 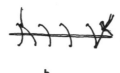 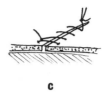

3. *Simple, Continuous Suture*

a) Initial part is identical to a simple, interrupted suture but the needle-loaded end is then inserted in a second pair of suture punctures, drawn through relatively tightly and then on diagonally to a third pair and so on.

b) To tie off at the last suture segment or pair of punctures, the needle is passed through the last pair of holes, *i.e.*, the thread is double and the free end of the suture is retained at the opposite side of the wound. The single end is then tied with the same double throw, reef knot as in the single, interrupted suture but with the double strand culminating in the needle.

c) A transverse section of the end of the wound with schematic perspective view of the closed wound.

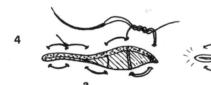 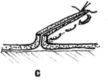

4. *Continuous, Mattress Suture*

a) The initial mattress is inserted and tied as in 2a (Interrupted Mattress) but the needle loaded end is carried along the knot side of the wound and inserted into, under and out on the opposite side, then along the same side, in, under and out on the knot side again, repeated according to the length of wound to be closed. The last section is also in a square pattern of 4 punctures, the single end being retained at the first of the four punctures and the double strand (loop) with needle attached tied off with a double throw reef knot at the fourth puncture.

b) Shows the completed surface view of the continuous, mattress suture.

c) Transverse section of end of sutured wound showing eversion of wound lips and tied off suture completed with schematic perspective of the remainder of the wound and suture line.

407

5

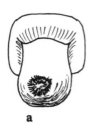 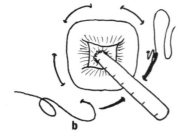 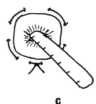

a   b   c

5. *Purse-string Suture* suitable for partial closure of cloaca after replacing prolapsed oviduct or rectum.

a) Insertion of suture in and out at approximately five points round the cloaca or wound, emerging near the original insertion with its suture tail.

b) Tying the first (and second) double throw, (reef) knot after gently drawing the suture onto the probe or thermometer to leave a small orifice after removal of the latter.

c) Completed purse-string suture in surface view. With an irregular wound closed by this method the probe is dispensed with for complete closure. (L. Arnall)

that part still attached are liable to die after being sutured into position, especially if badly bruised. It is therefore advisable to trim off and suture any excess over 1½ times the width of the base.

Large, deep wounds need only be treated as ordinary, simple, skin wounds from the point of view of repair, but infection must be prevented with the use of antibiotics, preferably by injection, but also orally or locally. The use of antibiotics in this way is particularly important in the case of puncture and ulcerated wounds. For further information see Chapter 21.

Treatment of Deep Open Puncture and Ulcerated Wounds

Crash landings or panicky flight can often produce fractures of the clavicle or wishbone and the air sacs in this region may be torn in the process. Less frequently, fracture of the skull may occur and this results in concussion which causes inco-ordination of the limbs, loss of balance and a dazed appearance. If bleeding occurs into the cranium, death may follow quickly or be delayed for a few hours, depending upon its severity. Fractures of the neck, other areas of the spinal column and bones of the pelvic region are less common. When they do occur, they are usually attributable to gunshot wounds or attacks by predatory animals. If birds are kept on a wire floor, their legs may become fractured or even amputated should a bird get caught up while in panic.

Fractures

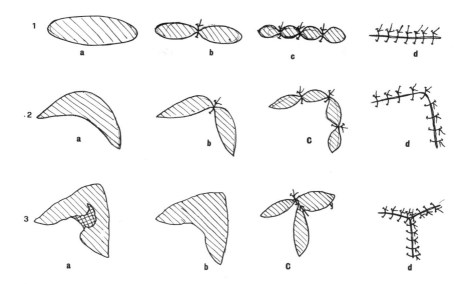

Figure 2/29. THREE METHODS OF WOUND CLOSURE

1. *Closure of a simple, straight, incised or small oval or round "skin-loss" wound.* Centre points of sides (1) are drawn together with forceps. At these points a simple interrupted suture is inserted (b) and tied with a double throw reef knot ("nylon knot"). If a standard reef is used, the first throw is liable to relax before the second is applied and drawn tight, thereby leaving a gap between the wound edges. Intermediate sutures (c) are placed midway along each half of the open wound. A third set can be infilled in larger wounds as necessary. The final wound is a straight or slightly curved line of sutures (d). Alternatively interrupted mattress sutures may be used in areas of loose skin to promote more rapid healing and a strong final result.

2. *Closure of a curved or L-shaped wound.* Centre of least curved side (a) or apex of the flap is drawn across to the centre or appropriate point of the more curved side of the wound (b) to produce equivalent relaxation of the two sides of the flap. A single interrupted, double reefed suture is placed at this point. Intermediate sutures (c) are inserted as in (1) above. The final wound presents an "L" or wide "U" suture line (d).

3. *Closure of a long flap or narrow V-shaped wound where the flap is severely bruised, "waisted," discolored or is more than 1½ times as long as its base.* (a) Appearance of the wound with narrow, wizened flap tip, and (b) with the damaged or excessive flap cut away. Sides of truncated flap are then both sutured to a comfortable point on the sides of the "V" wound so as not to stretch the flap tissues unduly (c). Intermediate sutures are placed on the sides of the flap and the remainder of the tip of the "V" sutured into a straight line, the leg of which is now becoming a Y-shaped suture line. Final appearance is of a Y-shaped, closed wound (d). (L. Arnall)

409

The most common fractures are those of the leg (Plate 2/29) and especially of the tibiotarsus. Fractures of the tarsometatarsus are much less frequent. Both are easy to recognize if the bird is held and examined carefully. A crackling sound or grinding sensation can be located at the site of the fracture when the limb is moved. Abnormal angling of the leg may often occur and, if it is freshly broken, there is exceptional and uncontrolled mobility. A fracture of the femur shows these signs less distinctly because the bone is more protected by muscle. In all fractures, some inflammation occurs and this results in the production of heat due to increased blood supply and loss or impaired use of the limb.

Fractured toes or phalanges are often not noticed until the bone heals, usually crookedly; by this time it is too late to treat the deformity satisfactorily.

Particularly difficult fractures to treat are those involving the joints. Sometimes it may not be possible to determine without an x-ray examination if the fracture is associated with dislocation. In skilled hands, however, a simple dislocation can sometimes be corrected by slipping the bone back into position under general anaesthesia.

Wing fractures (Plate 3/29) are less common than those of the legs. In the wild state, a fractured wing usually results in the bird's death from starvation if it lives long enough to escape the attention of a predator. Even if the wing is repaired by artificial means, satisfactory flight is seldom possible. Such a wild bird should not be given its freedom until it can fly strongly. To release a bird just after nursing it through the healing period of a fractured wing is about as kind as letting a lame fox free in front of a pack of foxhounds!

Wing fractures most frequently affect the humerus, ulna and radius, and here they produce the greatest deformity and loss of function of the wing. Although the wrist bones and those beyond, bear the bulk of the flight feathers, limited flying is often still possible even if these bones are quite badly damaged. A fractured wing is usually held low, most noticeably at its tip. Severe fractures to the humerus with angulation at the site of damage sometimes allow the carpal region to drop, but the wing tip to be raised. In all cases of wing fractures, however, diagnosis is relatively simple due to the unusual mobility of the wing, its limpness, an unusual crossing of the wing tips, and any of the other signs already mentioned with fractures of the leg. A word of warning is necessary because certain tumours of bone origin can cause weakness of the shafts of the long bones, cause proliferation of abnormal bone and show signs similar to those of fractures. The main difference is that the swelling is larger than that associated with a simple fracture, the skin shows no sign of damage, and mobility at the level of the swelling may not be accompanied by pain.

410

Sometimes nutritional diseases such as severe rickets or osteomalacia result in fractures of limb bones; in such cases the overlying skin may not show signs of damage.

Fractures or dislocations of joint surfaces are more difficult to diagnose because arthritis, gout and perosis (slipped gastrocnemius tendon) can show similar signs—evidence of pain and creaking or grinding sounds in the joints. The joints may also be swollen and lameness is nearly always present.

Bone usually heals quite rapidly, but the rate varies with the bone, somewhat with the species, and particularly the size of the bird. Those bones which are hollow since they contain part of the air sac instead of marrow, heal slowly because of the limited blood supply. The bones of small, passerine birds tend to heal more quickly than those of the larger species where the muscles exert more tension. If the two ends of the broken bone are brought closely together and kept in place, healing is usually rapid. If a gap is left or if there is an overlap, or if muscle lies between the fragments, healing is very slow or may not occur, especially where movement of the bones is possible. When the blood vessels are badly bruised or severed, not only may no bone be formed but it may actually be absorbed; the limb beyond the injury may also die. This is known as necrosis or death of tissue: infection hastens necrosis and if bacteria enter, gangrene may follow.

Fractures where the overlying skin is ruptured are known as "compound". Where the skin is intact the fractures are referred to as "simple", whether the bone is merely cracked in two or a dozen pieces. In the latter case, however, it is also called "comminuted". Several other types of fracture occur in the simple and compound groups.

A fractured leg is usually flexed and held up by the bird; as healing progresses it is gradually lowered onto the perch. Often, however, the foot is loosely clenched, the forward and backward pointing toes crossed and the muscles and tendons become set in an abnormal position during healing of the bone. If correct treatment is not given, the leg may remain permanently deformed. In cases of this type there may also be arthritis or damage to the nerves of the leg.

As with any serious wound, bathing with a 5 per cent sterile solution of common salt in water cleanses the tissues and helps to remove infection where the skin is broken. Antibiotics or sulphonamides should be given in these cases by mouth or by injection under the skin or into the thigh or breast muscle.

The simplest and often the most effective treatment of the actual fracture is to do nothing. The bird should be separated from its companions to prevent persecution and cannibalism and protection from its own frantic fluttering. A smooth-walled box with perches at floor level is best for wing and leg fractures. Wire netting should not be used except as a lid, because this material encourages attempts to climb.

So far we have dealt with the more straightforward leg fractures with fragments in contact. Marked inequality in length between each leg suggests over riding of the bones in the shorter limb. Repositioning the bones in these bad cases is painful, but the fragments must be brought as close as possible to their original position. Unless the manipulation can be easily and rapidly carried out, anaesthesia is necessary: inhalation of ether being satisfactory, using 1-2 ml. on cotton wool in a suitable sized cardboard funnel or mask. Repositioning generally consists of stretching the affected leg to the length of the normal one (Plate 4/29), then squeezing the fragments until they appear as one and in a straight line when felt through the layers of skin and muscle.

Splints for small birds may be made by padding a split portion of feather quill taken from a larger species. The splint is applied over the injured area and fastened with $\frac{1}{2}$ in. zinc oxide adhesive plaster strips down to and including the toes. The foot should be fixed in the fully open position with the knee and hock joints half flexed. Alternatively, match sticks, cardboard strips or wire can be used as a splint. Care must be taken in all cases to avoid chafing by the splints.

Plaster of Paris casts are too heavy and too cumbersome for any but the largest species. They are extremely difficult to remove safely, and in the experience of the author, seem to encourage chewing of the feet when used for parrots, whether or not the feet are included in the plaster.

In some birds a badly healed fracture or a piece of bone projecting from a wound may require an operation by a veterinarian before the bird can use the leg again.

The setting of wing fractures is particularly difficult because the position of the wing at rest is in a bent or flexed position. Pulling on the end of the wing in the case of overlapping or twisted fragments, therefore, separates rather than replaces the fractured bones. Even when they can be repositioned correctly, external splintings give little real support.

The best that can usually be achieved is to bring the fractured ends as nearly as possible into contact and be content with a reasonable alignment of the bones with the wing in the flexed position. This should be done under general anaesthesia. The tips of each wing, and preferably also the roots of the tail quills, are then fixed to each other with adhesive tape. A second circle of sticky tape around the front of the breast and encircling the shoulder joints prevents movement of the wings, dislodging the fracture and wing tip anchorage. According to the size and strength of the bird, a third circle of tape may be advisable between the first and second, its width depending also on the size of the patient. The third circle of tape must not be tight or it will restrict breathing. The dressings should be carefully removed after 7 to 28 days, depending upon the circumstances and activity of the bird.

Some success has been reported using internal stainless metal pins in fractures of the humerus, ulna and radius, femur, tibio-tarsus and even tarso-metatarsus, but this type of surgery is the province of the specialist veterinarian, and the methods are usually applicable only to larger birds. For fractures involving the elbow, carpus and hock, compression plates of moulded aluminium or plastic have been found very effective in immobilising these vulnerable areas. They should be made specially for the purpose, suitably padded and held in place by thread through holes in the edges.

Amputations   Amputation is often necessary when the fractured leg or wing is severely bruised and lacerated. The feathers of the wing or leg near the wound should be plucked and the skin cleansed. A ligature of cotton or synthetic thread is applied as a tourniquet above the injury, and the useless limb is amputated between the tourniquet and the injured zone with strong sterilized scissors or scalpel and sterilized hacksaw. Fine cotton should be used to suture through the flesh around the bony stump in such a way that the skin and muscle cover the bone. This operation should be carried out with the bird suitably anaesthetized, unless there is an emergency with danger of death from bleeding.

Pinioning   Pinioning to curtail the flight of birds by amputation of the wing at the level of the carpus or elsewhere and thus permanently removing the primary quills, is a practice that should be avoided. This type of mutilation is justified only when it is impossible to catch the birds regularly for the purpose of cutting wing feathers. If unavoidable, such amputation should be carried out by a veterinarian, as in the hands of the unskilled it is a barbarous procedure.

When flight must be curtailed, it is essential to remove half to two-thirds of each feather. Providing no more than two-thirds are cut, the bird will feel no pain. A few wing tip quills may be left to cover the ugly stumps in the folded wing. Normally little difficulty is experienced in shedding these at the moult, when new feathers will be grown necessitating further clipping if flight still needs to be impeded.

Re-shaping the Beak

The reasons which necessitate trimming and remodelling of the upper or lower mandibles have been discussed previously. The aim in re-shaping is to ensure adequate meeting and more normal wear of the opposing mandibles. Where beaks are over- or under-shot, trimming may be necessary at three monthly or even weekly intervals. Other deformities such as increased or shallower curvatures (Figure 3/29) or scissor beaks also need to be re-shaped repeatedly. It is insufficient to chop off the excessive growth from the tip; apart from being ugly in appearance, the exposed corium or living core is liable to bleed profusely.

Nail clippers are preferable to scissors for trimming beaks and the finer sculpturing is best achieved with scalpel and nail file or emery board. The surfaces of the beak must never be filed as this removes the protective covering of horn and leads to crumbling and splitting of the beak. Surfaces ruined by *Knemidocoptes* mite infestation can be coated with colourless nail varnish after removal of all mites and diseased tissue. Only the edges should be trimmed and, although this is potentially a dangerous procedure, it can be carried out safely with a scalpel by holding the head firmly against a cork or soft board; thin slices are then removed by cutting down onto the board, holding the clippers or scalpel obliquely, not at right angles to the beak, so as to retain the pointed ends of the mandibles. The mobile tongues of psittacine birds are particularly liable to be injured by this method, especially if the beak is not kept closed and restraint is not absloute.

When the beak is impacted with caked or sour food material it can be scraped clear with a suitable blunt, spoon-shaped probe or curette. The amputation of a necrotic or adherent tongue-tip and beak-tip in hummingbirds and similar species is sometimes necessary for the reasons discussed in Chapter 11.

Repair of the Damaged Beak

For repairing fractures, splints of plastic or fabric strips and a quick-setting glue can be used; nail varnish is useful for sealing small cracks. For wiring, it is necessary to drill very fine holes astride the fracture with the bird under general anaesthesia. An appropriate gauge of stainless steel wire (or in an emergency electric fuse wire) should be threaded through the beak and facial bones and gently twisted tight. Great care must be taken not to damage or obstruct the nasal passages. Healing is adequate in two to four weeks. Such operations can be very difficult and normally should be carried out only by a veterinarian.

Trimming Claws Normal claws turn down through a full right angle (see Figure 3/29), the "quick" or living portion extending for between two-thirds and three-quarters of the total length. These proportions go awry when claws are overgrown, shallowly curved, spiralled or distorted in other ways, and it is therefore easy for the blood supply to the claw to be accidentally cut and cause haemorrhage. Ferric perchloride ($FeCl_3$) or a silver nitrate stick may be used for cautery. In severe, continuous or recurrent haemorrhage, a touch with an electric soldering iron or darning needle made red hot in a gas flame, may be necessary to stem the flow of blood. When such thermocautery is used it is essential not to have ether in the room owing to the risk of fire. Immediate application of an antibiotic with corticosteroid cream minimises post-cautery pain.

Removal of Tumours and Cysts If ulceration or haemorrhage have occurred, it may be desirable to remove tumours or cysts at short notice. Before any operation is attempted the area should be plucked and cleaned with an antiseptic such as medicinal gentian violet or surgical spirit. Pedunculated tumours can be tied off or ligated, using strong cotton thread near the base, (see Figure 4/29). The swelling complete with the overlying skin is then severed at the neck just above the ligature to prevent bleeding. Dusting the ligated stump with a sulphonamide or antibiotic powder will check infection. It is unwise to attempt to remove sessile tumours (those without a stalk), especially if they are near joints or fixed immovably to underlying muscle or bone. This is particularly important when pain or disability of the joints near the growth is apparent. In some cases the contents of a sessile tumour (Figures 5/29 and 6/29) can be eased out whole as a core or picked out piecemeal, after which a suitable antibacterial cream should be thinly smeared into the cavity and the skin sutured using a sterilized needle and cotton thread.

Retained Eggs: Impacted and Prolapsed Oviduct, Rectum and Cloaca No attempt should ever be made to remove the reproductive tract (Plate 5/29), free eggs in the abdominal cavity or eggs impacted in the oviduct. This is essentially the province of the veterinarian.

If an impacted egg is visible during straining, when the bird relaxes the egg should be gently pushed back with a small loop of sterilized wire, small artery forceps or a blunt probe previously dipped in a mild antiseptic jelly or cream. The passage can be lubricated by a circular movement with the instrument around the egg. When the bird strains again, the instrument is introduced into the passage between the egg and the oviduct wall and used like a shoehorn. No pressure on the abdomen is desirable or necessary. When the egg is not visible and not prolapsing the oviduct, an oil which contains antibiotic should be inserted into the left side of the cloaca by a syringe with finest polythene tubing attached. After such treatment the egg may be laid within a quarter to half an hour, if the bird is quietly returned to its nest box.

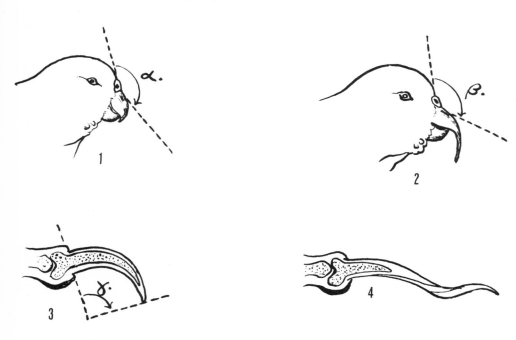

Figure 3/29. BUDGERIGAR: NORMAL AND OVERGROWN BEAKS AND CLAWS

1. The normal "set-on" angle (α) of beak. Circa 145-155°.

2. Reduced "set-on" angle (β). Circa 135°. The upper beak also shows a shallower curvature than normal and is overgrown at the tip.

3. The quadrant profile of a normal claw γ = 90°. The corium reaches to near the tip at this length.

4. Spiralled or ram's horn overgrowth—partially drawn in median longitudinal section to show the short corium and its contained os pedis (*i.e.*, pedal bone). (L. Arnall. Reproduced by courtesy of The Journal of Small Animal Practice).

416

Prolapse of the Oviduct

Often the fact that the bird is egg-bound is first noticed when the egg is outside the pelvic girdle enclosed in the everted cloaca and oviduct. As before, a pair of lubricated forceps or a probe should be inserted in the cloacal orifice in order to locate the egg if it is not visible. Such a prolapse may hang down behind the bird like a pendulous growth (Plate 3/16). It is red because of engorgement of the blood vessels and gradually over a few hours becomes a blackish red. If neglected, even for a few hours, the prolapse dries to such an extent that gangrene and inseparable adhesions form between the oviduct and the eggshell. If veterinary attention cannot be obtained very quickly, then the owner should soak and bathe the prolapse with *cold* 1 per cent saline solution and cotton wool. Using an antiseptic cream as a lubricant, gentle pressure with the fingers over the swollen end of the oviduct may reveal a portion of shell which can be removed by gently enlarging the cloacal orifice. If this is not possible, however, veterinary attention must be sought and a small puncture is made in the visible portion of the shell. One jaw of the forceps is inserted into this and the other jaw slowly pushed between the shell and the wall of the oviduct. The forceps are then closed around the shell and by rotating them the shell can be collapsed around the jaws and easily withdrawn. The contents of the egg will flow out during this procedure. The flaccid prolapsed oviduct is then further lubricated and replaced by means of a clean glass rod or thermometer, this being held in the replaced oviduct for one or two minutes, after which the rod can be safely withdrawn. Any tendency to further prolapse can be corrected by sewing up the vent with a purse-string suture around a glass rod: on its removal, a hole sufficiently large enough for passage of excreta remains. This procedure should normally be attempted only by a veterinarian. When kinking or valve-like folds occur in a prolapse and make it impossible to reach the egg by the method described, it is sometimes necessary for a veterinarian to cut down to the egg at the thinnest point of the prolapsed tissue and remove the egg through the incision. This leaves two wounds, one in the oviduct and the other probably in the cloaca. If these wounds are not instantly sutured (a difficult task in a contracting organ), peritoneal infection from the cloaca is likely to develop, impeding recovery. The alternative of an incision through the midline abdominal wall, opening the replaced oviduct and removing the egg, requires considerable surgical skill. Failures may often result from tearing the oviduct wall during or after suturing the incision.

Eggs partially visible at the vent with a dry, blackish, discoloured oviduct or cloacal wall adhering to them are best removed as soon as possible by immersing the tail and abdomen in warm 1 per cent saline for 1 to 5 minutes before

417

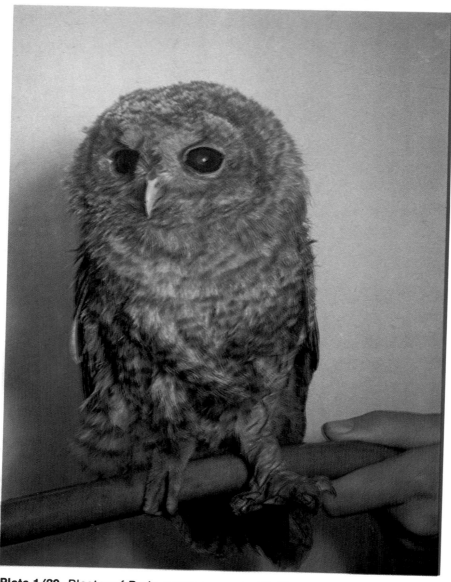

Plate 1/29. Plaster of Paris gauze covered with Zinc Oxide one inch plaster to support fracture of tibiotarsus. Tawny owl. (L. Arnall)

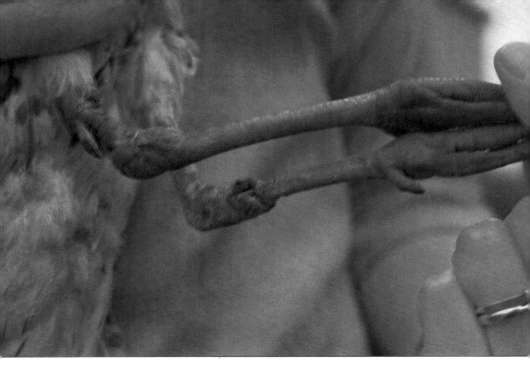

Plate 2/29. Fracture of right tarsometatarsus and left tibiotarsus in a snipe. (L. Arnall)

Plate 3/29. X-ray showing fracture of the radius with dislocation of the humero-ulna/radial joint in a pigeon. (L. Arnall)

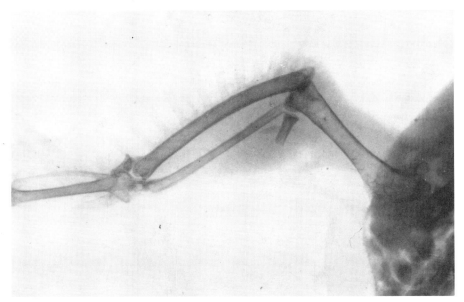

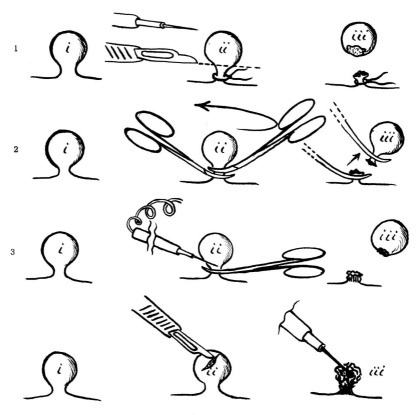

Figure 4/29. METHODS FOR REMOVAL OF SUPERFICIAL PEDUNCULATED TUMORS

1. Ligation and section distal to the ligature.

2. Double forceps clamps and torsion.

3. Single forceps clamp and cutting diathermy.

4. Ligation (incision optional) and coagulating diathermy or thermocautery. (L. Arnall. Reproduced by courtesy of The Journal of Small Animal Practice).

attempting to manipulate and remove the egg. For this type of impaction, oil should not be used for lubrication. Having succeeded in removing the cause of the prolapse, it can be completely replaced by careful manipulation. A soothing or anaesthetic cream should then be applied. If straining occurs then the cloaca will have to be partially closed by a veterina-

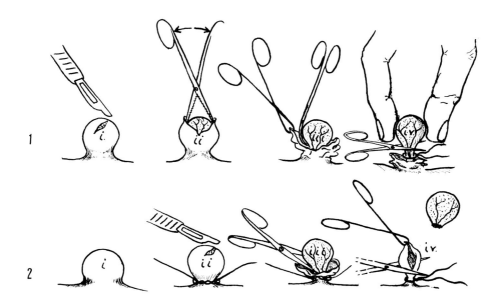

Figure 5/29. ALTERNATIVE METHODS FOR REMOVAL OF SESSILE, MORE VASCULAR OR LESS PEDUNCULATED TUMORS

1. Incision enlarged with forceps, blunt dissection of the skin flaps, ligation of the vascular pedicle and section distal to the ligature.

2. A variant of (1). A "running" ligature is slowly tightened round the tumor base, skin is incised and separated. Forceps or a second ligature is then placed round the vascular pedicle. The first ligature is finally tightened and the exposed contents are removed. The excess skin flaps can finally be trimmed. (L. Arnall. Reproduced by courtesy of The Journal of Small Animal Practice.

rian using a glass rod and purse-string suture which must be removed within 24 hours or excreta cannot be passed and straining may recommence. Twenty-four hours is usually long enough to allow most of the oedema and inflammatory swelling to subside in the replaced oviduct.

Relief of Crop Impaction After thoroughly plucking and cleaning the area, a longitudinal incision is made in the pendulous area of the neck through the skin and crop wall over the point of greatest

421

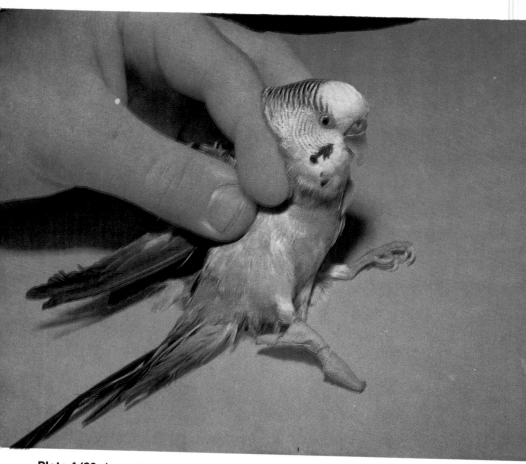

Plate 4/29. Leg strapped (or splinted) in extended position. Budgerigar. (L. Arnall)

Plate 5/29. Anesthetized parrotlet after laparotomy showing sutured wound and coils of dilated oviduct and ovary after removal. (L. Arnall)

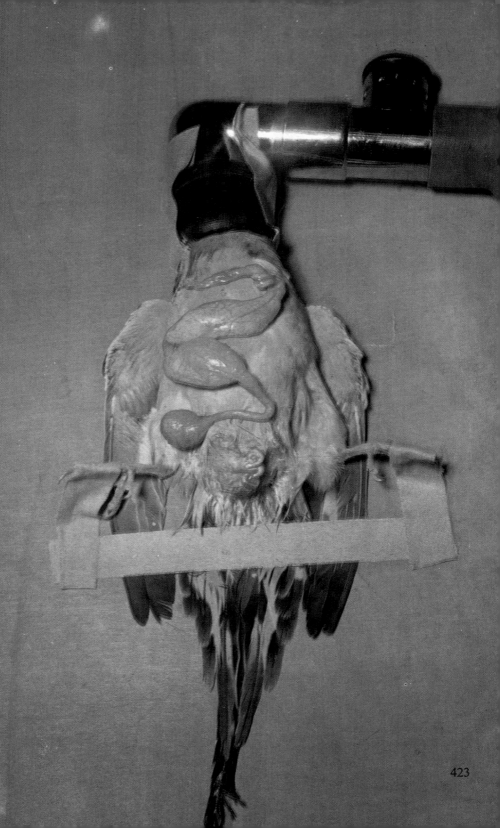

423

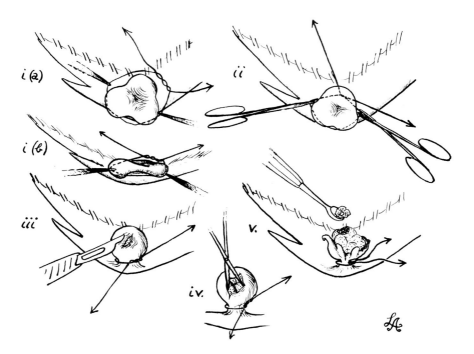

Figure 6/29. METHOD FOR REMOVAL OF SESSILE AND PLAQUE-LIKE LESIONS NEAR LIMB JOINTS

(ia) Application of "running" ligature around lesion held down by forceps (ii) while an assistant slowly tightens the ligature. This squeezes the mass (ib) so that the overlying skin becomes tense when the ligature has been drawn tight and the skin incised (iii and iv). The tumorous mass may then be moved piecemeal (v). The basal "running" ligature should be progressively tightened throughout the operation. (L. Arnall. Reproduced by courtesy of The Journal of Small Animal Practice).

swelling. The contents are then removed and the wound washed with 1 per cent saline solution. At this stage it is wise to test that the oesophagus below the crop is free of obstruction as far as the gizzard by probing with an instrument such as a length of round-ended stiff rubber tube. The crop wall and skin are each closed with a continuous suture of boiled cotton thread. An antibiotic, sulphonamide or other suitable antiseptic powder should be lightly dusted between the crop and skin before suturing the latter.

A light semi-liquid diet should be given at frequent intervals for the first three to five days after the operation, after which soaked and softened seed or finely minced foods can be given every three or four hours for a further week. Then normal food can be gradually resumed.

Removal of Leg Bands or Rings
If a ring is too tight, the bird may peck it in an attempt at removal. Even if it is the correct size for the species, it may become tight as the bird gets older since some birds develop thickened scales on the legs. Mite infestation of the legs also produces similar results. The ring then becomes a tourniquet and cuts off the blood supply. A swelling develops below it so that the ring becomes embedded in the tissues. The foot either dies and drops off later, or it becomes deformed if the ring is not rapidly removed, (see Plates 6/29 and 7/29).

To remove the embedded ring grasp it across its breadth with a pair of artery forceps, so that the points of a sharp pair of clippers can be placed astride it where it is least embedded. The artery forceps help to prevent it twisting and thus avoid fracturing the leg. The clippers are then slowly closed so as to cut through the ring. A second pair of artery forceps should be used to grip the ring on the opposite side of the split, so that it can be directly pulled or prized open against the first pair. At no stage must the ring be pulled against the leg. During the operation the bird should be either held by another person or anaesthetized. Unless great care is used the leg can be fractured easily whilst removing the ring.

A more efficient method of cutting the ring is to use a special jeweller's ring cutter instead of clippers—Figure 8/29.

If the leg has been badly damaged by the ring, dressings will be necessary and interference by the bird must be prevented. If there is swelling of the foot or leg below the ring this may persist for some weeks, or if it is long established, fibrous replacement of the damaged tissues will remain permanently.

Rings which are too large may cause trouble from chafing and need to be removed; they are also likely to get caught up in things and cause the bird to injure itself.

Rupture of the Abdominal Wall
If the rupture is soft and fluctuating and the contents can be pushed back into their normal position, plastic surgery can often be performed to remove the stretched and superfluous abdominal wall. Under anaesthetic a veterinarian can open the abdomen along the midline, with the bird on its back, and the displaced contents can then be replaced or "reduced". After a brief examination of the abdominal

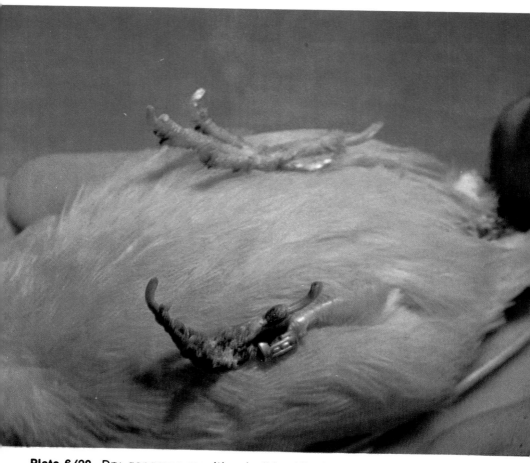

Plate 6/29. Dry gangrene resulting in "death" of the foot caused by the tourniquet effect of a ring following injury to the foot. Canary. (L. Arnall)

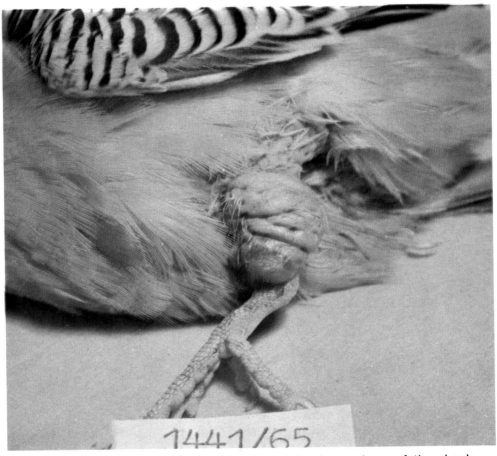

Plate 7/29. Chronic, fibrosed thickening following oedema of the shank region caused by a ring which tightened due to swelling associated with injury or growth. Budgerigar. (L. Arnall)

cavity to ensure that the duodenal loop or other organs are not remaining in the distension, he will clamp the base of the now empty sac with two parallel hair clips or by other means, cut off the spare flaps of abdomen which make up the sac, and suture the lips of the wound between the clamps with fine thread. The upper clamp should be removed immediately to avoid tissue necrosis; the lower one, outside the sutures, may remain for 12 to 24 hours. Healing is usually completed in about ten days and the eventual scar line gives midline support to prevent further rupture. Recovery and surgical success is usual in most cases.

If the rupture is tense, rubbery, or any colour other than pinkish-yellow, there may be a variety of causes such as an abdominal tumour, cyst or an egg developed outside the oviduct, retained tubal egg or eggs, or peritonitis. The prognosis for surgical correction in these cases is poor or in some instances hopeless.

Figure 7/29. MID-LINE LAPAROTOMY FOR THE REMOVAL OF SUB-LUMBAR INTRA-ABDOMINAL NEOPLASMS

(i) A small longitudinal incision is first made midway between the xiphisternum and the cloaca and this is then carefully extended. The abdominal, muscular wall is similarly opened to expose the viscera (iii). The healthy, normal organs are then moved aside and the sub-lumbar mass is isolated still on its vascular attachment by blunt dissection. Diathermy is preferable to forceps or ligature for section because of risk of hemorrhage. (L. Arnall. Reproduced by courtesy of The Journal of Small Animal Practice.)

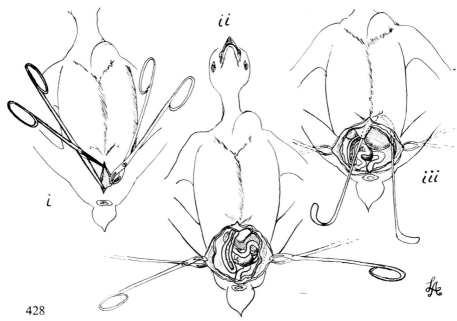

Removal of Fats, Oils, Tar and Greasy Medicaments from the Plumage	These are best removed by prolonged or repeated swabbing of the affected plumage with a shaving brush soaked in a dilute warm detergent solution. Afterwards the bird must be allowed to dry off in a heated hospital cage. When it is dry, the temperature of the cage should be lowered slowly to that of the environment before returning the bird to its own quarters. Methods of cleaning oiled seabirds are beyond the scope of this book, but special publications cover the subject fully (see selected bibliography).
Other Operations	Intra-abdominal operations or laparotomies for removal of tumours (Figure 7/29), eggs in the abdominal cavity and foreign bodies in the proventriculus or gizzard, should not be attempted by unqualified persons. These and the following procedures all belong strictly within the province of the veterinarian: paracentesis for sampling body fluids; the removal of diffuse or large sub-cutaneous fatty masses or neoplasms (Figure 9/29); high-level amputation of leg or wing; insertion of metal supports for fractured limb bones; "de-voicing" peacocks or other birds, and removal of an eye.
Haemorrhagic and Other Types of Post-operative Shock	Post-operative Shock which may follow surgery is discussed in Chapter 27.
Nursing and Post-operative Care	Sometimes birds become excitable when recovering from an anaesthetic and this can easily lead to damage of the plumage, skin or even the bones of the limbs. A simple method of preventing such damage is to enclose the anaesthetized bird in a roll of gauze, paper or thin card, and fix the edges with adhesive tape. Both ends of the cylinder are left open with the head free at one end. Most birds remain calm under these conditions and recover consciousness without damaging themselves. After recovery, sudden changes of temperature should be avoided and glucose saline or oxygen may sometimes be necessary to counteract shock (see Chapter 27).
Hospital Cages	(see Plate 8/29) Some birds appear to benefit from a period in a heated hospital cage after recovery from an anaesthetic, or if shocked, chilled, travel-weary or injured. Others unfortunately, seem to suffer more and may even die in such an environment. A sick bird takes in less food and burns its resources at a higher rate in order to maintain its raised temperature. One

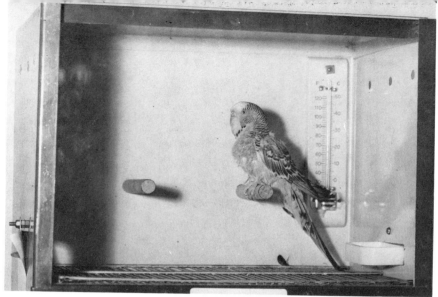

Plate 8/29. A commercially-produced hospital cage housing a sick budgerigar. Note the thermometer and electric fitting at the side to provide underfloor heating. (Central Photographic Dept. University of Liverpool)

Plate 1/30. Japanese quail prepared for *post-mortem* examination. The skin on the ventral surface of the body has been deflected to expose the pectoral (breast) and abdominal muscles. (I.F. Keymer and G. Dibley)

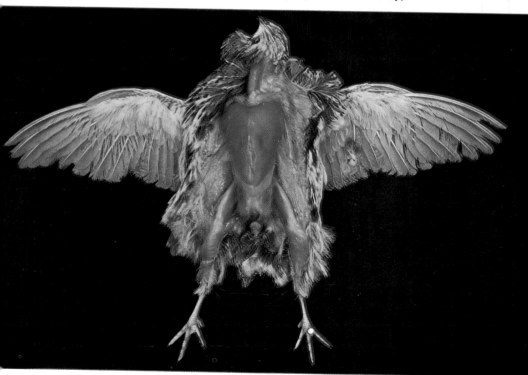

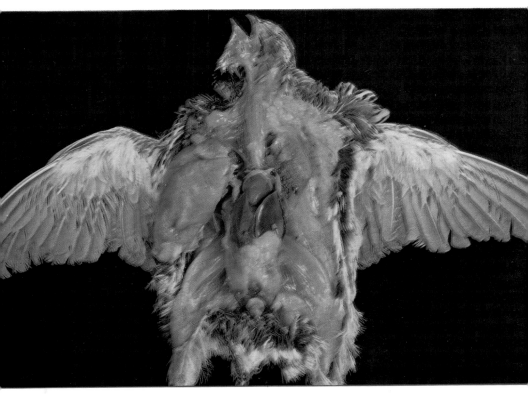

Plate 2/30. Healthy Japanese quail showing second stage of *post-mortem* examination with buccal cavity (mouth) opened, oesophagus and crop exposed and sternum with overlying pectoral muscles deflected to the right side by cutting through the ribs and clavicle on the opposite side. The heart is exposed lying in the anterior part of the thorax and immediately in front of the liver. The abdominal cavity has been left intact. (I.F. Keymer and G. Dibley)

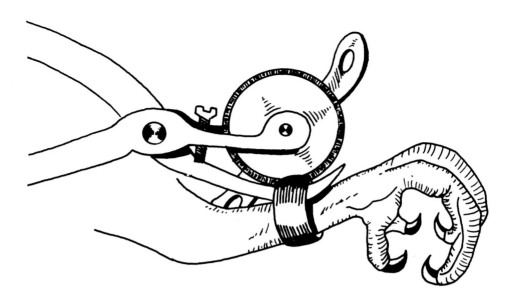

Figure 8/29. REMOVAL OF LEG RING USING JEWELLOR'S RING CUTTER.
The handles of the instrument are held in one hand, and with the other the wing nut and the fine-toothed cutting wheel are turned in the direction shown by the arrow. The screw allows for fine adjustment to the thickness of the ring. It is necessary for an attendant to hold the bird on its back. (L. Arnall)

or more of its organs will be functioning inefficiently and inactivity makes the bird more prone to further infection and chilling. All these factors amount to stress. If the stress of heat loss and the necessity for activity—jostling by other birds, looking for food, flight, etc.—is curtailed in a heated cage, the bird's resources can be put to better use in fighting the illness. The principle is the same as keeping an invalid in bed.

But the hospital cage can have other less desirable effects. If the thermostatic control is not sufficiently sensitive, over-heating or cooling, sometimes in alternation, may cause greater stress than an unheated cage. The small heated cage may sometimes be poorly ventilated, or the relative humidity so low that panting and fluid loss by evaporation can occur.

If the bird's blood pressure is low from inefficient heart action, or temperature control of the body is poor, a cage temperature of 28–34°C (85–95°F) may so increase the blood

432

Plate 3/30. Healthy Japanese quail showing third stage of *post-mortem* examination. The sternum and pectoral muscles have been completely removed. The cut surfaces of the pectoral muscles are situated either side and mainly anterior to the heart. The liver lies posterior to the heart, being partly in the thoracic cavity and partly in the abdomen. The posterior part of the liver covers the ventral surface of the gizzard, which is in contact with the large duodenal loop on the bird's right. (I.F. Keymer and G. Dibley)

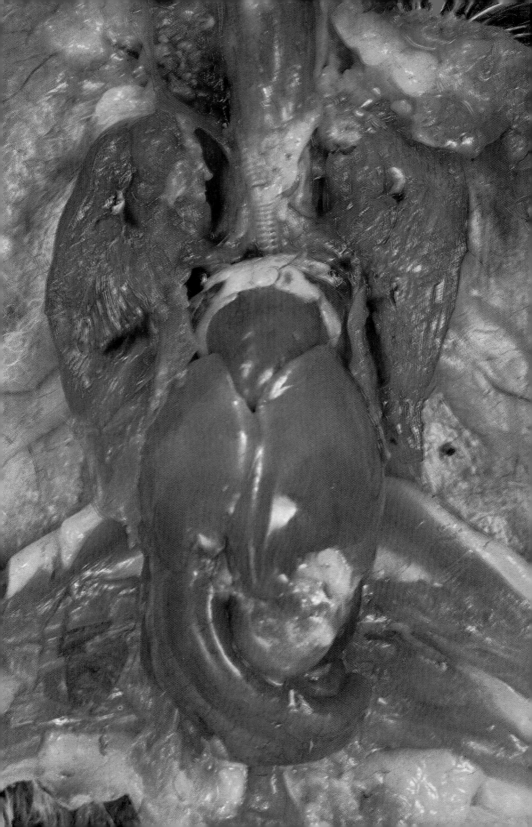

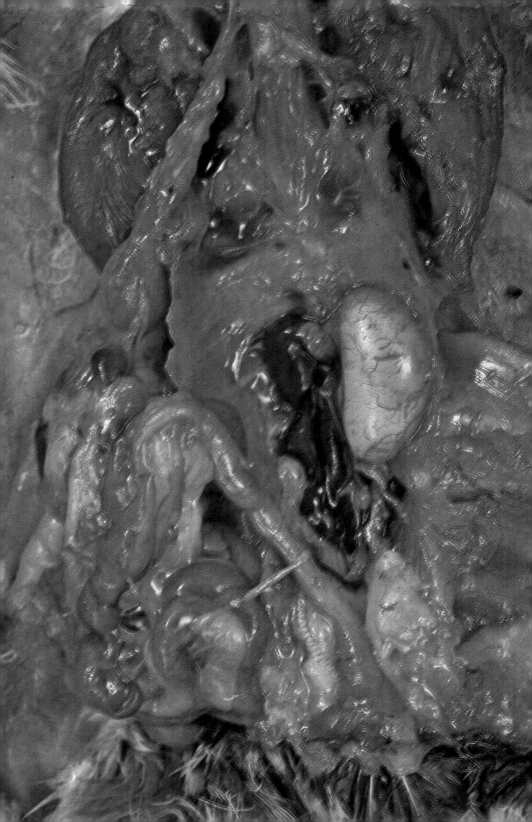

Plate 4/30. Healthy male Japanese quail showing further stage in *post-mortem* examination. The heart, liver and right testis have been removed. The alimentary tract has been deflected to the bird's right side and the rounded, normal, dark red spleen is visible lying close to the junction of the intact proventriculus and gizzard. Note the normal bright, reddish-pink lungs lying in the thoracic cavity. The air sacs are not visible because being healthy they were thin and transparent. The normal, dark, red kidneys lie in close apposition to the "roof" of the synsacrum immediately dorsal to the testes. The left testis is hypertrophied, whitish in colour and is the elongated organ lying in the abdominal cavity and concealing much of the left kidney. The right adrenal gland is just visible as a pale, yellowish-pink structure overlying the anterior pole of the right kidney. It was exposed when the right testis was removed. (I.F. Keymer and G. Dibley)

flow to the body surface and skin that blood pressure is further reduced, which can cause fainting, collapse and death. This is most likely to occur after surgical operations, anaesthesia and haemorrhage.

Although requirements vary, a hospital cage is of most use over a range of 22.5–28°C (75–85°F) with good ventilation and a moderate humidity. Higher temperatures are some-

Figure 9/29. METHOD FOR REMOVAL OF SESSILE DIFFUSE AND LIPOMATOSIS TYPE LESIONS OF THE BREAST AND BELLY

(i) Incision is made and enlarged by cutting between the two curved forceps clamps. (ii) Illustrates the incision and tumorous mass in cross section. The mass is removed by blunt dissection. The skin is then sutured (iii) with continuous mattress sutures using braided nylon, abralon or silk. (L. Arnall. Reproduced by courtesy of The Journal of Small Animal Practice.)

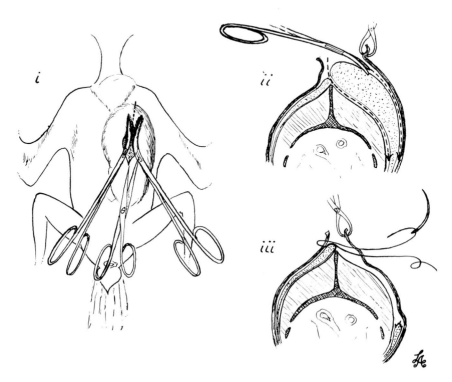

times needed, but the best guide is the posture and apparent comfort of the patient. Most veterinarians prefer to use an infra-red lamp or guarded electrical heating element instead of a hospital cage, the advantage being that the amount of heat on the bird can be controlled more easily. The bird can also move away from the source of heat if it becomes too hot. The hospital cage or any other cage in which a sick bird has been kept, must be scrupulously cleaned between patients, any of which may be the first case of a subsequent epidemic. Most hospital cages on the market are almost impossible to sterilize and are fitted with electric light bulbs as a source of heat, so that in order to keep the bird warm it is necessary to subject it to continuous light. which is bad for it and tends to prevent it resting properly. Since electrical parts are liable to damage by sterilization, and the metal parts are subject to chemical corrosion, poisonous gas sterilization is preferable to hot water and detergents. The entire cage can be put in a plastic bag for several hours with the source of gas. Sulphur dioxide, chlorine and ammonia are suitable, although the first two form acids in moist air and can also corrode.

Plate 5/30. Healthy female Japanese quail showing similar stage of *post-mortem* examination to that depicted in the male quail (Plate 4/40). Below the lungs the active ovary is visible comprising well developed, rounded yolks on the left side. The hypertrophied oviduct is visible extending posteriorly below the ovary. The alimentary tract has been deflected to the other side and shows the proventriculus overlying the right lung, followed by the gizzard, the duodenal loop enclosing the dark red pancreas, beneath and below which are the coils of the intestinal tract obscuring the kidneys. (I.F. Keymer and G. Dibley)

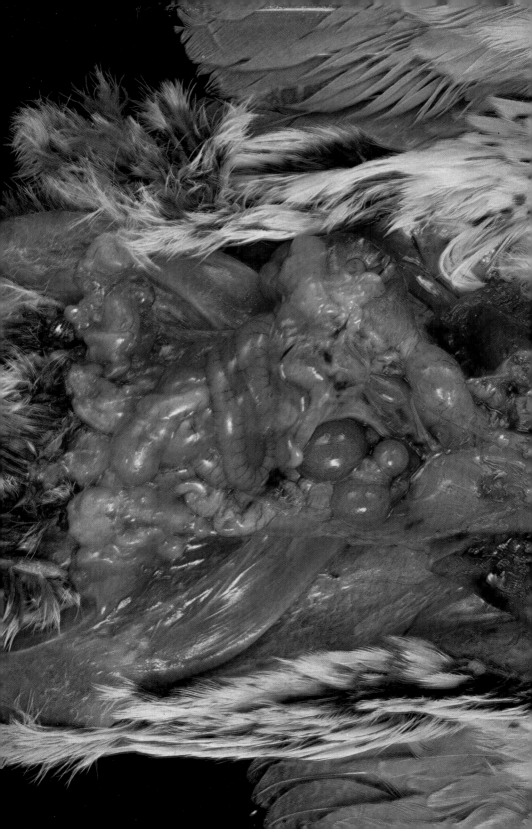

SELECTED BIBLIOGRAPHY

ANONYMOUS (1972). *Recommended treatment of oiled sea-birds.* Advisory Committee on Oil Pollution of the Sea, Dept. of Zoology, University of Newcastle-upon-Tyne, England, 10pp. Price £0.25.

ARNALL, L. A. (1960). *Some common surgical entities of the budgerigar.* Vet. Rec. *72*, 888–890.

ARNALL, L. A. (1966). *The Clinical Approach to Tumours in Cage Birds*—IV. Treatment of Cage Bird Tumours. J. small anim. Pract. *7.*, 241–251.

GANDAL, C. P. (1969). Surgical Techniques and Anaesthesia. In *Diseases of Cage and Aviary Birds,* p.217–231. Ed. Petrak, M. L., Philadelphia. Lea and Febiger.

SCHWARTE, L. H. (1965). Poultry Surgery. In *Diseases of Poultry,* p.1149–1161. Eds. Biester, H. E. and Schwarte, L. H. 5th Ed. Ames, Iowa. State University Press.

SAMPLING AND NECROPSY

Ideally all birds which die or are destroyed should be submitted to a veterinary laboratory for *post-mortem* examination. When this is impracticable, the following brief description of necropsy techniques may help the unqualified person with no knowledge of pathology to grasp the cause of trouble and to understand the layout and colour of organs in healthy and diseased birds.

Materials
Pair of rubber gloves.
Bowl of cold water and disinfectant.
Waste container—to be incinerated with carcase and remains.
Small screw-top, water-tight jars.
Cork mat or board 6 in. square or bigger.
Stout pins or small nails.
Scalpel or other sharp knife.
Dissecting forceps: one pair with plain ends and another pair
    with "rat-tooth" ends.
Fine pointed scissors about 5 in. long.
Strong scissors or bone forceps.

Blood Sampling
Samples may be collected from either live or dead birds as explained below.
   A layman should not attempt to take blood from the wing or other large veins of a living bird by hypodermic needle and syringe; in unskilled hands a subcutaneous haemorrhage thus induced may be difficult to control. If a foot is carefully washed and then rubbed with cotton wool soaked in surgical or methylated spirits, a minute nick of a toe pad with a clean scalpel will produce several drops of blood. These can be dropped directly into a sterilized 5 ml. screw-topped bottle or small, rubber-corked, test tube, or they may be drawn up by a sterilized eye dropper or pipette. A little sticking plaster around the toe will stop further bleeding. In birds which have died recently, blood can be taken from the heart—after the

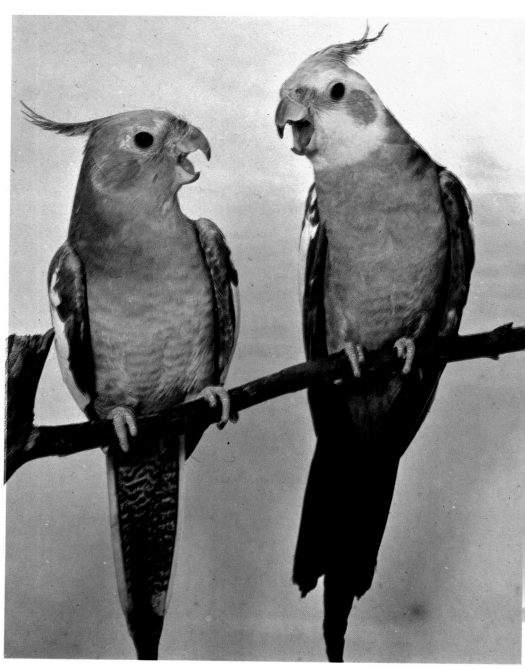

Cockatiels (*Nymphicus hollandicus*). This small Australian psittacine is a popular aviary bird, being hardy and a prolific breeder.

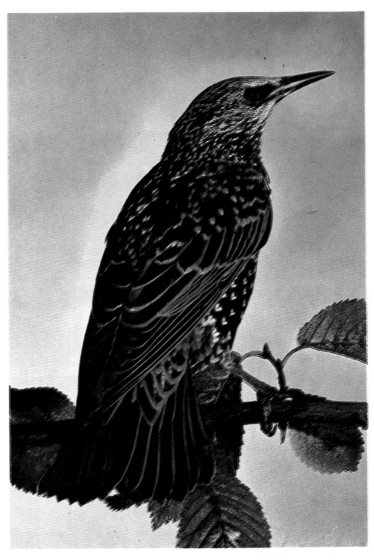

The starling (*Sturnus vulgaris*) is a pest to bird keepers in many parts of the world. It steals the food of aviary birds and can transmit diseases such as pseudotuberculosis (Chapter 7) and "gapes" or syngamiasis (Chapter 10).

pericardial sac is opened—by inserting a hypodermic needle and syringe into the middle of the heart. Alternatively a pipette can be used after cutting across the auricles of the heart. Pipette, syringe and blades, however, must be sterilized before use.

Smears for microscopical examination can be made satisfactorily only by veterinarians or experienced technicians. Smears may be taken before or after death, the latter being unsuitable for haematological purposes but suitable to examine for blood parasites.   **Blood Smears**

Ascitic or other peritoneal fluids should be removed only from live birds by qualified persons as great care is necessary to avoid puncturing gut, liver, oviduct or airsacs with the needle.   **Abdominal Fluid**

Swellings which are rubbery, fluctuate owing to the presence of fluid and lie immediately under the skin, can be drained safely by using a sterile syringe and needle. Swellings in the lower neck, however, should not be punctured by the inexperienced because they are often filled with blood and haemorrhage may result.   **Cystic Fluids**

Creamy swellings around various joints, especially of the limbs, may be deposits of urates or may be pus arising from bacterial infection. Samples can be obtained from the live bird by cleansing the affected area with spirits, nicking the swelling with a scalpel and picking up the material on a twist of cotton wool or a matchstick, all suitably sterilized; the sample should then be placed in a sterile corked tube or small bottle. This type of sterile swab is useful for bacteriological investigations and swabs can also be used for blood, pus, excreta or body fluids obtained from elsewhere. The cotton-wool and stick probes used for cleaning infants' noses are ideal and a readily-obtainable alternative to the home-made swab.   **Pus and Exudates**

These should be collected directly from the bird and can usually be obtained by gently pressing the abdomen. The droppings should be allowed to fall into a sterile, screw-topped small jar. Excreta taken from the floor of the cage, or even from a sheet of paper on it, are likely to be contaminated and dehydrated. If the bird is too sick to handle, however, then the latter method of collection is better.   **Droppings or Excreta**

444

Nasal, Ocular and other Discharges	A sterile swab is the best means of obtaining samples of discharges. The swab must be placed immediately in a sterile tube or bottle.

Skin Scrapings, Scabs, Feather Cysts and Damaged Feathers

These can be obtained by scraping the skin with a blunt scalpel or small knife. The samples should be placed in a sterile bottle when being sent to a laboratory for examination for fungi or parasites.

The contents of feather cysts or necrotic fatty tumours may be scraped out with a curette or similar blunt instrument. Sometimes tissues suspected of being infected with avian pox virus can be taken in this way, or with a swab.

Biopsies

The removal of a slice of living or necrotic tissue from a live bird for microscopic examination is essentially a task for the veterinarian and may require the administration of an anaesthetic. Unless the tissue is removed correctly, severe haemorrhage may occur. Small stalked (pedunculated) tumours can, however, be safely removed by ligaturing, or tying a piece of thread around the stalk-like attachment. The tumour eventually dies from lack of blood and falls off. Feather cysts and other similar structures can be removed similarly.

***Post-mortem* Examination**

If a necropsy is attempted, the bird should be placed on its back with wings and legs extended by transfixing them with pins to the board. The feathers of the neck, breast and belly should be dampened and removed by plucking to avoid their dispersal in the air. This also lessens the risk of spreading infections such as psittacosis. The skin should be incised from throat to vent and dissected sideways from the midline to expose the muscle layers, (Plate 1/30).

A small incision in the abdominal wall near the vent should be made with scissors and then enlarged forward and out to one side behind the ribs. Cutting through the ribs, clavicle and pectoral muscles, the entire sternum with overlying muscles can be lifted and deflected to one side; a similar cut on the other side will allow complete removal of the sternum. With strong scissors or scalpel, the jaw can be deflected similarly by cutting longitudinally through the angle between upper and lower jaws, (Plate 2/30 and 3/30).

At this stage the tongue, glottis, inner nares, trachea, syrinx, oesophagus and crop can be inspected. Then the trachea and oesophagus can be split open to examine their lining and contents. Abnormalities include growths, parasites, impactions, foreign bodies and inflammatory reactions.

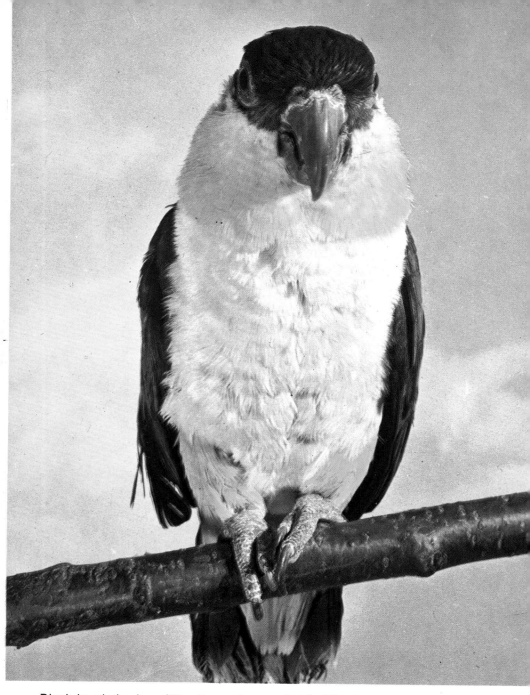

Black-headed caique (*Pionites melanocephala*). All caiques as well as lories and conures need large quantities of fruit which results in watery excreta. This is not therefore abnormal for these species and should not be regarded as a sign of kidney disease or confused with diarrhoea.

446

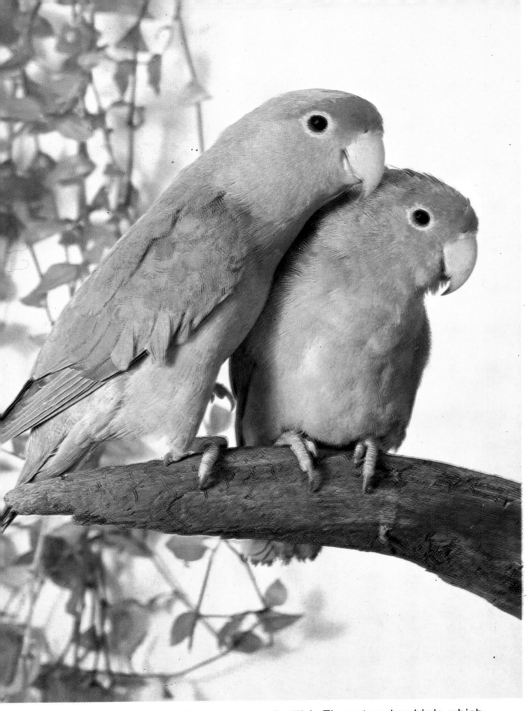

Peach-faced lovebirds (*Agapornis roseicollis*). These true lovebirds which, unlike parakeets have short tails, are very popular aviary birds. In common with all psittacine birds they are highly susceptible to psittacosis (Chapter 6).

Inside the chest can be found the bronchi, lungs, heart within its pericardinal sac, the great blood vessels and also the lower part of the oesophagus and the proventriculus.

Further back lie the gizzard, duodenum and loops of small intestine, the caeca (when present), rectum, the liver, oviduct and ovaries or testes. The gonads and kidneys, and much of the liver if normal, can be adequately seen only when the intestine has been removed, (Plate 4/30 and 5/30).

When the surface of each organ has been carefully examined, the cut surface should be inspected similarly, care being taken to spill as little blood as possible when removing heart and liver. Any organs suspected to be abnormal can be put in a screw-topped, sterilized jar and placed in a refrigerator or in a solution of 10 per cent formol saline. The refrigerated tissue will be suitable for bacteriological examination for about 72 hours if the bird died within a few hours of the necropsy. However, it is much more satisfactory to submit the carcase intact to a laboratory for bacteriological examination.

The next step is to strip the skin entirely from the carcase. Then skeleton, bones, joints and muscles can be examined for injury, deformity, swelling or discolouration.

It must be remembered that the natural colours of tissues persist for only a few hours after death, especially at room or nest-box temperatures. Bluish-black, green or other hues develop within about 24 hours in muscles and organs in contact with the gut, liver and especially the gall bladder, due to bacterial action. Within an hour of death, blood seeps into the bony substance of the cranium and is frequently mistaken for evidence of head injury by the inexperienced; merely rubbing with a finger greatly accentuates this effect.

Packaging

When it is necessary to send an entire carcase or samples to a veterinarian or laboratory, knowledge of a few rules will make all the difference between the specimens arriving fresh or only fit for the garbage bin.

All containers must be clean and sterilized before use, especially in the case of samples for bacteriological and virological examination. A satisfactory way of achieving this is to place them in an ordinary domestic pressure cooker for 20 minutes under 15 lb. pressure.

Carcases of birds suspected of carrying disease transmissible to human beings such as ornithosis should be dipped in a reliable disinfectant, packed whilst damp, insulated with paper and despatched in a strong water-tight tin to the nearest laboratory. Carcases or specimens should never be posted in an envelope or in flimsy boxes. The parcel should always be clearly labelled "URGENT: PATHOLOGICAL SPECIMEN".

No preservatives should be used with specimens or carcases on which bacteriological examination or chemical tests of any kind are required. Carcases for *post-mortem* examination should not be deep frozen, but placed in a refrigerator and kept at just over freezing point for about 12 hours before despatch. If specimens are likely to be in transit for more than 36 hours (or merely a few hours in hot climates), then they should be packed in ice or solid carbon dioxide within a thermos flask. The flask must be very well padded to avoid breakage.

An adequate history of all events leading up to the trouble, including diet, source of food, details of recently acquired birds, visits to shows, as well as a description of the clinical signs, must accompany a description of the specimen. In most cases your veterinarian will despatch the specimen and request the appropriate examinations and tests by the laboratory. He will also interpret the laboratory report and advise the owner accordingly.

Usually a list of local veterinarians can be obtained from the telephone directory, police or from the local cage-bird society.

SELECTED BIBLIOGRAPHY

HUNGERFORD, T. G. (1969). Post-mortem examination. In *Diseases of Poultry including Cage Birds and Pigeons,* p.548–549. 4th Ed. Sydney, London, Melbourne. Angus and Robertson.

KEYMER, I. F. (1961). *Post-mortem examinations of pet birds.* Mod. Vet. Pract, *42* (23), 35–38 and *42* (24), 47–51.

CLASSIFICATION OF BIRDS
AND HOST LIST OF IMPORTANT DISEASES

The system of scientific classification of living things which is in universal use today was developed by the Swedish naturalist Carl Linnaeus in the 18th century. It is a convenient method of arranging related plants and animals which is unlikely to be supplanted. The system is based on seven main groupings, commencing with the broadest distinctions between living organisms —the Plant and Animal Kingdoms— down to the individual units or species. There are a number of other subdivisions such as sub-genera, sub-families and super-families. All these are spelt with a capital letter and many can be recognised by their spelling, *e.g.,* family names all end in "ae" and names of orders end in "formes". Except for sub-genera these names are not printed in italics and a sub-generic name is placed in brackets after the name of the genus.

As an illustration, the classifications of Man and the Budgerigar are set out below:

	Man	*Budgerigar*
Kingdom	Animalia	Animalia
Phylum	Chordata	Chordata
Class	Mammalia	Aves
Order	Primates	Psittaciformes
Family	Hominidae	Psittacidae
Genus	*Homo*	*Melopsittacus*
Species	*sapiens*	*undulatus*

Although there are only two kinds of Kingdom, it will be appreciated that the numbers of other groups increase progressively with each subdivision.

In the Animal Kingdom in addition to Mammalia (mammals) and Aves (birds) there are three other important classes, namely Pisces (fishes), Amphibia (amphibians—frogs, toads, newts) and Reptilia (reptiles). The class Aves contains 27 Orders, many more Families and Genera and approximately 8,600 species. The phylum Arthropoda is by far the largest group in the Animal Kingdom. It includes over a million species comprising the well known invertebrates such as insects (class Insecta), spiders, ticks and mites (class Arachnida), some of which are parasites and have been dealt with in this book.

Every species of animal and plant when it is first described is given a scientific name, usually derived from Latin or Greek. Many are also given a common or vernacular name. Although a bird has only one scientific name which is used throughout the world, it may have many vernacular names. For example, in Australia everybody has heard of the budgerigar, which was originally named by the aboriginals. It is known by the same name in Great Britain, but in North America the bird is often referred to as a "shell parakeet" or simply a "parakeet". The French call it "la perruche ondulé" and the Germans "Der Wellensittich", but the scientific name used by ornithologists and other biologists, is *"Melopsittacus undulatus"*. The first or generic name shows the genus and the second name the species. It is customary to use

451

a capital for the first letter of the generic name and a small letter for the specific name and to print both in italics.

A great deal of confusion can arise if only the vernacular name is used in referring to a bird, because sometimes the same name may be used for more than one species. A good example is the robin, which in North America is a type of thrush with the scientific name *Turdus migratorius*, whilst in Great Britain it is the small warbler *Erithacus rubecula*. In this book the correct scientific name for each specific bird mentioned in the text has been given in the glossary, to prevent this type of misunderstanding.

Taxonomists have divided many species into sub-species, these being designated by the addition of a third scientific name following the specific one. Sub-species are also printed in italics and begin with a small letter. Sub-species of a species differ only very slightly from each other and can interbreed.

Under normal circumstances birds of one species cannot breed with birds of other species, but only amongst individuals of their own kind. Some species, although not being able to breed with each other, may nevertheless be closely related in many respects. For example, there are a number of very similar South American Amazon parrots. These species therefore have been grouped together in one genus, in this case *"Amazona"*. *Amazona aestiva* is the blue-fronted Amazon and *A. ochrocephala* is the yellow-fronted Amazon parrot.

Birds were originally classified by taxonomists purely on the basis of clearly visible anatomical features, such as beak and feet structure, skeletal and plumage features. More recently it has been realized that certain physiological and biochemical characteristics, such as the different types of amino acids present in egg proteins, can be used as an aid to determining the relationships of various species. Susceptibility to various diseases may be yet another factor to consider, although as yet it has received scant attention, because so little is known about the subject.

An attempt has been made here (it is believed for the first time) to analyse the susceptibility of birds in various orders to the most important diseases, especially those which are infectious. It is based on a review of the scientific literature and personal experience, and in the present state of knowledge can be regarded as a rough guide only to the types of diseases to which species in the various orders are susceptible. For the sake of simplicity and because the disease/host list refers to orders and not species, only the vernacular names of species are given. The first order, Struthioniformes, contains only one family Struthionidae and one living species, namely, the Ostrich, *Struthio camelus*, so that examples of diseases listed under this Order have obviously all been recorded in the Ostrich. The last order, Passeriformes, however, is the largest order of birds and contains more than half of all the species in existence. It is split into many families which, although considered to be related, contain a diverse range of species differing considerably in appearance, behaviour, feeding habits and probably in their susceptibility to disease. Under this heading, therefore, it does not necessarily mean that all diseases which are listed are capable of infecting every species in the Order, indeed there may be differences in the susceptibility of species in different families. Ideally, the order Passeriformes and the other large orders should be divided into families for the purpose of listing the diseases, but this is not yet worthwhile because there is insufficient information at present regarding the susceptibility of most species to various diseases. It will be noted that for a few orders no information is recorded, mainly because the members are seldom kept in captivity, and therefore seldom examined. There is a considerable amount of information available concerning the order Galliformes because this order contains domestic poultry. The susceptibility to disease of some other species, such as game birds, has also been studied intensively.

In addition to lack of information, this host list of diseases is incomplete because only naturally-occurring diseases, as opposed to experimental infections, are included. Many species are simply healthy carriers of some infectious organisms, especially parasites, and these also have not been included. Indeed, all species harbour parasites of some kind and therefore these are listed only when there is evidence that they may be pathogenic.

So little is known about the diseases of non-domesticated birds, and so few have been examined by veterinary pathologists, that it is seldom possible to suggest the prevalence of various diseases in different orders or other groups; nevertheless, an attempt has been made in a few cases.

Infectious diseases which occur in both the free-living and captive states are included, although those listed under the heading of "Nutritional/Metabolic Diseases" are almost entirely confined to birds in captivity. If incorrectly fed, all species become susceptible to the wide range of nutritional deficiency diseases, and therefore only those are listed which are commonly met with under conditions of captivity. As more is learned about nutrition of birds, these deficiences will of course become rare.

STRUTHIONIFORMES. Ostriches. (Figure 8/2).

Viral/Rickettsial Infections: Newcastle Disease (rare).

Bacterial Infections: Anthrax, tuberculosis, *Edwardsiella tarda* infection (probably rare), pseudomoniasis, salmonellosis, staphylococcosis, *Escherichia coli* septicaemia.

Fungal Infections: Aspergillosis.

Helminth Infestations: Tapeworms (relatively common), *Libyostrongylus* (Syn. *Ornithostrongylus*) *douglassi* infestation of proventriculus (young birds), *Houttuynia struthionis* infestation of small intestine (young birds).

Nutritional/Metabolic Diseases: Rickets and similar nutritional bone diseases. Probably vitamin and/or protein deficiencies, especially in growing birds, causing degenerative disease of the heart (cardiomyopathy).

Others: Ingestion of foreign bodies causing impaction or perforation of proventriculus and gizzard and peritonitis. Intestinal disorders probably common. **Atherosclerosis and arteriosclerosis.**

RHEIFORMES. Rheas. (Figure 1/AP).

Viral/Rickettsial Infections: Pox. Newcastle Disease.

Bacterial Infections: Tuberculosis.

Fungal Infections: Candidiasis, aspergillosis.

Helminth Infestations: *Houttuynia* sp. infestation of small intestine.

Nutritional Metabolic Diseases: Vitamin deficiencies in growing birds. Perosis.

Others: Atherosclerosis, arteriosclerosis, gizzard and intestinal impactions with grass or foreign bodies causing perforation and peritonitis (probably common).

CASUARIIFORMES. Cassowaries and Emus. (Figure 8/2).
Viral/Rickettsial Infections: Newcastle Disease (Cassowary).
Bacterial Infections: Tuberculosis.
Protozoan Infections: *Trichomonas gallinae* associated with enteritis.
Nutritional/Metabolic Diseases: Perosis.
Others: Arteriosclerosis.

APTERYGIFORMES. Kiwis. (Figure 2/AP).
Pneumoconiosis (in captivity).

TINAMIFORMES. Tinamous. (Figure 1/AP).
Bacterial Infections: Tuberculosis.
Fungal Infections: Aspergillosis.

SPHENISCIFORMES. Penguins. (Figure 1/AP).
Viral/Rickettsial Infections: Newcastle disease (rare).
Bacterial Infections: Salmonellosis, tuberculosis (rare), erysipelas (rare), pasteurellosis, *Vibrio* sp. infection (rare; king penguin).
Fungal Infections: Aspergillosis (very common), candidiasis.
Protozoan Infections: Malaria (in warm climates).
Nutritional/Metabolic Diseases: Vitamin A deficiency may be relatively common in captivity.
Others: Heat stroke (Antarctic penguins in warm climates).

GAVIIFORMES. Divers or Loons. (Figure 1/AP).
Viral/Rickettsial Infections: Ornithosis.
Bacterial Infections: Salmonellosis, Tuberculosis.
Fungal Infections: Aspergillosis.

Others: Common victims of oiling at sea; botulism.

PODICIPEDIFORMES. Grebes. (Figure 1/AP).
Viral/Rickettsial Infections: Pox.
Bacterial Infections: Pasteurellosis, erysipelas.
Others: Botulism.

PROCELLARIIFORMES, Albatrosses. Petrels, Shearwaters. (Figure 11/2).
Viral/Rickettsial Infections: Ornithosis, puffinosis or vesicular dermatitis (Shearwaters, fulmar petrels).
Fungal Infections: Aspergillosis.
Protozoan Infections: Renal coccidiosis (so-called "limey-disease"), Shearwaters.

PELICANIIFORMES. Tropic birds, Pelicans, Cormorants, Darters, Frigate birds, Gannets. (Figure 8/2).
Viral/Rickettsial Infections: Ornithosis, Newcastle disease (shags, cormorants and gannets), pox (cormorants).
Bacterial Infections: Salmonellosis, tuberculosis, pasteurellosis, erysipelas
Fungal Infections: Aspergillosis.
Helminth Infestations: *Contracaecum* infestation of proventriculus (pelicans).
Nutritional/Metabolic Diseases: Vitamin E deficiency has been suspected in pelicans, causing steatitis.
Others: Atherosclerosis, susceptible to foot injuries such as arthritis in captivity (especially gannets), botulism.

CICONIIFORMES. Egrets, Herons, Bitterns, Storks, Hammerkop, Ibises, Flamingos, Shoebills, Spoonbills. (Figure 11/2).
Viral/Rickettsial Infections: Ornithosis (relatively resistant), pox (storks and flamingos), avian leucosis complex (egret), Newcastle disease (storks,

herons, ibises and flamingos).

Bacterial Infections: Localised Staphylococcal infections of the feet ("bumblefoot"), pasteurellosis, erysipelas, tuberculosis, anthrax (flamingos), streptococcosis, salmonellosis.

Fungal Infections: Aspergillosis (common), candidiasis.

Protozoan Infections: *Haemoproteus* infection (spoonbill).

Helminth Infestations: Nematode infestations of proventriculus and gizzard.

Arthropod Infestations: Lice (common).

Nutritional/Metabolic Diseases: Rickets and similar nutritional bone disease. Vitamin A and B deficiencies.

Others: Botulism, susceptible to all kinds of foot injuries including frost bite and arthritis, atherosclerosis (old birds in close captivity), intestinal disorders including impactions, nephrosis of various types.

ANSERIFORMES. Screamers, Swans, Geese, Ducks. (Figure 1/AP and 11/2).

Viral/Rickettsial Infections: Ornithosis (relatively resistant), Newcastle disease (relatively resistant), duck virus hepatitis, duck plague or duck virus enteritis, eastern encephalitis arbovirus, Marek's disease (rare), fowl plague (rare), aegyptianellosis (geese).

Bacterial Infections: Salmonellosis, staphylococcosis, pasteurellosis, tuberculosis (common), anthrax (rare), pseudotuberculosis, spirochaetosis, listeriosis, erysipelas, vibriosis or *Vibrio metchnikovi* infection (geese), goose influenza or infectious myocarditis, streptococcosis, duck septicaemia (*Pasteurella*[Syn. *Pfeifferella* or *Moraxella*]*anatipestifer* infection).

Fungal Infections: Aspergillosis (common), candidiasis (geese).

Protozoan Infections: Leucocytozoonosis, renal coccidiosis (mainly young geese), intestinal coccidiosis caused by various species of coccidia (rare).

Helminth Infestations: Gizzard worms (*Amidostomum* spp. common especially in young geese), thorny-headed worms (*Polymorphus boschadis*—mainly in young birds), trichostrongylosis (*Trichostrongylus tenuis* infestation—especially in goslings), echinuriasis (*Echinuria* spp. infestation) of proventriculus, tetrameriasis (*Tetrameres* spp. infestation) of proventriculus, avioserpensiasis (*Avioserpens taiwana* infestation) of mouth, gapeworms (*Syngamus trachea* until recently called *Cyathostoma bronchialis* in waterfowl), trematode *Cyathocotyle bushiensis* infestation.

Others: Botulism, leech infestations (usually secondary to diseases such as botulism), atherosclerosis.

FALCONIFORMES. Vultures, Secretary birds, Hawks, Eagles, Ospreys, Falcons, Falconets, Caracaras. (Figure 11/2).

Viral/Rickettsial Infections: Newcastle disease (highly susceptible), *Herpes* virus hepatitis, pox, Marek's disease, ornithosis (rare).

Bacterial Infections: Tuberculosis (common), salmonellosis, *Escherichia coli* infections, pseudomoniasis (*Pseudomonas aeruginosa* infection), pasteurellosis, staphylococcosis, erysipelas, listeriosis, *Corynebacterium ovis* infection (rare), pseudotuberculosis (rare), anthrax (rare), *Mycoplasma* infections of eyes, "bumblefoot" infections due to *Staphylococci, Streptococci* or *Escherichia coli* (common).

Fungal Infections: Aspergillosis (common in captivity).

Protozoan Infections: Trichomoniasis of crop, malaria (rare).

Helminth Infestations: Filarial worms (*Serratospiculum* spp.), Capillariasis of oesophagus and intestine.

Arthropod Infestations: Lice appear to be the most common ectoparasites.

Nutritional/Metabolic Diseases: Rickets and osteomalacia (common in pet birds and those belonging to inexperienced falconers), Vitamin A and B deficiencies in captivity.

Others: Atherosclerosis. (Incidence is higher than in any other Order of birds or mammals; mainly old birds in Zoological Gardens). Botulism; turkey vultures are stated to be resistant.

GALLIFORMES. Brush turkeys, Curassows, Guans, Grouse, Ptarmigans, Pheasants, Partridges, Domestic Fowls, Quails, Guinea Fowls, Turkeys, Hoatzins. (Figure 3/2).

Viral/Rickettsial Diseases: Newcastle disease (most species highly susceptible), fowl plague, pox, infectious laryngotracheitis (domestic fowl and pheasants), ornithosis (especially turkeys), infectious bronchitis (domestic fowl), leucosis complex including Marek's disease or fowl paralysis or neurolymphomatosis and osteopetrosis (mainly domestic fowl), encephalomyelitis or epidemic tremor (domestic fowl), infectious synovitis (domestic fowl and turkeys), avian monocytosis (domestic fowl and turkeys), avian viral arthritis (domestic fowl), Gumboro disease (domestic fowl), eastern encephalitis arbovirus, rabies (domestic fowl; very rare), quail bronchitis (apparently confined to bobwhite quail), aegyptianellosis (domestic fowl).

Bacterial Infections: Tuberculosis, salmonellosis including pullorum disease or bacillary white diarrhoea (B.W.D.) and fowl typhoid, pasteurellosis or fowl cholera, erysipelas (especially turkeys), listeriosis (uncommon), pseudotuberculosis (especially turkeys), *Escherichia coli* infections, streptococcosis, staphylococcis, mycoplasmosis (infectious sinusitis and air-sacculitis), "bumblefoot" infections due to *Staphylococcus* spp., *Streptococcus* spp. and *Escherichia coli*, infectious coryza caused by *Haemophilus gallinarum* (mainly domestic fowl), vibriosis or *Vibrio metchnikovi* infection (domestic fowl), vibrionic hepatitis (domestic fowl), anthrax (domestic fowl; very rare), spirochaetosis (poultry and pheasants). *Pasteurella* (Syn. *Pfeifferella* or *Moraxella*) *anatipestifer* infection (quail and pheasants).

Fungal Infections: Aspergillosis (common), candidiasis (mainly turkeys and partridges), favus due to *Trichophyton* infection (uncommon).

Protozoan Infections: Histomoniasis or "blackhead" (common in turkeys, peafowl and game birds), intestinal and caecal coccidiosis caused by *Eimeria* spp. (common in poultry, peafowl and game birds), hexamitiasis (turkeys), malaria (domestic fowl, turkeys and partridges), *Haemoproteus lophortyx* infection (Californian quail).

Helminth Infestations: Roundworms (*Ascaridia galli*), capillariasis of crop and intestine due to *Capillaria contorta* and *C. obsignata*, trichostrongylosis due to *Trichostrongylus tenuis* especially in grouse and partridges, syngamiasis due to *Syngamus trachea* especially in game birds, diapharynxiasis due to *Dyspharynx nasuta* especially in young grouse and other game birds.

Arthropod Infestations: Red mites (*Dermanyssus* and *Ornithonyssus* spp.) *Knemidocoptes mutans* causing scaly-leg disease (occasional).

Nutritional/Metabolic Diseases: Vitamin A deficiency (nutritional roup), Vitamin E deficiency (nutritional encephalomalacia), rickets and osteomalacia (rare with improved poultry diets).

Others: Botulism, atherosclerosis.

GRUIFORMES. Bustard quail, Plains-wanderer, Cranes, Limpkin, Trumpeters Rails, Gallinules, Coots, Crakes, Sun-bitterns, Cariamas, Bustards. (Figure 1/AP).

Viral/Rickettsial Infections: Pox (Great bustards and Cranes), ornithosis, Newcastle disease, (Cariama and Cranes. Rare).

Bacterial Infections: Salmonellosis, tuberculosis, erysipelas, pasteurellosis, "bumblefoot" infections due to *Staphylococcus, Streptococcus* spp. and *Escherichia coli*, pseudotuberculosis (apparently rare), listeriosis (rare) and *Escherichia coli* infection of internal organs.

Fungal Infections: Aspergillosis, candidiasis.

Protozoan Infections: Hexamitiasis (Cranes).

Helminth Infestations: Gizzard worms, syngamiasis.

Nutritional/Metabolic Diseases: Nutritional bone disease.

Others: Atherosclerosis, rather susceptible to foot injuries including arthritis.

CHARADRIIFORMES. Jacanas, Waders (Snipes, Sandpipers, Curlews, Godwits, Plovers, etc.), Phalaropes, Pratincoles, Coursers, Sheathbills, Skuas, Gulls, Terns, Skimmers, Auks, Guillemots, Razorbills. (Figure 1/AP, 8/2 and 11/2).

Viral/Rickettsial Infections: Ornithosis (relatively resistant), puffinosis or vesicular dermatitis (gulls), fowl plague (terns), pox (rare). Newcastle disease (gull, rare).

Bacterial Infections: Tuberculosis, pasteurellosis, staphylococcal, streptococcal and *Escherichia coli* infections of the joints, pseudotuberculosis, salmonellosis (especially gulls), erysipelas, listeriosis.

Fungal Infections: Aspergillosis, candidiasis (apparently rare).

Helminth Infestations: Gizzard worms (kittiwakes), *Contracaecum* infestations of oesophagus and proventriculus (common in the auks), syngamiasis (some waders).

Others: Waders are susceptible to all kinds of foot injuries including frost bite and arthritis, oiled auks in captivity being particularly susceptible to arthritis of the hock joint. Auks, including guillemots and razorbills are the main victims of oiling at sea. Botulism, atherosclerosis (uncommon).

COLUMBIFORMES. Sand grouse, Pigeons, Doves. (Figure 11/2).

Viral/Rickettsial Infections: Ornithosis, Newcastle disease (rather resistant), *Herpesvirus* infection or inclusion disease, pox, eastern encephalitis arbovirus, Marek's disease (rare), fowl plague (rare).

Bacterial Infections: Salmonellosis, pasteurellosis (rare), pseudotuberculosis, tuberculosis, erysipelas, localised staphylococcal infections of the feet ("bumblefoot"), listeriosis (rare), *Haemophilus* infection and/or mycoplasmosis causing infectious sinusitis, streptococcosis.

Fungal Infections: Aspergillosis, candidiasis.

Protozoan Infections: Trichomoniasis (common), coccidiosis (uncommon), hexamitiasis (rare), malaria (rare).

Helminth Infestations: Ornithostrongylosis, capillariasis, ascaridiasis, dispharynxiasis (*Dispharynx nasuta* infestation of proventriculus).

Arthropod Infestations: Lice (common).

Nutritional/Metabolic Diseases: Goitre (Carneaux and Tippler breeds of *Columba livia* mostly affected), rickets.

Others: Botulism, atherosclerosis.

457

PSITTACIFORMES. Parrots, Parakeets, Lories, Lorikeets, Lovebirds, Macaws, Cockatiels, Cockatoos, Conures, Parrotlets, Budgerigars. (Figure 11/2).

Viral/Rickettsial Infections: Psittacosis (common; all spp. probably highly susceptible), Pacheco's parrot disease (rare), Newcastle disease (fairly susceptible), pox (rare), avian influenza, leucosis complex including Marek's disease (suspected in budgerigars), aegyptianellosis (Nyasa lovebirds).

Bacterial Infections: Salmonellosis, pasteurellosis (rare), pseudotuberculosis (uncommon), erysipelas, tuberculosis (rare; parrots susceptible to human and bovine strains), *Mycoplasma* infection of respiratory tract, listeriosis (rare), *Escherichia coli* infection, *Klebsiella pneumoniae* infection (rare).

Fungal Infections: Aspergillosis, candidiasis (mainly parrots).

Protozoan Infections: Trichomoniasis (rare), coccidiosis (rare), leucocytozoonosis, giardiasis (rare), *Haemoproteus* infection (only rarely pathogenic).

Helminth Infestations: Filariasis, ascaridiasis (especially common in Australian parakeets), capillariasis, nematode infestations of proventriculus.

Arthropod Infestations: *Knemidocoptes* mites causing scaly-face disease (common in budgerigars), red mite infestations (uncommon; budgerigars resistant).

Nutritional/Metabolic Diseases: Rickets, osteomalacia, goitre due to iodine deficiency (common in budgerigars unless on supplemented diet).

Others: Neoplasms (very high incidence in budgerigars), atherosclerosis (common in old parrots), articular gout (common in older budgerigars),

oesophageal and crop necrosis of unknown aetiology (common in budgerigars). French moult (mainly budgerigars). Feather plucking (mainly parrots).

CUCULIFORMES. Touracos, Cuckoos, Coucals, Roadrunners. (Figure 1/AP).

Viral/Rickettsial Infections: Newcastle disease (cuckoos).

Bacterial Infections: Tuberculosis, pseudotuberculosis, erysipelas, Salmonellosis.

Fungal Infections: Candidiasis.

Nutritional/Metabolic Diseases: Rickets and similar nutritional bone diseases.

STRIGIFORMES. Owls. (Figure 8/22).

Viral/Rickettsial Infections: Newcastle disease (highly susceptible), *Herpes* virus hepatosplenitis, ornithosis (rare), Marek's disease (rare).

Bacterial Infections: Pasteurellosis (relatively common), tuberculosis (common), salmonellosis, fowl typhoid, erysipelas, pseudotuberculosis, listeriosis, *Escherichia coli* infections.

Fungal Infections: Aspergillosis.

Protozoan Infections: Leucocytozoonosis, malaria.

Nutritional/Metabolic Diseases: Rickets and osteomalacia (common in pet birds).

Others: Atherosclerosis (common in old birds in zoological gardens), disorders of the alimentary tract and urinary system (relatively common), botulism.

CAPRIMULGIFORMES. Goatsuckers, Frogmouths, Nightjars. (Figure 8/2). No information.

APODIFORMES. Swifts, Hummingbirds. (Figure 2/AP, 11/2).

Viral/Rickettsial Infections: Ornithosis.

Bacterial Infections: Salmonellosis, staphylococcosis, tuberculosis, (rare).
Fungal Infections: Candidiasis (hummingbirds), pulmonary mycosis (rare).
Helminth Infestations: Tapeworms (relatively common in hummingbirds).
Others: Hummingbirds especially susceptible to nephrosis and visceral gout in captivity.

COLIIFORMES. Mousebirds or Colies. (Figure 1/AP).
No information.

TROGONIFORMES. Trogons, Quetzals. (Figure 2/AP).
Bacterial Infections: Pseudotuberculosis.
Fungal Infections: Aspergillosis.

CORACIIFORMES. Kingfishers, Todies, Motmots, Bee-eaters, Rollers, Hoopoes, Hornbills. (Figure 2/AP and 11/2).
Viral/Rickettsial Infections: Newcastle disease (hornbills and kingfishers), ornithosis.
Bacterial Infections: Salmonellosis, tuberculosis, pseudotuberculosis.
Fungal Infections: Aspergillosis.
Helminth Infestations: Gizzard worms (hornbills).
Arthropod Infestations: Red mite, (*Ornithonyssus sylviarum*).
Others: Atherosclerosis (hornbills).

PICIFORMES. Jacamars, Puffbirds, Barbets, Honeyguides, Toucans, Toucanets, Woodpeckers, Wrynecks. (Figure 8/2 and 11/2).
Viral/Rickettsial Infections: Newcastle disease (toucans and toucanets), pox (flickers), ornithosis.
Bacterial Infections: Salmonellosis, pseudotuberculosis (probably common in toucans and toucanets), tuberculosis.

Fungal Infections: Candidiasis (toucan).
Protozoan Infections: Giardiasis (toucan).
Helminth Infestations: Capillariasis (toucan).
Arthropod Infestations: Red mite, (*Ornithonyssus sylviarum*).
Others: Atherosclerosis (common in old toucans in confined captivity).

PASSERIFORMES. Antbirds, Broadbills, Ovenbirds, Cotingas, Manakins, Pittas, Wrens, Lyrebirds, Larks, Swallows, Martins, Wagtails, Pipits, Bulbuls, Shrikes, Waxwings, Dippers, Thrushes, Flycatchers, Warblers, Tits, Nuthatches, Treecreepers, Flowerpeckers, Sunbirds, Zosterops, Buntings, Tanagers, Sugarbirds, Vireos, Hangnests, Canaries, Finches, Waxbills, Weavers, Starlings, Mynahs, Orioles, Drongos, Bower birds, Birds of Paradise, Crows. (Figure 2/AP, 8/2 and 11/2).
Viral/Rickettsial Infections: Ornithosis, pox (relatively common in canaries; also common in many other species), Newcastle disease (mostly relatively resistant), Marek's disease suspected (canary, rare), Pedal papilloma common in wild chaffinches.
Bacterial Infections: Salmonellosis (common), pseudotuberculosis (relatively common), pasteurellosis, erysipelas, spirochaetosis (canaries), streptococcosis, tuberculosis (relatively rare), listeriosis (rare), vibriosis due to *Vibrio metchnikovi* infection (sunbirds), pseudomoniasis (*Pseudomonas aeruginosa* infection), *Escherichia coli* and Paracolon infections.
Fungal Infections: Aspergillosis (relatively uncommon), favus caused by *Trichophyton* infections (uncommon).
Protozoan Infections: Trichomoniasis (canaries and other finches), lankesterellosis (especially common in canaries and house sparrows), malaria (canaries).

459

Helminth Infestations: Syngamiasis (common, especially in "softbills"), capillariasis.
Arthropod Infestations: Red mites (*Dermanyssus* and *Ornithonyssus* spp.) attack canaries (commonly) and many other species. *Knemidocoptes* mites, causing "scaly leg" and "tasslefoot" diseases, *Sternostoma tracheacolum* infestation of lungs (mainly canaries and Gouldian finches).
Others: Botulism, atherosclerosis (probably uncommon).

SELECTED BIBLIOGRAPHY

AUSTIN, O. L. (1962). *Birds of the World.* A survey of the twenty-seven orders and one hundred and fifty-five families. Ed. Zim, H.S., Feltham, Middlesex, England. The Hamlyn Publishing Group Ltd., pp.317.

PETERS, J. L. (1931–60). *Check List of Birds of the World.* Cambridge. Mass. Harvard University Press. 8 Vols.

WETMORE, A. (1960). *A Classification for the Birds of the World.* Smithsonian Misc. Coll. Vol. 139 (11), 1–37.

SCIENTIFIC NAMES OF BIRDS MENTIONED IN THE TEXT

The following list refers to all birds mentioned in the book except those species classified under orders in Chapter 31. The following list specifies to which order the bird or group of birds belongs. The relationship of the various species to each other can be roughly judged by referring to the list of orders in Chapter 31, where a list of the diseases to which birds in different orders are susceptible is also given.

AUK. A name for three species of the family Alcidae, order Charadriiformes.

AVADAVAT, Red. *Estrilda amandava*, order Passeriformes.

AVOCET. *Recurvirostra avocetta*, order Charadriiformes.

BIRD of PARADISE, King of saxony. *Pteridophera alberti*, order Passeriformes.

BIRD of PREY. The term is usually reserved for birds in the order Falconiformes but can also include the Strigiformes (owls).

BLACKBIRD, European. *Turdus merula*, order Passeriformes.

BUDGERIGAR. *Melopsittacus undulatus*, order Psittaciformes.

BULBUL. Substantive name of most species in the family Pycnonotidae, order Passeriformes.

BUSTARD. A species in the family Otididae, order Gruiformes.

BUSTARD, Great. *Otis tarda*, order Gruiformes.

CANARY. *Serinus canaria*, order Passeriformes.

CARDINAL. Usually *Pyrrhuloxia* spp. especially, *P. cardinalis*, order Passeriformes.

CASSOWARY. *Casuarius* spp. order Casuariiformes.

CASSOWARY, Australian. *Casuarius casuarius*, order Casuariiformes.

CHAFFINCH. *Fringilla coelebs*, order Passeriformes.

CHLOROPHONIA, Blue-backed. *Chlorophonia cyanea*, order Passeriformes.

COCKATIEL. *Nymphicus hollandicus*, order Psittaciformes.

COCKATOO. A psittacine bird, usually a *Kakatoe* sp. in the subfamily Kakatoeinae, order Psittaciformes.

COCKATOO, Leadbeater's. *Kakatoe leadbeateri*, order Psittaciformes.

COCKATOO, Sulphur-crested. *Kakatoe galerita*, order Psittaciformes.

CONURE, Blue-crowned. *Aratinga acuticaudata haemorrhous*. A subspecies of the sharp-tailed conure, *A. acuticaudata*.

COOT. *Fulica* spp., order Gruiformes.

CORMORANT. *Phalacrocorax* spp., order Pelecaniiformes.

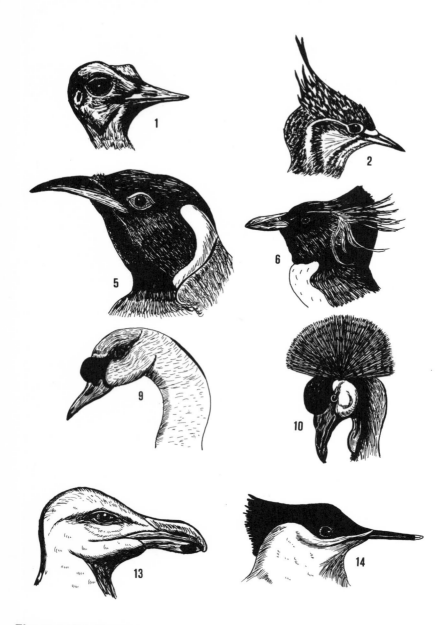

Figure 1/AP. Further representatives (see also Figs. 8/2 and 11/2) of various biological orders. 1. Common rhea (Rheiformes). 2. Common Tinamou (Tinamiformes). 3. Great-crested grebe (Podicipediformes). 4. Great northern diver (Gaviiformes). 5. King penguin (Sphenisciformes). 6. Rock hopper penguin (Sphenisciformes). 7. Crested screamer (Anseriformes).

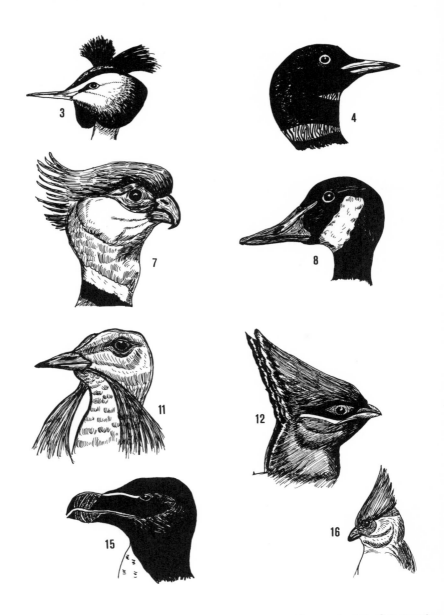

8. Canada goose (Anseriformes). 9. Mute swan (Anseriformes). 10. Crowned crane (Gruiformes). 11. Great bustard (Gruiformes). 12. Common touraco (Cuculiformes). 13. Greater black-backed gull (Charadriiformes). 14. Sandwich tern (Charadriiformes). 15. Razorbill (Charadriiformes). 16. Blue-naped mouse-bird (Coliiformes). (Janet Keymer)

CRAKE. An alternative name for a rail in the family Rallidae, order Gruiformes.

CRANE. A species in the family Gruidae, order Gruiformes.

CRANE, Crowned. *Balearica pavonina*, order Gruiformes.

CROSSBILL. *Loxia curvirostra*, order Passeriformes.

CUCKOO. A member of the family Cuculidae in the order Cuculiformes, *e.g.*, *Cuculus canorus* the common European species.

CURASSOW. A substantive name for some species in the family Cracidae, order Galliformes.

CURASSOW, Great. *Crax rubia*, order Galliformes.

CURLEW, Common. *Numenius arquata*, order Charadriiformes.

CUTTHROAT. *Amadina fasciata*, order Passeriformes.

DIVER, Great northern. *Gavia immer*, order Gaviiformes.

DOVE. A common name usually confined to smaller species of the pigeon family Columbidae, order Columbiformes.

DOVE, Stock. *Columba oenas*, order Columbiformes.

DUCK. A substantive name for most of the smaller members of the family Anatidae, order Anseriformes.

DUCK, Domestic. Probably derived from the Mallard, *Anas platyrhynchos*. Order Anseriformes.

EAGLE. A name given to some of the large members of the subfamily Accipitrinae, especially the genus *Aquila*, order Falconiformes.

EAGLE, Golden. *Aquila chrysaetos*, order Falconiformes.

EAGLE, Verreaux's. *Aquila verreauxi*, order Falconiformes.

EGRET. Name given to several species of the family Ardeidae, order Ciconiiformes.

EGRET, Little. *Egretta garzette*, order Ciconiiformes.

EMU. *Dromaius novae-hollandiae*. Syn. *Dromiceius novae-hollandiae*, order Casuariiformes.

FALCON. Substantive name usually given to *Falco* spp. in the order Falconiformes.

FINCH. Substantive name given to many species of the family Fringillidae, order Passeriformes.

FINCH, Cutthroat. *Amadina fasciata*, order Passeriformes.

FINCH, Gouldian. (Syn. *Cholebia*) *Poephila gouldiae*, order Passeriformes.

FINCH, Zebra. *Poephila guttata*, (Syn. *Taeniopygia castanotis*), order Passeriformes.

FLAMINGO. A bird belonging to the family Phoenicopteridae in the order Ciconiiformes. Some authorities classify the birds in a separate order Phoenicopteriformes.

FLAMINGO, Greater. *Phoenicopterus ruber*, order Ciconiiformes.

FLICKER. A *Colaptes* sp. belonging to the family Picidae, order Piciformes.

FLOWERPECKER. Substantive name of some species in the family Dicaeidea, order Passeriformes.

FLYCATCHER, Pied. *Ficedula hypoleuca*, order Passeriformes.

FOWL, domestic. *Gallus gallus* (Domestic variety), order Galliformes.

FULMAR, Giant. *Macronectes giganteus,* order Procellariiformes.

FULMAR petrel or Fulmar. *Fulmarus glacialis,* order Procellariiformes.

GAME BIRDS. A vague term to describe birds used for sport, mainly shooting. It includes grouse (family Tetraonidae), pheasants and partridges (family Phasianidae) as well as other birds in the order Galliformes. In some areas bustards (family Otididae of the order Gruiformes), tinamous (order Tinamiformes), certain waders (order Charadriiformes) and ducks, geese and swans (order Anseriformes are also included.

GANNET. *Sula bassana,* order Pelecaniformes.

GOLDFINCH. *Carduelis carduelis,* order Passeriformes.

GOOSE. A name given to many of the members of the family Anatidae, these usually being larger than ducks and often grazers. Order Anseriformes.

GOOSE, Ashy-headed. *Chloephaga polio,* order Anseriformes.

GOOSE, Canada. *Branta canadensis,* order Anseriformes.

GREBE, Great-crested. *Podiceps cristatus,* order Podicipediformes.

GREENFINCH. *Chloris chloris,* order Passeriformes.

GROUSE. A fowl-like "game bird". Substantive name of many species in the family Tetraonidae, order Galliformes.

GUILLEMOT. A bird mainly of the genus *Uria,* order Charadriiformes.

GUINEA FOWL. Name given to several species in the order Galliformes, the domesticated species being *Numida meleagris.*

GULL. A substantive name of nearly all the species in the subfamily Larinae, family Laridae of the order Charadriiformes.

GULL, Herring. *Larus argentatus,* order Charadriiformes.

GULL, Greater black-backed. *Larus marinus,* order Charadriiformes.

HARDBILL. Fanciers' and aviculturists' term for a bird of the order Passeriformes with a small, conical bill adapted for seizing and shelling seeds.

HAWFINCH. *Coccothraustes coccothraustes,* order Passeriformes.

HAWK. Name given to many members of the family Accipitridae, order Falconiformes.

HERON. Name given to most species of the subfamily Ardeinae, family Ardeidae, order Ciconiiformes.

HERON, Eastern purple. *Ardea purpurea,* order Ciconiiformes.

HERON, Great blue. *Ardea herodias,* order Ciconiiformes.

HOATZIN. *Opisthocomus hoazin,* order Galliformes.

HONEYCREEPER. Substantive name of some species in the family Drepanididae, (order Passeriformes) and also some species in subfamily Coerebinae, many of which are called sugarbirds; order Passeriformes.

HONEYEATER. Substantive name of many species in the family Meliphagidae, order Passeriformes.

HOOPOE. *Upupa epops,* order Coraciiformes.

HORNBILL. Name for all species of the family Bucerotidae, order Coraciiformes.

HORNBILL, Silvery-cheeked. *Bycanistes brevis,* order Coraciiformes.

HUMMINGBIRD. Name given to many species of the family Trochilidae, order Apodiformes. All New World species.

HUMMINGBIRD, Bee. *Calypte helenae,* order Apodiformes.

KINGFISHER. A name for all species in the family Alcedinidae, order Coraciiformes. The Common European kingfisher is *Alcedo atthis.*

KITTIWAKE. *Rissa tridactyla,* order Charadriiformes.

KIWI. *Apteryx* sp., order Apterygiformes.

LORIKEET. A name for some of the small species of lory, order Psittaciformes.

LORIKEET, Ornate. *Trichoglossus ornatus,* order Psittaciformes.

LORY, Substantive name of species in the subfamily Loriinae, order Psittaciformes.

LOVEBIRD. Name for one of the *Agapornis* spp. (African) and sometimes the Budgerigar, *Melopsittacus undulatus* (Australian), order Psittaciformes.

LOVEBIRD, Masked. *Agapornis personata,* order Psittaciformes.

LOVEBIRD, Nyasa. *Agapornis lilianae,* order Psittaciformes.

MACAW. Substantive name of *Ara* spp. and *Anodorhynchus* spp., order Psittaciformes.

MACAW, Hyacinth. *Anodorhynchus hyacinthus,* order Psittaciformes.

MAGPIE. *Pica pica,* also substantive name of species of several genera in the family Corvidae, order Passeriformes.

MANNIKIN. Substantive name of various species in the genus *Lonchura* (Syn. *Spermestes*). Family Estrildidae, order Passeriformes.

MARTIN. Substantive name of some species of the family Hirundinidae, order Passeriformes.

MERGANSER, Red-breasted. *Mergus serrator,* order Anseriformes.

MOORHEN. *Gallinula chloropus,* order Gruiformes.

MOUSEBIRD, Blue-naped. *Colius macrourus,* order Coliiformes.

MYNAH. Substantive name of species of *Acridotheres, Gracula* and *Sturnus,* order Passeriformes.

MYNAH, Hill. *Gracula religiosa,* order Passeriformes.

MYNAH, Greater Indian hill. *Gracula religiosa intermedia,* order Passeriformes.

NIGHTJAR. Substantive name of the Old World members of the family Caprimulgidae, order Caprimulgiformes.

NIGHTJAR, European. *Caprimulgus europaeus,* order Caprimulgiformes.

NUN, Substantive name of a *Lonchura* sp., order Passeriformes.

NUN, Tricoloured or Three-coloured mannikin. *Lonchura malacca,* order Passeriformes.

NUTHATCH, Corsican. *Sitta whiteheadi,* order Passeriformes.

OIL BIRD. *Steatornis caripensis*, order Caprimulgiformes.

OSTRICH. *Struthio camelus*, order Struthioniformes.

OWL. Substantive name of all the species in the order Strigiformes, most of which are nocturnal birds of prey.

OWL, Collared scops. *Otus bakkamoena*, order Strigiformes.

OWL, Eagle. *Bubo bubo*, order Strigiformes.

OWL, Tawny. *Strix aluco*, order Strigiformes.

PARAKEET. Name given to some of the smaller species of psittacine birds *i.e.*, those belonging to order Psittaciformes. They are usually slim birds with long pointed tails. Alternative spelling "Parrakeet".

PARAKEET, New Zealand or Redfronted. *Cyanoramphus novae-zelandiae*, order Psittaciformes.

PARAKEET, Pennant's. *Platycercus elegans*, order Psittaciformes.

PARAKEET, Quaker. *Myiopsitta monachus*, order Psittaciformes.

PARAKEET, Shell. Another common name for the budgerigar *Melopsittacus undulatus*, order Psittaciformes.

PARROT. Name given to many species in the order Psittaciformes, especially the larger ones, without crests and with relatively short tails.

PARROT, African grey. *Psittacus erithacus*.

PARROT, Amazon. Blue-fronted Amazon *Amazona aestiva*, Yellow-fronted Amazon, *Amazona ochrocephala*, order Psittaciformes.

PARROT, Eclectus. *Lorius roratus*, order Psittaciformes.

PARROTLET. A small psittacine bird of the genus *Forpus*, order Psittaciformes.

PARTRIDGE. Substantive name of species of several genera in the family Phasianidae, order Galliformes. The species most widely used for sport is the common or so-called Hungarian or grey partridge, *Perdix perdix*.

PEAFOWL. *Pavo cristatus*, order Galliformes.

PELICAN. Substantive name of all species of the family Pelecanidae, order Pelecaniformes.

PELICAN, Brown. *Pelicanus occidentalis*, order Pelecaniformes.

PENGUIN. Name for any species in the order Sphenisciformes.

PENGUIN, King. *Aptenodytes patagonica*, order Sphenisciformes.

PENGUIN, Rock hopper. *Eudyptes crestatus*, order Sphenisciformes.

PETREL. Name given to many species of marine birds (so-called Tubinares) in the order Procellariiformes.

PHEASANT. Substantive name of many species of the family Phasianidae, order Galliformes. The species most widely kept in captivity and for sport is the common or ring-necked pheasant *Phasianus colchicus*.

PIGEON, domestic. *Columba livia*, order Columbiformes. Feral pigeons are this species.

PIGEON, Pouter. *Columba livia* (domestic variety), order Columbiformes.

PIGEON, Racing. *Columba livia* (domestic variety), order Columbiformes.

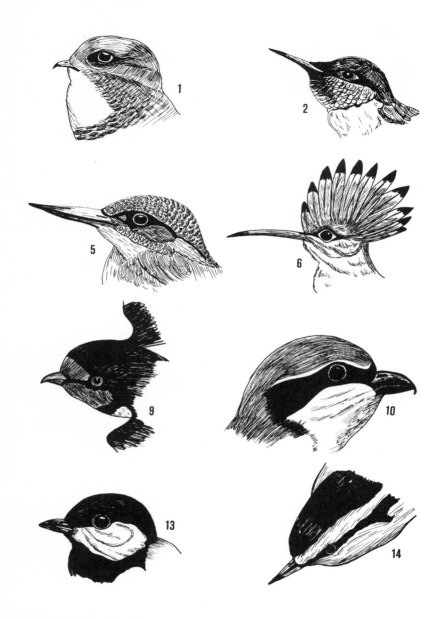

Figure 2/AP. Further representatives (see also Figs. 8/2, 11/2 and 1/AP) of various biological orders. 1. Alpine swift (Apodiformes). 2. Bee humming bird (Apodiformes). 3. Kiwi (Apterygiformes). 4. White-tailed trogon (Trogoniformes). 5. Common kingfisher (Coraciiformes). 6. Hoopoe (Coraciiformes). 7. Pied flycatcher (Passeriformes).

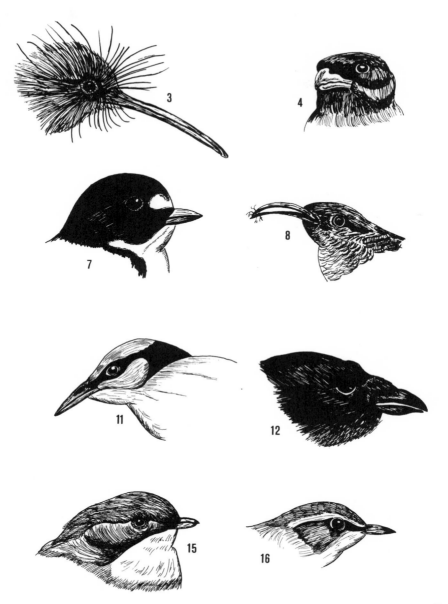

8. Variable sunbird (Passeriformes). 9. Swallow (Passeriformes). 10. Red-backed shrike (Passeriformes). 11. Black-naped oriole (Passeriformes). 12. Raven (Passeriformes). 13. Great tit (Passeriformes). 14. Corsican nuthatch (Passeriformes). 15. Pekin robin (Passeriformes). 16. Willow warbler (Passeriformes). (Janet Keymer)

POCHARD. *Aythya ferina,* order Anseriformes.

POULTRY. A collective term for domesticated species, especially those of agricultural importance and bred for the table. *i.e.,* the domestic fowl, turkey and duck.

PUFFIN. *Fratercula arctica,* order Charadriiformes.

QUAIL. Substantive name of species of mainly game birds belonging to groups in the family Phasianidae, namely the American quails (subfamily Odontophorinae) and the Old World Quails which include mainly *Coturnix* spp.

QUAIL, Bobwhite. *Colinus virginianus,* order Galliformes.

QUAIL, California. *Lophortyx californicus,* order Galliformes.

QUAIL, Chinese painted. *Excalfactoria chinensis,* order Galliformes.

QUAIL, Japanese. *Coturnix coturnix japonica,* order Galliformes.

RAIL. Substantive name of any species of the family Rallidae in the order Gruiformes.

RAPTOR. A bird of prey, the word being derived from the obsolete order Raptores, comprising diurnal birds of prey and owls, now represented by the Falconiformes and Strigiformes.

RAVEN. *Corvus corax,* order Passeriformes.

RAZORBILL. *Alca torda,* order Charadriiformes.

RHEA. *Rhea americana* (Common rhea) and *Pterocnemia pennata,* order Rheiformes.

ROBIN, European. *Erithacus rubecula,* order Passeriformes.

ROBIN, North American. *Turdus migratorius,* order Passeriformes.

ROBIN, Pekin. *Leiothrix lutea,* order Passeriformes.

RUFF. *Philomachus pugnax,* order Charadriiformes.

SANDGROUSE, Black-bellied. *Pterocles orientalis,* order Columbiformes and not the order Galliformes as the common name suggests.

SCREAMER, crested. *Chauna torquata,* order Anseriformes.

SHAG. A name almost synonymous with Cormorant, meaning a species of *Phalacrocorax.* The British shag is *P. aristotelis,* order Pelecaniformes.

SHEARWATER. Substantive name of some species in the family Procellariidae, especially in the genera *Puffinus* and *Procellaria,* order Procellariiformes.

SHELDUCK. Substantive name of *Tadorna* spp. The European shelduck is *Tadorna tadorna.* Order Anseriformes.

SHRIKE, Red-backed. *Lanius collurio,* order Passeriformes.

SICKLEBILL, White-tipped. *Eutoxeres aquila,* order Passeriformes.

SNIPE, Common. *Gallinago gallinago,* order Charadriiformes.

SOFTBILL, A vague term used by fanciers and aviculturists for predominantly insectivorous, frugivorous and nectar-feeding birds. Included are numerous species which mainly but not entirely, belong to the order Passeriformes.

SPARROW, House. *Passer domesticus,* order Passeriformes.

SPARROW, Java. *Padda oryzivora,* order Passeriformes.

470

SPOONBILL. Substantive name of the species in the subfamily Plataleinae, family Threskiornithidae, order Ciconiiformes. The European spoonbill is *Platalea leucorodia*.

SPOONBILL, Roseate. *Ajaia ajaia*, order Ciconiiformes.

SQUAB. An unfledged nestling pigeon or dove (order Columbiformes), under approximately one month of age.

SQUEAKER. A young pigeon or dove (order Columbiformes) between the ages of about 1–2 months, so-called because of its characteristic squeaking call.

STARLING, Glossy. A species of *Lamprotornis* or *Spreo*, order Passeriformes.

STORK. Substantive name of most species in the family Ciconiidae, order Ciconiiformes.

STORK, Marabou. *Leptoptilos crumeniferus*, order Ciconiiformes.

SUGAR BIRD. Name for the two species of the genus *Promerops* in the family Meliphagidae, order Passeriformes. All Old World species.

SUNBIRD. Substantive name of most species of the family Nectariniidae. All Old World species. Order Passeriformes.

SUNBIRD, Variable. *Cinnyris venustus*, order Passeriformes.

SWALLOW. Name given to most species of the family Hirundinidae, order Passeriformes. The European swallow is *Hirundo rustica*.

SWAN, Mute. *Cygnus olor*, order Anseriformes.

SWIFT. Substantive name of species in the families Apodidae and Hemiprocnidae, order Apodiformes.

SWIFT, Alpine. *Apus melba*, order Apodiformes.

TANAGER. Substantive name of many species in the family Emberizidae, order Passeriformes.

TERN. Substantive name of most species of the subfamily Sterninae of the family Laridae, order Charadriiformes. Mostly coastal species.

TERN, Sandwich. *Sterna sandvicensis*, order Charadriiformes.

THORNBILL, Herran's. *Chalcostigma herrani*, order Passeriformes.

THRUSH. Name given to some species of the subfamily Turdinae in the family Muscicapidae, order Passeriformes.

THRUSH, Song. *Turdus philomelos*, order Passeriformes.

TINAMOU, Common. *Eudromia elegans*, order Tinamiformes.

TIT. An abbreviated and more common version of "titmouse" which includes most species in the family Paridae, order Passeriformes.

TIT, Great. *Parus major*, order Passeriformes.

TOUCAN. Substantive name of species in the family Ramphastidae, order Piciformes.

TOUCAN, Red-billed. *Ramphastos tucanus*, order Piciformes.

TOUCAN, Sulphur-breasted. *Ramphastos sulfivatus*, order Piciformes.

TOUCANET. Name given to all species in the genus *Aulacorhynchus* being mainly green-coloured birds. Belong to the family Ramphastidae in the order Piciformes.

TOURACO, Common. *Touraco corythaix*, order Cuculiformes.

471

TROGON, White-tailed. *Trogan viridis,* order Trogoniformes.

TROUPIAL. *Icterus icterus,* order Passeriformes.

TURKEY, Common or Domestic. *Meleagris gallopavo,* order Galliformes.

VULTURE. Substantive name for some species of the families Cathartidae (New World Vultures) and Accipitridae which includes the Old World Vultures. Order Falconiformes.

VULTURE, Turkey. *Cathartes aura,* order Falconiformes.

WADER. This is a general term commonly used, especially in Great Britain for members of the sub-order Charadrii of the order Charadriiformes.

WARBLER, Willow. *Phylloscopus trochlus,* order Passeriformes.

WATER BIRD. A rather vague but popular term which includes aquatic (but mainly freshwater) birds in the orders Anseriformes, Gaviiformes, Podicipidiformes, Pelecaniiformes, Ciconiiformes, Gruiformes and Charadriiformes.

WATERFOWL. A rather vague term mainly for birds in the order Anseriformes, especially ducks.

WAXBILL. Name given to various species of small seed-eating passerines mainly in the genus *Estrilda.* Order Passeriformes.

WAXWING, Bohemian. *Bombycilla garrulus,* order Passeriformes.

WEAVER. A general name given to many species of the families Ploceidae and Estrilidae. They are mainly small, seed-eating birds and include so-called buffalo weavers, the true weavers (subfamily Ploceinae) and the weaver-finches known as waxbills, grass-finches and mannikins. Order Passeriformes.

WHITE-EYE. Substantive name of many species in the family Zosteropidae, order Passeriformes.

WHYDAH, Giant. *Coliuspasser* (Syn. *Euplectes*) *progne.* The whydahs are also called Widow-birds. There is some confusion regarding their taxonomic position, but the term usually refers to a species in the family Ploceidae, order Passeriformes. The present species is also called the Long-tailed widow bird. Whydah is also sometimes spelt "Wydah" or "Whidah".

WOODPECKER, Black. *Dryocopus martius,* order Piciformes.

WOODPIGEON *Columba palumbus,* order Columbiformes.

WRYNECK. A substantive name of species of *Jynx,* order Piciformes.

APPENDIX

SELECTED BIBLIOGRAPHY

General

ARNALL, L. A. (1958). *Experiences with cage-birds.* Vet. Rec. *70,* 120–128.

ARNALL, L. A. (1961). *Further experiences with cagebirds.* Vet. Rec. *73,* 1146–1154.

BEACH, J. E. (1962). *Diseases of budgerigars and other cage birds.* A survey of post-mortem findings. Vet. Rec. *74,* 10–17 (Part I), 63–68 (Part II) and 134–140 (Part III).

BIESTER, H. E. & SCHWARTE, L. H. (1965). *Diseases of Poultry.* 5th Ed. Ames. Iowa, State University Press, 1,382pp.

BLOUNT, W. P. (1949). *Diseases of Poultry.* Baillière, Tindall & Cox, London. 562pp.

DAVIS, J. W., ANDERSON, R. C., KARSTAD, L. & TRAINER, D. O. Eds. (1971). *Infectious and Parasitic Diseases of Wild Birds.* Ames, Iowa, State University Press 344pp.

GRAY, H. (1936). *The diseases of cage and aviary birds with some reference to those of furred and feathered game.* Vet. Rec. *16,* 343–352, 377–386 and 417–427.

HUNGERFORD, T. G. (1969). *Diseases of Poultry including Cage Birds and Pigeons.* 4th Ed. Angus and Robertson Sydney, 672pp.

KEYMER, I. F. (1958). *Some Ailments of Cage and Aviary Birds.* Proc. 1st. Ann. Congr. Br. small Anim. vet. Ass., 18–24.

KEYMER, I. F. (1962). *Ornithology and the veterinary profession.* In *The Veterinary Annual,* p.28–34. Fourth Year. Ed. Pool, W.A., John Wright Bristol.

LESBOUYRIES, G. (1941). *La Pathologie des Oiseaux.* Vigot Frères. Paris 868pp.

MVP REDBOOK (1965). *A handbook on cage birds.* Mod. Vet. Pract. *46* (12), 176–198.

REINHARDT, R. (1950). *Lehrbuch der Geflugelkrankheiten.* M-H Schaper, Hannover. 384pp.

SENEVIRATNA, P. (1969). *Diseases of Poultry* (including cage birds). John Wright, Bristol. 229pp.

STARTUP, C. M. (1970). *The Diseases of Cage and Aviary Birds* (Excluding the specific diseases of the Budgerigar) p.46–58. In Rutgers, A & Norris, K.A. Eds. Encyclopedia of Aviculture, Vol. I. Blandford Press, London.

THOMSON, SIR A. LANDSBOROUGH, (1964). *A New Dictionary of Birds.* Thomas Nelson, London and Edinburgh. 927pp.

VAN TYNE, J. & BERGER, A. J. (1959). *Fundamentals of Ornithology.* John Wiley & Sons, New York. 624pp.

WALLACE G. J. (1955). *An introduction to ornithology.* Macmillan, New York. 443pp.

Waterfowl

HUMPHREYS, P. N. (1973). *Some veterinary aspects of maintaining waterfowl in captivity.* In *International Zoo Yearbook.* Vol. 13. p.87–94. Ed. Duplaix-Hall, N. Zoological Society of London.

Birds of Prey

COOPER, J. E. (1973). *Veterinary Aspects of Birds of Prey.* Hawk Trust, Newent, Gloucestershire, England. 112pp.

KEYMER, I. F. (1972). *Diseases of Birds of Prey*. Vet. Rec. *90*, 579–594.

Pigeons

BRITISH VETERINARY ASSOCIATION (1964). *Handbook on the Treatment of Exotic Pets*. Part One. Cage Birds, p.48–65. British Veterinary Association, London.

HUNGERFORD, T. G. (1969). Pigeons, p.586–602. In *Diseases of Poultry including Cage Birds and Pigeons*. 4th Ed. Angus and Robertson, Sydney.

Psittacines

BLACKMORE, D. K. (1969). *Diseases of Larger Parakeets*. In *Proceedings of the British Veterinary Zoological Society* 1961–1970, p.22–30. Eds. Keymer, I. F., Irvin A. D. and Cooper, J. E. (Sept. 1972). Price £1, British Veterinary Association, London.

BRITISH VETERINARY ASSOCIATION (1964). *Handbook on the Treatment of Exotic Pets*. Part One. *Cage Birds*, p.28–47. British Veterinary Association, London.

COFFIN, D. L. (1954). *Diseases of Parrots*. In *Parrots and Parrot-like Birds*, p.24–44. By Duke of Bedford, All-Pets Books, Fond du Lac, Wis. Inc.

FROST, C. (1961). *Experiences with pet budgerigars*. Vet. Rec. *73*, 621–626.

KEYMER, I. F. (1958). *The diagnosis and treatment of common psittacine diseases*. Mod. Vet. Pract. *39* (21), 22–30.

Canaries and Other Passerine Birds

BRITISH VETERINARY ASSOCIATION (1964). *Handbook on the Treatment of Exotic Pets*. Part One: *Cage Birds*, p.12–27 British Veterinary Association, London.

KEYMER, I. F. (1959). *Specific diseases of the canary and other passerine birds,* Mod. Vet. Pract. *40* (17), 32–35; *40* (18), 45–48 and *40* (24), 16.

KEYMER, I. F. (1959). *The diagnosis and treatment of some diseases of seed-eating passerine birds.* Mod. Vet. Pract. *40* (7), 30–34 and *40* (8), 34–37.

KEYMER, I. F. (1973). *Diseases of Passerine Birds,* The Vet Review, XXIII, (3), 47–52. May & Baker Ltd., Dagenham.

GLOSSARY

ACARICIDE. Substance capable of killing acarine arthropods, *i.e.,* 8-legged creatures known as mites, belonging to the Class Arachnida, order Acari.

ACUTE. An illness which has a short and relatively severe course. Not chronic.

ALOPECIA. Baldness—patchy or general loss of feathers or hair without their immediate replacement.

AMOEBA. A single-celled microscopic form of animal life belonging to the phylum Protozoa, which is the lowest division of the animal kingdom. In spite of its primitive form, it moves, eats, voids waste products and avoids enemies by changing shape and flowing from one point to another.

ANAEMIA. (See also Haemoglobin). A state in which the blood is deficient either in quantity or in quality. In the latter case, this is due to a diminution of the amount of haemoglobin or of the number of red cells which contain it.

ANOREXIA. Lack of or drop in appetite.

ANOXIA. Oxygen deficiency.

ANTIBODY. (See also Antigen). A specific chemical substance produced in the body by higher forms of animal life in response to the presence of an antigen and which reacts specifically with the antigen in some observable way. The antibody for example may inactivate the antigen by "dissolving" it or "clumping" (*i.e.,* precipitating or agglutinating) it.

ANTIGEN. (See also Antibody). Any substance which when introduced either naturally or artificially into the blood or tissues of the body stimulates the formation of antibody.

ATAXIA. Failing powers of locomotion, unsteadiness, weakness, inco-ordination.

ATROPHY. (See also Hypertrophy). Decrease in size of a cell, an organ, tissue or part of, or the whole body.

AVITAMINOSIS. (See also Hypovitaminosis). Any disease due to absence of a vitamin in the diet, *e.g.,* Avitaminosis A. Often used incorrectly instead of hypovitaminosis.

BLEPHARITIS. Inflammation or dermatitis of the eyelids and their margins.

BREED. To induce reproduction, produce offspring. A domesticated strain or race of certain species, which produces offspring of a similar physical and genetic type.

CARDIAC. Relating to the heart; in the direction of the heart.

CARDIOMYOPATHY. Disease process occurring in or involving heart muscle.

475

CARNIVOROUS. Feeding on predominantly animal matter: flesh-eating—including insects, molluscs, etc.

CERE. Means wax or waxy; hence the fleshy area round the nostrils of such birds as budgerigars and certain birds of prey, which has a waxy bloom and is not covered with feathers. The term is also used by pigeon breeders for the fleshy area round the eyes.

CHRONIC. Long continued. The opposite to acute.

CILIA. Eyelashes; vibrating or rhythmically sweeping hair-like appendages in unicellular forms of life also in more advanced creatures in organs including mucous cells of bronchi and trachea. (Longer "hairs" are often called flagellae).

CONJUNCTIVITIS. Inflammation of the mucous, conjunctival membrane lining the eyelids and covering the membrana nictitans (third eyelid) and the front of the eyeball.

CONTAGIOUS. Capable of being contracted or "caught" by touch or contact, especially a disease.

CRUSTACEAN. Large class of mainly aquatic animals characterised by a shell or exoskeleton, e.g., crabs, lobsters, crayfish, prawns, shrimps, daphnia (waterfleas), belonging to the phylum Arthropoda.

DIRECT LIFE CYCLE. Applies to a parasite or other pathogen which spends its whole life in the same host species, although usually a short period is spent free living, in order to ensure perpetuation of the species by transference to another host. (See, e.g., Figures 1/9, 5/10).

DORSAL. Related or directed towards upper or vertebral surface, the "back" of the body or neck.

DROPPINGS. The body's waste products which fall from mammals, birds, etc. In birds, droppings consist of two fractions: one from the bowels (the faeces), which is grey, green, brown, black, reddish or yellow, and the other from the kidneys (urine) which is white or creamy coloured and also semi-solid. Clearish, watery urine is normal in certain fruit-eating birds.

DROPSY. The abnormal accumulation of watery body fluid in tissue or in a body cavity. It is always a serious sign of kidney, lung or heart disease, wasting due to cancer, debility, malnutrition or certain poisonings.

DUCTLESS GLANDS. Glands which disseminate their secretion via the blood and body tissues generally and not through special tubes or direct to the organs which the secretions control. Also known as endocrine glands.

DYSPLASIA. Abnormal development of a tissue or organ, usually an underdevelopment.

EMPHYSEMA. A swelling or inflation due to the presence of air in the interstices of connective tissue (e.g., beneath the skin) or in the tissues between the air cells of the lungs.

EXUDATE. Outflowing of body fluids, such as plasma or serum. The protein and mineral, soluble or colloidal elements of blood excluding the red cells.

FAECES. Waste material from the gut ejected from the large intestine and cloaca. Comprises the darker fraction of bird droppings.

FERAL. Literally wild or untamed. In ornithological terminology, applied to populations of domesticated species of birds such as pigeons or waterfowl that have reverted to the wild, free-living state.

FRUGIVOROUS. Fruit-eating.

GALLINACEOUS. Belonging to the order of birds Galliformes, which include domestic and jungle fowl, pheasants, grouse, partridges, peafowl, etc.

GENUS. A group of animals (including birds) or plants having common structural characteristics distinct from other groups. It may contain one or several species.

GOITRE. Pathological enlargement of the thyroid gland, showing in advanced cases as a prominent or pendulous swelling in the throat.

GRANULATION TISSUE. Fleshy, usually rounded, mass of tissue which forms in wounds. It consists of new blood capillaries and fibroblasts, which give rise to fibrous tissue within the connective tissue.

GRANULOMA. A localised tumour-like growth found in chronic inflammations, which consist of granulation tissue.

HAEMOGLOBIN. The oxygen-carrying red pigment of the blood, consisting basically of protein and iron.

HISTOLOGY. Study of the microscopic anatomy of normal tissues.

HISTOPATHOLOGY. Study of microscopic anatomy of abnormal tissues.

HYPERSENSITIVE. Excessively sensitive, over-reacting to a drug, protein, allergen or other substance or stimulus by an organism. The reaction may be local, e.g., by the skin or other tissue, or general by the whole body, producing shock.

HYPERTROPHY. Enlargement or overgrowth of an otherwise normal organ or tissue due to increased size of its component cells.

HYPERVITAMINOSIS. (See also Hypovitaminosis). A disease produced by an excessive amount of a specific vitamin in the diet, e.g., hypervitaminosis D. The opposite of hypovitaminosis.

HYPOVITAMINOSIS. (See also Avitaminosis). Any disease due to a deficiency or lack of a specific vitamin in the diet, e.g., Hypovitaminosis B.

INDIRECT LIFE CYCLE. Applies to a parasite which spends part of its life in a main or definitive host and part in one or more intermediate hosts, there also usually being a free living stage outside the body of a host. (See e.g., Figures, 2/9, 1/10, 2/10, 4/10, 6/10, 9/10).

INFECTIOUS. (See also Contagious). Capable of infecting or invading another species of animal or plant. An infectious disease is one caused by parasites such as bacteria, protozoa or fungi. It may also be contagious.

INGEST. Take in food via the mouth or similar orifice and alimentary tract. To eat.

INSECTICIDE. Substance capable of killing insects (6-legged arthropods).

INSECTIVOROUS. Eating insects and other small arthropods as the primary diet.

INVERTEBRATE. Animal possessing no vertebral column or backbone. Includes animals in groups Protozoa (Chapter 9), Parazoa or Porifera (sponges), Coelenterata (sea-anemones, etc.), Platyhelminths (Chapter 10), Acanthocephala (Chapter 10), Nematoda (Chapter 10), Mollusca (snails), Annelida (*e.g.* leeches), Arthropoda (Chapter 10) and several other less well known groups.

KERATIN. Hard wearing and relatively inert protein which forms horny layers of skin, feathers, nail and beak. Made up of sulphur-containing amino acids, hence the sulphurous smell when these substances are burnt.

LAPAROTOMY. The operation for or process of opening the abdominal cavity.

LATERAL. At or to the side of; towards or of the side.

LESION. Any abnormality caused by disease of a cell, tissue, organ or limb. A diseased or damaged area with changes of colour, size, texture, structure or function.

LIPOMATOSIS. Disease process involving excessive, widespread or generalised deposits of fat; generalised, diffuse obesity.

LUMEN. Cavity of or interior of tube or hollow organ, *e.g.,* the lumen of the small intestine or blood vessels.

MEDIAL. Towards the mid-line or middle of the body, inward facing; inside (*e.g.,* of a leg). Opposite: lateral (outward facing) surface of limb.

METABOLIC RATE. Speed of living of an organism. Rate of build-up and breakdown of cells expressed in calories of energy used in relation to body surface and weight.

METABOLISM. The sum of all the chemical and physical processes by which living organised substance is produced and maintained; the transformation by which energy is made available for the uses of the organism.

MOLLUSC. A member of the group or phylum Mollusca. Soft-bodied (without internal skeleton) and generally hard-shelled animals; including slugs, snails, oysters, mussels, limpets, etc., which comprise a large part of the diet of many fresh and salt water, as well as land birds. They are frequently the intermediate hosts of parasites, particularly trematodes or flukes: See Chapter 10.

MYCOSIS. A disease caused by infection with fungi, *i.e.,* Mycotic or fungal infection.

NECROPSY. *Post-mortem* examination; autopsy.

NECROSIS. Death of a clearly delineated area of the body involving one or more tissues. A lesion comprising dead cells, with clear outline caused by change of colour and consistency relative to the surrounding living tissue.

NECROTIC. Dead. Refers to a part or area of the whole organism; from the Greek NEKROS, a corpse.

NEMATODE. Worm of a cylindrical or thread-like form.

NEPHRITIS. Inflammation of the kidneys.

NEPHROSIS. Non-inflammatory, degenerative, disease process or affection of the kidneys. (This general term is not acceptable to all pathologists.)

OEDEMA. The presence of an abnormally large amount of fluid in the space between tissues.

OMNIVOROUS. Capable of eating anything. An adjective describing a bird, mammal or other animal whose digestion can deal with both animal and various types of vegetable food.

PARACENTESIS. Drainage of dropsical fluid, pus or other fluid from body cavities. Tapping fluid from the abdominal or chest cavity with a cannula or large calibre hypodermic needle.

PARALYSIS. Impairment or complete loss of motor (power of movement) and/or sensory (power of sensation) nervous functions.

PARENTERAL. Administration by any route other than via the alimentary tract. By injection (of medicament, vaccine, etc.).

PARESIS. Incomplete paralysis.

PASSERINE. A bird of the order Passeriformes. Usually a perching bird, as opposed to a bird which sleeps on the ground.

PATHOGEN. Invasive organism capable of causing disease or suffering, especially bacterium, virus, protozoan, fungus, helminth, arthropod or chemical.

PATHOGENIC. Capable of causing disease.

PATHOGENICITY. Power of pathogen to cause disease or suffering; virulence.

PATHOLOGIST. A person who specialises in pathology.

PATHOLOGY. The branch of medicine (including veterinary) which deals with the study of disease, especially the structural and functional changes caused by disease.

PESTICIDE. Pest killer. The pests may be molluscs, insects or arthropods, rodents, or other living organisms considered to be harmful to man, his domestic animals or possessions.

PRECOCITY. State of early or premature development in some respect, *e.g.*, physical, sexual or mental.

PREMEDICATION. Literally, "beforehand treatment". Often refers to preliminary drugs given before anaesthesia to produce tranquillization. This usually lowers the amount of anaesthetic needed and reduces such side effects as excitability during recovery.

PRIMATES. The order of mammals which include man, apes, monkeys and lemurs.

PROGNOSIS. Forecast of the course and outcome of a disease, prediction of future health of the individual or flock affected.

PSITTACINE. A bird of the order Psittaciformes, which consists of the family Psittacidae, *e.g.*, the parrots, macaws, cockatoos, lorys, conures, parakeets, etc.

PURULENT. Consisting of, or containing pus.

PUS. A liquid product of inflammation made up of dead or dying white corpuscles, yielding a sticky whitish, or yellowish fluid. At some stage it contains bacteria or other pathogenic organisms. The contents of an abscess; the product of suppuration.

PYGOSTYLE. The fused tail portion of the backbone.

SEBACEOUS. Fatty or greasy. Secreting or conveying oily substance (gland, duct, follicle).

SEPTICAEMIA. Septic or poisoned blood. Circulation of pathogenic organisms and their associated poisons in the blood, resulting in generalised illness, high temperature and frequently death.

SPASTIC. Subject to involuntary muscular contraction—clonic (jerky), tonic (prolonged); spasms of extension or rigid flexion of muscles especially the limbs.

SPECIES. A genetically similar group of organisms, differing in minor details only. A classification, subordinate to the larger group, the genus.

Abbreviation: singular = sp.

plural = spp.

STEATITIS. Inflammation of fat or adipose tissue.

SUBACUTE. Neither acute nor chronic, but with some of the characteristics of both.

SUTURE. A stitch. To join two edges of wound with stitches of thread, gut, wire, etc. Also line of union between the skull bones.

TITRE. The level or quantity of a substance (*e.g.,* antibodies in blood or other body fluids) required to produce a reaction with a given volume of another substance.

VARIETY (of bird). A variant form within a species or population which is otherwise alike. Synonymous with a "breed" of a domesticated species.

VECTOR. An animal (usually an invertebrate) which is a carrier of parasites or infections to another species.

VENTRAL. Of or towards the lower surface of the body or belly. The under surface as opposed to the upper dorsal or vertebral surface.

VERTEBRATE. Animal possessing vertebral column. A member of the animal kingdom Vertebrata, to which belong mammals, birds, reptiles, amphibians and fish.

VISCERA. The plural of viscus. The internal organs of any species, but usually of vertebrates: lung, heart, liver, kidney, intestinal tract and brain.

APPENDIX

KEY TO ABBREVIATIONS IN THE TABLES

g.	—	gram(me)
i/m	—	intramuscular
i/p	—	intraperitoneal
i.u.	—	international units
i/v	—	intravenous
kg.	—	kilogram(me)
mg.	—	milligramme
ml.	—	millilitre
s/c	—	subcutaneous
μg.	—	microgram(me)
wt.	—	weight

WEIGHTS, HEART RATES, Etc.

Order	Popular name Species	Body Weight	Heart rate (beats per minute)	Respiratory rate (beats per minute)	Daytime body temperature (Night 2–4°C less)
ANSERIFORMES	Domestic Duck	2–3.5 kg	180–230	♂30–50, ♀45–95	41°C
	Domestic Goose	4–5 kg			41°C
GALLIFORMES	Japanese Quail	18–42 g			
	Bob White Quail	c. 150 g			44°C
	Domestic Fowl	1.75–4 kg	250–340	♂10–20, ♀20–40	41.5°C
	Domestic Turkey	4.0–15.0 kg	80–100	10–38	41°C
GRUIFORMES	Crowned Crane	3.5–4.0 kg	220–240	64	
COLUMBIFORMES	Domestic Pigeon	260–350 g	180–250	20–35	41°C
PSITTACIFORMES	Budgerigar	30–60 g Up to 100 g if obese	240–600	75–96	42°C
	Love Birds, various species	50–70 g	220–300	120–140	
	Red-crowned Parakeet	60–75 g	300–400	88	
	Blue Crowned Conure	84–96 g	220–300	36–48	
	Cockatiel	100–140 g	360–420	100–120	
	Pennant's Parakeet	180–200 g	380–440	120	
	African Grey Parrot	300–380 g	120–200	32–42	
	Blue-Fronted Amazon Parrot	320–460 g			
	Leadbeater's Cockatoo	c. 500 g			
	Eclectus Parrot	600 g	300–350	28	
	Hyacinth Macaw	c. 4·0 kg	180–250	18	
APODIFORMES	Humming Birds	2.5–5.0 g		160–400	42–44.5°C
PASSERIFORMES	Zebra Finch	10–16 g	c.850–1200	140–200	40–42°C
	Goldfinch and Greenfinch	15–20 g	320–900	110–136	
	English Robin	20–30 g	550–700		
	Java Sparrow	24–30 g	c.600–900		
	Canary	12–29 g	c.700–1000	90–125	41–42°C
	House Sparrow	25–30 g	350–900		41–44°C
	Cardinal	c. 40 g			41–43°C
	Glossy Starling	74–82 g	180–220	60–76	
	Greater Indian Hill Mynah	180–240 g	120–200	24–48	

DRUGS AND DOSAGES

The administration of drugs, particularly by injection, is always an experiment in all species of animals, as well as man. No one can foretell with certainty the therapeutic effect of any drug in any individual at any given time. Still less can the unwanted side effects be prophesied. For this reason it has been decided to omit dosages of the potentially more dangerous drugs from the following tables.

Where dosages are listed they should be regarded as suggestions only. With a species in which the drug (except antibiotics) is not known to have been used before, it is wise to try a fractional test dose at first, e.g. 1/10 to 1/2 of the calculated therapeutic dose—and to increase the amount according to the response obtained. The list of drugs given below is by no means complete but does cover most of those which can be used for birds.

Oral dosage in food or drinking water is generally unreliable, and depends upon the extent to which the bird is feeding; it should be avoided whenever possible. This is particularly the case with grain-eating birds, such as budgerigars or canaries. However, as canaries usually have a relatively high intake of water, administration via the drinking water may be effective for this species when a drug of low toxicity is used. The soft-feeders such as nectar and fruit eaters, with a more regular and larger water consumption, may also benefit from medication of the fluid diet—provided the drug of choice is innocuous in doses 5-10 times the estimated normal quantity. Oral dosage should ideally be carried out by means of a "stomach tube".

The tube should be made of metal, with a rubber extension for large parrots because their powerful beaks may damage plastic or glass. Prior tranquillisation by injection may sometimes be necessary because there is a real danger of accidentally passing the tube into the trachea of a frightened vociferous bird.

Subcutaneous, intramuscular, and in some instances intravenous injections for small birds, require the use of 1 ml syringes graduated in hundredths of a ml. These are usually made entirely of glass or plastic, with a metal ferrule for the needle (23-25 gauge). Microlitre syringes are manufactured in 0.1 ml and 0.05 ml capacity and graduated in 0.002 ml and 0.001 ml divisions, but are so delicate that any grease or viscous fluid will cause damage. Only true solutions and not suspensions can be used in microlitre syringes. Doses, however, must be accurate and dilution of drugs makes it possible to use millilitre syringes with quite small birds of only 10 or 20 g body weight.

Dosages calculated on a body weight basis, but also bearing in mind the age and condition of the bird, are likely to be effective and safe for most species including budgerigars, parrots, canaries, pigeons, falcons, hawks, gallinaceous species (e.g. poultry and game birds), ducks, geese and swans. For the smaller passerine birds, treatment by injection is liable to be a hazardous adventure. In all species care must be taken when injecting into the pectoral muscles not to penetrate them too deeply (max. 0.5 cm in a budgerigar), otherwise the needle may enter the large venous sinus in these muscles and cause haemorrhage.

ANTIBIOTICS

Trade names	Short chemical names and preparations available	Manufacturer or distributor
Penbritin	Ampicillin Suspensions 150 mg/ml Injectable Powder plus diluent 100 mg/ml	Beecham
Crystapen	Penicillin: Crystalline sodium benzylpenicillin for injection	Glaxo
Streptopen	Dihydrostreptomycin sulphate and procaine penicillin G ALSO Streptomycin in all forms	Glaxo
Aureomycin and others	Tetracyclines Chlortetracycline hydrochloride Soluble Powder Ophthalmic ointment spray and Capsules	Cyanamid G.B. (UK) Lederle, (USA)
Terramycin and others	Oxytetracycline, Injectable Sol. Tablets Ophthalmic (see polymyxin B below)	Pfizer and others
Terramycin Ophthalmic	Oxytetracycline hydrochloride and Polymyxin B Ophthalmic ointment	Pfizer
Doctor Marten's Avicur	Chlortetracycline (C.T.C.) in the form of medicated seed	Oberhausener Kraftfutterwerk W. Germany
Nebacetin	Spray powder containing neomycin and bacitracin	Intervet

Uses and Special indications	Comments and special precautions
Broad spectrum antibiotic active against a wide range of Gram positive organisms, *e.g. Streptococci, Staphylococci.* Also several important Gram negative organisms, *e.g.* some strains of *Escherichia coli, Pasteurella,* and *Salmonella.*	Low incidence of shock or other side effects.
Diseases due to penicillin-sensitive bacteria, i.e. *Erysipelothrix,* almost all *Streptococci* and a few *Staphylococci.* Crystalline P. gives very high levels for few hours. 4 day, low level treatments available.	The first antibiotic. Safe in normal dosages. Many strains of bacteria resistant to penicillin have developed throughout the world. Largely replaced by Ampicillin for birds. PROCAINE penicillin for injection is NOT RECOMMENDED FOR BIRDS because of toxicity.
Effective against Gram positive and many Gram negative organisms.	NOT RECOMMENDED FOR INJECTION: MAY BE LETHAL. Oral and topical forms (mixtures and ointments) *may be* tolerated by some species.
Broad spectrum antibiotics effective against almost all Gram positive and a high proportion of Gram negative organisms including *Mycoplasma* and Psittacosis—lymphogranuloma group of organisms. Useful in septicaemias, respiratory, alimentary, urinary and wound infections.	Prolonged treatment should be avoided, otherwise fungal infections may develop. Use max. 5 days treatment then min. 3 days without, before starting a second course. These antibiotics are *not* likely to be effective if administered by dilution in the drinking water. Injections with some oxytetracycline preps. may be painful.
Very effective eye ointment against many pus forming organisms including Gram negative bacteria such as *Pseudomonas aeruginosa.* Useful for sinusitis.	Apply to the eye or wound 2–4 times daily after salt water bathing.
Psittacosis/Ornithosis. For treatment and prevention.	Necessary to feed continuously at appropriate dosage levels for 45 days as only source of food. Vitamin supplements should be given in conjunction with the treatment.
Powder for dusting wounds and opened "bumblefoot" lesions. Non-irritant, dissolves in tissue fluids. Wide antibacterial spectrum of activity.	Appears to be of low toxicity. Use sparingly.

485

Chloromycetin and others	Chloramphenicol Palmitate suspension, Ophthalmic ointment	Parke-Davis, and others
Orbenin	Cloxacillin for injection	Beecham
Erythrocin	Erythromycin for injection	Abbott
Fulcin Grisovin	Griseofulvin tablets	ICI Glaxo
Linco-Spectin	Lincomycin + Spectinomycin soluble powder for oral administration	Upjohn
Spectam	Spectinomycin dihydrochloride for injection	Abbott
Neomycin 5	Neomycin sulphate for oral administration	Bayer
Nystan ointment and suspension ready mixed	Nystatin: Ointment and Oral Suspension Feed Supplement	Squibb
Mycostatic 20	Feed Supplement	

486

Broad spectrum antibiotic particularly of use against gut organisms, *Listeria* and for treatment of crop necrosis in budgerigars.	Safe in budgerigars. Tendency to produce resistant strains of bacteria such as *Salmonellae* and *Escherichia coli*. Therefore its use is being restricted in UK to cases where it is likely to be the only effective antibiotic available. The antibiotic is not recommended for injection, especially of falcons and hawks.
Injectable broad spectrum antibiotic effective against penicillin resistant *Staphylococci*.	Use with care and give test doses in resistant "bumblefoot," septic arthritis, infected torn crop, airsac infections etc.
Moderately broad spectrum antibiotic particularly effective against Gram positive cocci and *Mycoplasma*.	Found safe by intra muscular injection in budgerigars.
Fungicidal antibiotic. May be tried against ringworm fungi (rarely seen) and *Candida*.	Tablets are too large for small birds so have to be broken up. This may make the drug less effective by hastening absorption.
Valuable for upper respiratory tract infections (*Mycoplasma* and *E. coli*) of gallinaceous birds.	Promising antibiotic suitable for birds which will take the drug in food or by a "stomach" tube.
Effective against *Mycoplasma* and a wide range of Gram negative bacteria, *e.g. Salmonella* and *Pasteurella*.	Particularly recommended for gallinaceous birds.
Effective against many gut bacteria. Poorly absorbed into bloodstream. Best used with Kaolin, Magnesium trisilicate or chalky base.	Parenteral preparations not tested in cagebirds, but side effects likely.
Fungicidal ointment for cutaneous mycoses Effective against *Candida* causing crop mycosis.	Not effective against *Aspergillus* species.

ANTI-PROTOZOAL DRUGS

Trade names	Short chemical name and preparations available	Manufacturer or distributor
Emtryl	Dimetridazole soluble powder, tablets and Premix	May & Baker
Mecryl	Mepacrine hydrochloride tabs. and solution	May & Baker
Neftin Premix	Powder containing furazolidone 4.4%	Smith Kline
Sulphamezathine	Sulphadimidine sodium powder, solution, and tablets	ICI
Embazin	Sulphaquinoxaline solution	May & Baker
Saquadil	Sulpha-quinoxaline plus diaveridine solution	May & Baker
Tribrissen oral suspension	Trimethoprim and sulphadiazine	Wellcome

Uses and special indications	Comments and special precautions
Blackhead (*Histomonas meleagridis* infection) in pheasants and other game birds. *Trichomonas gallinae* infection or "Canker" (pigeons); "Frounce" (birds of prey).	Liable to be toxic in usual therapeutic doses for some small species. Administered in the drinking water, by medication of food or directly by mouth. As a prophylactic for blackhead in pheasants, use half the therapeutic dose and give continuously during periods when birds most likely to be at risk.
Plasmodium spp. (malaria). Other blood-borne protozoa and Coccidia.	———
Histomoniasis and hexamitiasis, also bacterial gut infections including salmonellosis and *Escherichia coli*.	Powder for incorporation in the food. Too toxic at levels required for treatment of *Trichomonas* infection. Must be used with care and only under veterinary supervision.
Used for treatment of coccidiosis and some bacterial infections of gut.	Inactive in presence of pus and para-amino-benzoic acid. For the treatment of birds, it is usually given in the drinking water.
Coccidiosis, especially game birds.	Both these drugs are administered via the drinking water.
A new anti-bacterial treatment: two drugs acting at two stages in bacterial metabolism. Therefore very little tendency to drug resistance. Active against wide range of Gram-negative and Gram-positive bacteria.	Non-irritant. Minimal side effects. High therapeutic index.

DISINFECTANTS AND ANTI-

Common Name	Chemical Name	Uses and Special indications
Coal Tar Derivatives Various names	Cresols in soap-base	Variable disinfecting value. More effective and less toxic than phenol-based disinfectants.
Instrument Dettol	Active ingredient chloroxylenol BPC 6.25%	Useful disinfectant for food utensils, equipment and surgical instruments. Few non-sporing organisms survive immersion in appropriate solution.
Liquefied Phenol Carbolic Acid	Phenol liquefactum Phenol	Powerful disinfectant. Fairly expensive. Used as a standard for disinfectants. 5% is maximum for general purposes of disinfection. Not an antiseptic for skin use.
Reducing Agent Formalin	Liquor Formaldehydi	Powerful disinfectant even in the presence of organic matter; does not corrode utensils or instruments. Gas not effective unless premises made virtually airtight. In 4% liquid form, a tissue preservative and effective bacteriostat.
Quaternary Ammonium Compounds Numerous		Widely used general antiseptic and disinfectant for utensils, instruments and even eggs. Not effective against viruses, some Gram negative bacteria and fungi. Activity reduced by pus.
Physical Agents	Sunlight	Very effective against viruses: less against bacteria. Use limited to cages, utensils and movable equipment.
	Heat	Temperatures of 80°C for a few minutes kill all viruses and bacteria except heat tolerant spores, which may need 35 min. at 120°C.
U.V. Light or rays	Ultraviolet Light	As sunlight—but can be used also inside premises.
Other Agents Washing Soda	Sodium Carbonate	Degreasing agent. Dissolves keratin—a cleansing disinfectant. Effective against reasonable range of non-sporing bacteria. The alkalinity of 4% solution makes it effective against some viruses.
Alcohol	Ethyl Alcohol 70%	Precipitates protein, kills viruses and most bacteria but some spores survive.
Medicinal Gentian Violet or Crystal Violet	Violacrystallina Methylrosaniline chloride	A powerful non-irritant antiseptic active against Gram positive bacteria.

490

SEPTICS (MOSTLY AVAILABLE TO THE PUBLIC)

Modes of use	Comments. Special precautions
Must be adequately diluted and used on premises, perches, nest boxes etc. only, according to manufacturers' instructions.	Cresols mix with, but are only slightly soluble in water. Coal tar saponified products form milky emulsion with water.
Not to be used on birds. For most purposes use 2% aqueous solution.	Pleasant to use.
Use manufacturers' recommendations for general disinfectant purposes. Phenol liquefactum (80%) is applied on "baby cotton wool buds" to cauterise ulcers.	80% solution is corrosive to tissues. A penetrating and local anaesthetic. Greatly diluted for general disinfectant purposes.
Used as a spray (10%) or fumigation with Formaldehyde gas produced by mixing 35 ml Formalin with 17.5 g potassium permanganate.	Unpleasant to use (can cause conjunctivitis, excessive tears and hardening of the skin). Some people allergic or hypersensitive to formalin. Birds should be removed during fumigation or spraying but vapour soon disperses.
Use manufacturers' recommendations.	Colourless, odourless, deodourizing, non-irritant to normal skins. Inactivated by soap, but can be mixed with alcohol.
Ad libitum.	Ultraviolet light not very penetrating. Therefore organic debris reduces the effect of the rays.
Moist steam heat 120°C for 20 min. Dry heat (oven) 180°C for 20–30 min. or 280°C for 15 min.	Sterilization in a pressure cooker (10 lb pressure) for 20 min. kills all significant pathogens. *Pseudomonas* may need over 30 min.
Equipment must produce rays of wavelength of 2800 to 2600 Angstrom Units.	Requires expensive equipment which must be replaced periodically. Dangerous to eyes. Burns skin if bird or man excessively exposed to rays. Remove birds from cage before use.
4% solution for premises only; best scrubbed in or pressure-sprayed.	Good and cheap cleansing disinfectant for general use. 1% in water in a sterilizer prevents rusting of non-stainless metal instruments.
Immerse instruments for at least 1 hour.	Useful to maintain cleanliness of instruments and suture materials but does not necessarily sterilise them.
For external use only on burns, chronic ulcers and fungal skin affections.	Preferable to commercial gentian violet and methyl violet.

491

ANTI-PARASITIC DRUGS OR

Group	Trade names	Chemical names	Manufacturer or distributor
ORGANO-PHOSPHORUS COMPOUNDS		Malathion 4% and 5% powders	Murphy Chemical Ltd. and others
	Vapona Flykiller	Dichlorvos	Shell
	Dylox	Metriphonate	Chemagra Corp. Kansas City, USA
ORGANIC SULPHUR CONTAINING COMPOUND	Tetmosol solution	Monosulfiram 25% w/v solution in methylated spirits	ICI
PLANT PRODUCTS	None	Prepared Derris Powder Rotenone 4–6% is active principle	
		Nicotine Sulphate solution	Campbell & Sons
	Aerosol Flyspray	Pyrethrins plus piperonyl butoxide 2%	Wellcome
	Veterinary Insecticide (Pybuthrin), Cooper	Dusting powder. Pyrethrins 0.25% Piperonyl butoxide 2.5%	Wellcome

PESTICIDES

Uses and special indications	Dosage and route of administration	Comments and special precautions
Although toxic, less so than other organo-phosphorus comps. Use against airsac mites in canaries, finches, lovebirds and others.	As a 5% or 4% dust inhaled for 5 mins. as a dense fog in box $10 \times 10 \times 15$ cm repeated every 1–6 weeks.	These are maximum concentrations. Risk of toxicity if exceeded. Powder usually sold only in bulk.
In the form of a solid plastic, resin, vapour strip for hanging in buildings.		Danger of toxicity to some species, but may be used on vacated premises for 1–4 days.
Respiratory acariasis (airsac mites). May be tried against Gapeworms.	0.2 ml of a 1:500 suspension in distilled water i/m for canaries with respiratory acariasis. Equivalent to 10 mg/kg body wt. of active principle. Repeat in 10 days.	A toxic drug. Needs to be used with great care and under veterinary supervision.
May be tried for mites such as *Knemidocoptes* spp., (scaly face and scaly leg disease).	Dilute 1:25 to make 1% sol. with water and use as a wash or paint.	Toxic if used in too strong a solution or on large and especially inflamed areas. The solution is stable for only a few hours and should be freshly prepared as required.
Safe and moderately effective insecticide for wide range of parasites including mites.	Dusting powder for birds and nests.	Only mild toxicity, may occur with recommended treatment levels.
Insecticide largely superseded by newer agents.	Use for premises when required, at dilution recommended by makers.	MUST NOT BE USED DIRECTLY ON BIRDS. 40% solution highly toxic to all species by contact absorption. Use only for pressure spraying of empty cages, aviaries and premises.
For blowflies, fleas, lice and red mites.	Spray birds and nests and premises lightly according to manufacturers' instructions.	Piperonyl butoxide assists the action of pyrethrum.
For control of fleas, lice and ticks.	Powder should be used dry. Use at weekly intervals.	Safe for small birds under ordinary circumstances.

MISCELLANEOUS	No common name	Benzyl Benzoate 25% Emulsion	Various
	Nemecide	Levamisole hydrochloride 7.5%	ICI
	Coopane	Piperazine adipate. Tablets or powder	Wellcome
	Game bird Wormer	Soluble Powder containing Tetramisole hydrochloride 10% w/w	ICI
	Thibenzole	Thiabendazole 13.3% suspension, water-dispersible powder 58.4% with cobalt sulphate 1.8%	Merck Sharp & Dohme
	Dicestal	Dichlorophen Tablets 0.5 g	May & Baker
	Alugan	Bromocyclen 1.4 g in each 170 g container of aerosol spray 42.5 g in 100 g conc. powder 4.25 g in 100 g dusting powder	Hoechst

Knemidocoptic mange.	10% emulsion applied to lesions on 3 occasions at 24 to 48 hour intervals.	May be very toxic at 25%, but diluted to 10% appears well tolerated for small areas.
Effective against a range of roundworms including *Ascaridia*, *Capillaria* and *Heterakis* species.	Oral dose: 0.25–0.5 mg/kg body wt. Can be injected in mammals but no recommendations for birds except gamebirds. For oral use dilute to give adequate volume.	Has been used successfully in a range of gamebirds and both larger and smaller psittacines. Fairly safe, but test dose with valuable birds or flocks.
Effective in paralysing *Ascaridia* and other intestinal worms.	Powder or Tablet. 1.0 g/kg body wt. in divided small doses during the day. 500 mg/kg body wt. single dose, Orally, followed by liquid paraffin every 2–3 weeks.	
Gapeworms, roundworms, hair worms and caecal worms.	Give in food or drinking water at an average dose level of 50 mg/kg body wt. (See also manufacturer's instructions).	
Gape worms in many species and Ornithostrongylosis in pigeons. Can also be used against gizzard and thorny-headed worms.	Powder. 44 mg/kg body wt. orally equivalent to 0.25 ml/kg of 13.3% suspension.	Reportedly successful in a raven, pheasants and mynahs.
For treatment of tapeworms.	3 mg/10 g body wt. orally, after feeding.	Although little is known about the susceptibility of various species of avian cestodes to this drug, it is worth trying.
For control of fleas, lice, louse flies and mites such as *Knemidocoptes*. Powder and spray suitable for use on birds.	For Knemidocoptic mange paint area with 0.2% suspension of powder.	Use with care on small birds. Avoid spraying eyes.

ANAESTHETICS, SEDATIVES &

Group	Trade Names	Short chemical names	Manufacturer or distributor
ANAESTHETICS **INHALATION** (Gaseous)	—	Cyclopropane	British Oxygen
	"Laughing Gas"	Nitrous Oxide	British Oxygen
INHALATION (Volatile)	Chloroform	Chloroform	Several
	Ether (Anaesthetic)	Diethyl Ether B.P.	Several
	Fluothane	Halothane	ICI
	Penthrane	Methoxyflurane B.P.	Abbott
PARENTERAL	Nembutal Sagatal	Pentobarbitone Sodium	Abbott May & Baker
	Equithesin	Pentobarbitone Sodium 9.6 g with Chloral Hydrate 42.6 g and Magnesium Sulphate 21.2 g per litre	Jensen-Salsbery

TRANQUILLIZERS

Special indications and uses	Dosage and route of administration	Comments and special precautions
Excellent, controllable and safe anaesthetic. Gaseous.	Inhalation 20–25% with oxygen for induction. Then add oxygen to maintain anaesthesia in closed circuits.	Anaesthetic dangerous to operator in confined or unventilated spaces. Inflammable. Explosive in low concentration, especially with oxygen.
Partial or incomplete gaseous anaesthetic.	Inhalation 90% with 10% oxygen reducing to 80% in 20% oxygen.	Must be used with oxygen. Non-inflammable.
FOR EUTHANASIA ONLY.	Kills canaries within 3 seconds and budgerigars within 10 seconds.	Lethal, hepatotoxic and cardiatoxic. Unsuitable for anaesthesia.
Safe and "flexible" anaesthetic when volatilized with oxygen blown over or through liquid. Also with air via an ether-impregnated pad in movable mask. Up to 90 min. safe anaesthetic.	Inhalation of oxygen bubbled through for induction and blown over ether in a Boyle's ether bottle for maintenance. Be prepared to give pure oxygen if deep anaesthesia is reached.	HIGHLY INFLAMMABLE. Explosive in certain concentrations. Floor level vapour can be ignited by spark from electric socket or switch, cigarette end or steel shoe stud on a concrete floor.
Potent, poorly volatile anaesthetic can often be used for long periods up to 90 min. Flexible but slower induction than ether.	Up to 3% in oxygen. For safety a special vapourizer is needed.	Not resented. Apparently toxic to some species. Non-inflammable.
Less potent than halothane, poorly volatile but very safe anaesthetic for long periods. In some birds premedication may be necessary to induce and/or maintain beyond light level of anaesthesia.	Maximum concentration is obtainable by bubbling oxygen through liquid at room temp. in a Boyle's Trilene bottle. Is entirely safe.	Very safe, non-inflammable, non-explosive.
Variable depth and duration with same dose in birds of similar weights. Short, light to medium anaesthesia of 3–15 min. in a total period of 30–90 min. from administration to recovery.	Dilute to suitable volume. Give subcutaneously at back of neck or intramuscularly into breast or thigh at the rate of 20–40 mg per kg body wt. The higher dosage-level to be used in smaller birds and by subcutaneous route.	Unsafe beyond light to medium anaesthesia. Preferably give test dose first (e.g. half computed dose i/m to assess effect) and add part or all remainder after 10 mins.
Primarily an equine anaesthetic. Comments as for Pentobarbitone but less variable and longer useful effect.	Dilute 1 part to 5 or 10 of water to obtain measurable volume for use in small birds. Use centilitre syringes. If undiluted: 2–2.5 ml/kg body wt.	As for pentobarbitone sodium. Useful duration 10–30 mins. A further 25% of anaesthetic dose may be given after 45–60 mins. if required. Danger of overdosage and cooling (hypothermia) as with all parenteral anaesthetics.

497

	Saffan	Alphaxalone and Alphadolone acetate steroid anaesthetic.	Glaxo

LOCAL, TOPICAL and REGIONAL ANAESTHETICS	Xylocaine with or without adrenalin	2% Xylocaine hydrochloride	Astra
	Ophthaine	Proxymetacaine hydrochloride, plus glycerine and preservative	Squibb

SEDATIVES and TRANQUILLIZERS (Premedicants)	Acetyl promazine	Acetyl promazine injection 2 mg/ml	Crookes
	Largactil	Chlorpromazine hydrochloride 10 and 25 mg tablets	May & Baker
	Themalon	Diethylthiambutene hydrochloride, 50 mg tablets for injection	Wellcome
	Hypnodil	Metomidate hydrochloride	Crown Chemical and Janssen Pharmaceutica
	Avicalm	Metoserpate hydrochloride soluble powder in dextrose base	Squibb

Tranquillizer sedative. Light to fairly deep anaesthetic. Useful for operations involving the head. Anaesthetic period 3–15 mins. according to depth of anaesthesia and species. Prolonged tranquillization 20 mins. to 1 hr. with subcutaneous dosage route. Useful for dressings and nervous birds. Used in budgerigars, pigeons, poultry, gamebirds, hawks and falcons.	1–1.5 ml/kg body wt. subcutaneously, intramuscularly or intraperitoneally in mid-line near cloaca. Premedication may increase anaesthetic safety. Higher dose given s/c seldom produces more than light anaesthesia.	Respirations do not get slower before death during deep anaesthesia. Pedal and palpebral reflexes are weak in medium anaesthesia. Danger signs of transition from deep anaesthesia to death are not noticeable. Antidotes Bemegride (Megemide ICI) and Millophylline (Dales Pharms) reverse anaesthesia to medium or light in 30–60 secs.
Local or regional anaesthesia of skin.	1–20% solution by local infiltration subcutaneously. Maximum dose 10 mg/kg body wt. No entirely safe dosage level.	Danger of convulsions, coma and death if injected in high doses or in vascular areas.
Surface-absorbable, 0.5% aqueous, local anaesthetic for fresh skin wounds or for eyes.	0.5% solution. Spray or paint lightly.	Toxic side effects possible in some species. Use with care. Local anaesthesia occurs in less than 30 secs. and persists for about 15 mins.
Premedicant. Tranquillizer and sedative in higher doses. Use parenterally.	0.025–0.05 ml/kg body wt. 0.05–0.10 mg/kg body wt. By intramuscular injection.	Lowers anaesthetic dosage required. Contra-indicated where liver damage suspected.
ditto	1.0–2.0 mg/kg body wt. by mouth.	ditto
Analgesic, hypnotic, sedative, premedication narcotic.	2–5 mg/kg body wt. The higher dose is for birds with body wt. below 100 g (i/m for lower doses, s/c for higher doses).	Narcotic. Hyperaesthesia to sound is common side effect. Partial antidote and resuscitator. Nalorphine ("Lethidrone," Wellcome). Good therapeutic index in budgerigars.
Hypnotic and analgesic. Can be used alone for minor surgery or in conjunction with a volatile anaesthetic.	Dosage rate varies for different species. Normally give 10 mg/kg or 15 mg/kg for small birds by i/m injection.	Use 0.1% solution for birds under 100 g body wt. and 1% for heavier species. For very large spp. such as cranes and ostriches use 5% solution. Very safe for all species.
A tranquillizer to facilitate handling for minor procedures.	Administered in the drinking water at concentration of 0.015%. Degree of tranquillization is directly dependent upon the amount of drug ingested.	The product is manufactured for poultry but there appears to be no reason why it should not be used for other species.

VACCINES AND RELATED

Group	Common name	Chemical name	Manufacturer
ANTITOXINS	Type C Mink Vaccine	*Clostridium botulinum* type C Antitoxin	*Clostridium* C Adsorbat Vaccine, Marburg. Probably obtainable in most countries through Department of Health or Agriculture.
ANTISERA		Antibacterial, antiviral hyper-immune sera.	Can be produced on a small scale for some pathogens which are resistant to drugs. Provided by some private laboratories.
VACCINES	Erysorb. Swine Erysipelas Vaccine	*Erysipelothrix insidiosa* (Syn *E. rhusiopathiae*) Vaccine	Hoechst
	Newcastle Disease vaccines	Contain La Sota or Hitchner B. strains of Newcastle Disease virus	Hoechst
	Pox vaccine	Attenuated pigeon pox vaccine	Not yet available in U.K. Used in U.S.

BIOLOGICAL PRODUCTS

Uses and special indications	Dosage and route of administration	Comments and special precautions
Antitoxin will neutralize toxin in the general circulation, but is effective for only a short time.	Normally to be given intra-peritoneally at dosage as recommended by supplier	Botulism. Administration of fresh water orally helps to flush out and dilute toxin.
Serum containing antibodies in high concentration for injection into birds at risk.	To be used only under veterinary supervision.	Since the introduction of antibiotics and other antibacterial drugs, the use of antisera has fallen. The only commercial antiserum regularly available in the U.K. is an Erysipelas Antiserum. Conceivable use in birds as an alternative to Penicillin therapy.
Relatively few outbreaks of Erysipelas infection have been reported. To date, only sporadic deaths recorded but vaccination advisable with birds in contact.	Maker's recommendations are for turkeys only.	A combined Pasteurellosis-Erysipelas vaccine for turkeys is also produced, but nothing is known concerning the effectiveness of any of these vaccines for other birds.
The vaccines are manufactured for poultry and game birds. Some have been tried on other species including birds of prey and pigeons. For prevention of pigeon pox.	Dosage for species other than poultry are still in experimental stage.	

HORMONES AND ENZYMES

Group	Trade name and preparations	Chemical or proper name	Manufacturer or distributor
HORMONES	Female hormone	Stilboestrol Diproprionate in oil for injection. Also Implant Tabs. 10 mg and 5 mg	Various manufacturers
	Male hormone	Testosterone esters or salts e.g. Testosterone phenyl propionate 10 mg/ml in oil for injection	Ditto
	Thyroid	Thyroxine Thyroid tabs. (crude) 60 mg/Tabs. Thyroid extract	Ditto
ANABOLIC STEROIDS	Vebonol Laurabolin Retarbolin	Boldenone undecylenate Nandrolone laurate Nandrolone cyclo-hexylpropionate	CIBA Intervet Berk
PANCREATIC EXTRACT (Digestive enzyme)	Chymar (5000 Armour units of proteolytic activity)/in 5 ml vial—soluble crystals.	Chymotrypsin	Armour Pharmaceutical Co. Ltd.
CORTICOSTEROIDS	Betsolan Injection	Betamethasone 2.0 mg/ml	Glaxo
	Depo-Medrone for injection	Methylprednisolone acetate 40 mg/ml	Upjohn

(ORGANIC CATALYSTS)

Uses and special indications	Comments and special precautions
For reproductive problems in females and plumage problems in both sexes. Used for chemical caponization.	Sex hormones should be used only under strict veterinary supervision.
Effective in reaffirming lost male libido. Improves colour of male plumage. Used also in immaturity, senility, debility and other retarded sexual states.	
For slow delayed moult, poor quality plumage. Hypothyroidism: fat, sluggish, constipated bird, with low levels of activity. Correct dose promotes moult in a few weeks and growth of new plumage. *Single. injection. Duration of Effectiveness*	Overdose produces palpitation of heart, hyperaesthesia, loss of weight, and may precipitate heart attacks.

3 weeks ⎫
3 weeks ⎬ Accelerate build-up of cells and
3–4 weeks ⎭ tissues, while slowing down
breakdown of tissues. Aid
retention of calcium. Help
increase appetite and weight.
Digests extra-cellular protein—blood and
protein in bruises, wounds and abscesses.
Removes swelling, pain, and oedema. This
allows other drugs such as antibiotics to
penetrate diseased tissue and act effectively.
Given by i/m injection.

Contra-indicated in renal disease or major liver damage. Useful after recovery from prolonged or serious illness. Marked improvement in general condition. Different (synthetic) group from corticosteroids.
Tends to dissolve sutures in the gut more quickly than in other areas. Therefore danger of gut-sutured abdominal wounds breaking down. Use antibiotic at same time as this enzyme.

| For reduction of inflammatory reactions due to allergy, infection or injury. For shock and circulatory collapse. | Contra-indicated in some kidney and heart diseases. Always use with an antibiotic, particularly where infection exists. |

NUTRITIONAL ADDITIVES:

Group	Trade name	Chemical name	Manufacturer or distributor
VITAMINS: FAT-SOLUBLE	Vitamin A	Vitamin A 10,000–100,000 iu/ml in oil	Various
	Vitamin D	Vitamin D3 20,000–1,000,000 iu/ml	Ditto
	Vitamin E	Vitamin E Alpha-tocopherol Acetate or Succinate 10, 50, 100, 200 and 1,000 mg Tabs. Also, injection-form in A, D3 and E mixtures	Ditto
VITAMINS: WATER-SOLUBLE	Vitamin B1	Aneurine hydrochloride (thiamine) 1, 3, 10 and 20 mg Tabs. Also injectable solution	Various
	Vitamin B12	Cyanocobalamin 250 µg–1,000 µg/ml Hydroxycobalamin 250 µg–1,000 µg/ml	Ditto

VITAMINS, MINERALS, AMINO-ACIDS AND MIXTURES

Uses and special indications	Dosage and route of administration	Comments and special precautions
Except for fish and seed-eaters additional Vitamin A is rarely required. Sources readily available in most diets. Deficiency affects health of skin and mucous membranes.	Single dose of 1–2,000 iu/kg body wt. i/m.	Too much Vitamin A may be a contributory cause of French Moult of budgerigars; an excess (as in cod liver oil) destroys Vitamin E, especially if oil is rancid. Therefore preferably used in conjunction with Vitamin E therapy.
Essential for normal bone growth especially in birds used to much sunshine. Aids calcium and phosphorus retention. Prevents soft-shelled eggs and some nervous disorders. See also Vitamins of B group, e.g. Aneurine.	10,000–50,000 iu/kg body wt. i/m. Repeat weekly if required.	Synthesised in the skin by the ultra-violet fraction of sunlight. High level of phosphorus or phosphates in the diet increase the need for Vitamin D.
Maintains and augments heart and skeletal muscle power and development. Maintains health of male and female gonad function. Vitamin E deficiency may permanently impair female reproductive organs. With anabolic steroids Vitamin E helps to reverse debility and to rejuvenate old birds.	High therapeutic index, a safe drug. 5–50 iu/kg body wt., orally.	Excess Vitamin A in the diet and rancid oils oxidise Vitamin E and make it unavailable for absorption.
Essential in conversion of carbohydrate to give energy. Recreates appetite, maintains digestive functions, corrects certain types of nerve/muscle weakness such as loss of grip when perching.	1–2 mg/kg body wt., orally.	Grain is a good source of Vitamin B1 provided it is fresh
Involved in metabolism of carbohydrate fat and protein; its use therefore maintains general health, breeding potential, bone growth and energy. One of the best and safest general tonics available.	High therapeutic index: safe and apparently non-toxic. 250–5,000 µg/kg body wt. The lower levels are probably adequate.	Droppings may become pink a result of high doses. Vitamin probably produced in the gut many birds; broad spectrum antibiotics if fed to birds for periods will inhibit its production and deficiency may result.

VITAMINS: MULTIPLE, WATER AND FAT-SOLUBLE PREPARATIONS	Several types available.	Vitamins A, D2, D3 + E often together with other vitamins and minerals	Various
	Crookes Multi-Vitamin Injection	Vits. A, D3, Tocopheryl acetate B.P.C., selection of Vit. B group etc.	Crookes Veterinary
	Abidec drops	Vit. A, Calciferol B.P., Thiamine hydrochloride, Riboflavine, Pyridoxine, Nicotinamide, Ascorbic acid	Parke-Davis
VITAMINS: MULTIPLE, WATER-SOLUBLE PREPARATIONS	Several types available	Riboflavin (B2), Nicotinamide (Niacin), Pyridoxine (B6), Pantothenic Acid, Biotin, Choline, Folic Acid, Ascorbic Acid. Often together with other vitamins and minerals	Various
VITAMINS and MINERALS	Powder, e.g. Vionate	Multi fat- and water-soluble vitamins plus numerous minerals.	Squibb
VITAMINS (±MINERALS) FATTY ACIDS ETC.	e.g. Norderm	Linoleic acids, other glycerides, Vit. A and E and other constituents	Smith Kline and others
AMINO-ACIDS and other breakdown products of muscle protein	Ovigest Elixir and Protogest	About 8% protein digest and 10% glucose	Wellcome
AMINO-ACIDS, SORBITOL VITAMINS and MINERALS	Trophysan	Complex composition. Produced for i/v injection of humans	Servier

According to individual ingredients.	Oral—according to makers' recommendation. Usually given in drinking water.	In some products the ratios of some Vitamins is unsuitable for birds. Seek veterinary advice before use.
For all stress conditions and to hasten convalescence.	By s/c or i/m injection, 2 ml/kg body wt.	Some species may show allergic or hyper-sensitivity reactions following the injection.
As supportive treatment for debilitated or convalescent birds.	Orally; by direct administration, in food or water. For budgerigars or birds of similar size, give 0.3 ml every 3rd day.	Do not use in galvanised drinking vessels. Excessive doses can lead to hypervitaminosis A and D.
Prevention of curled toe paralysis in chicks, perosis, inhibited growth, poor feathering, dermatitis, loss of weight, poor appetite. Also, poor egg production and hatchability, foot and mouth necrosis, spinal cord lesions, anaemia, fading of plumage and paralysis.	Orally or by injection according to manufacturers' recommendations for small animals. Usually 0.1–1.0 ml/kg body wt. No injectable product contains all constituents.	Impossible to tell clinically which vitamin is deficient, therefore a full range is preferable to a single vitamin. Vitamin C probably not needed by birds, except some nectar an fruit eaters.
Combines all the theoretically essential vitamins plus calcium, phosphorus, sodium chloride, iodine, iron, cobalt, copper, magnesium and manganese. Useful for geriatric, post-operative, convalescent, breeding and nutritionally deprived birds.	Oral administration as food supplement. Canaries, budgerigars and species of similar size: 25 mg each. Pigeons, etc. 250 mg each.	A useful supplement for soft feeders.
Particularly useful for recuperation in convalescence and re-establishment of good body and plumage condition.	Orally once daily—small doses best injected into a suitable piece of food. "Norderm" 0.025–0.1 ml/kg body wt.	These supplements sometimes give very good results.
Provides pre-digested protein food, absorbable directly by the gut or on i/p injection, by the peritoneum, thereby resting an irritated gut.	Oral i/p injection can be used. 2.5 ml/kg body wt.	Must be sterile, therefore use within 24 hours (3 days if kept a refrigerator).
Used in conjunction with Norderm, this is almost a complete diet for weak, anorectic birds.	By i/v injection or oral administration.	Expensive, because these products are only available in sterile 500 ml bottles and are only fractionally used.

VARIOUS PREPARATIONS

Common name	Chemical name	Uses and special indications
Liquid paraffin	Paraffinum Liquidum	A bland laxative. Suitable lubricant for egg-binding.
Potassium iodide	Potassii Iodidum	For prevention of simple goitre, hypothyroidism and iodine deficiency. In birds it may possibly help to prevent Aspergillosis.
Calcium gluconate and Calcium lactate tablets	Calcii Gluconas Calcii Lactas	Can be used as an extra source of calcium when this mineral is deficient and causing diseases such as rickets.
Lunar caustic or Silver nitrate stick	Argenti Nitras	Has astringent, antiseptic, caustic and styptic properties. When applied to living tissue it combines with the protein, giving tissue a brownish black appearance.
Epsom salts or Magnesium sulphate	Magnesii Sulphas	Given by mouth it is a powerful saline purgative.

(MOSTLY READILY AVAILABLE TO THE PUBLIC)

Dosage and route of administration	Comments and special precautions
As a laxative: 5 ml/kg body weight by mouth (via "stomach" tube if necessary). Cloacal injection for faecal impaction of rectum and for egg binding.	Safe preparation, but regular use interferes with absorption of fat soluble vitamins and carotene.
For pigeons add 10 mg to one kg of mineral mixture. Estimated to give each bird 0.1–0.2 mg per week. Alternatively 150 mg dissolved in 60 ml of the drinking water daily or every other day.	Efficiency for fungal infections is doubtful, but drug is relatively harmless providing it is not given continuously for periods longer than one week.
Only to be used under veterinary supervision. Given by mouth.	Absorption from the intestines is slow, but can be increased by administering Vitamin D.
For external use only. 2–6% aqueous solution is used for cauterising ulcers and granulation tissue.	Needs to be protected from light. Solutions should be freshly prepared and stored in glass stoppered bottles.
May be added to drinking water to give a 5% solution or birds may be dosed individually at rate of 0.5–1.0 g/kg.	

POISONS

Toxic substance/source or use	Signs of poisoning
PESTICIDES	
Chlorinated hydrocarbons: DDT, DDD (TDE), Aldrin and BHC (Gammexane) Endosulphur or Lindane. Chlordane Dieldrin Heptachlor Endrin Methoxychlor	Apprehension, jumpiness, twitching, inco-ordination, convulsions, death due to lack of oxygen when respiratory mechanism paralysed. DDT and DDD among the least toxic; BHC vapour toxic to budgerigars; Aldrin fatal to pheasants at rate of 5 p.p.m. in feed; Dieldrin less toxic but powder absorbed via the skin. All are general stimulants of nervous system with effects observed within 24 hours.
Mercury: Seed dressings (with or without lead). Also in organo-mercury compounds.	Mainly in wild birds, e.g. pigeons eating quantities of dressed seed. Gut lesions (enteritis) and kidney damage.
Monosulphiram (Tetmosol)	Depression and death in hens when applied as a dressing over entire body at strength of 1 part monosulphiram to 4 parts water. Depression only is caused, when treatment confined to shanks.
Organophosphorous compounds: Chlorthion Diazinon Dipterex Malathion Parathion Schradan HETP DFP Dichlorvos (DDVP) Fenchlorvos	Individual drug differences occur, but usually excessive digestive secretion, diarrhoea, vomiting, abdominal pain, mucus from eyes and respiratory tract. Twitching and involuntary muscle movement, weakness of voluntary muscles. With some, drowsiness occurs prior to convulsions and death.
Veterinary Mange Dressings. Benzyl benzoate (emulsion)	Can be fatal to budgerigars if used topically on extensive lesions of Knemidocoptic mange, or if used in too great concentration, *i.e.* exceeding 10%.

510

Treatment/antidote	Comments
Use depressants to counter excitability, e.g. barbiturates or pentobarbitone. Birds should be washed free of remaining insecticides. Glucose and calcium borogluconate intravenously 5% and 10% respectively in larger birds.	Some are long and slow acting; others readily absorbed and quick acting, but excreted quickly. Many banned because they are too persistent in soil, or animal tissues. In an oily base, all can penetrate intact skin. Little absorbed by the gut.
Raw white of egg. Sodium thiosulphate—Hypo. Treatment generally ineffective if delayed 15 minutes or more after ingestion.	Geese are susceptible to poisoning from calomel (mercurous chloride).
No specific measures.	Use with caution. Test reaction by treating small area: for example *Knemidocoptes* infestation in budgerigars.
Atropine parenterally (s/c or i/m) also, 2-PAM (2-hydroxyimino-methyl-N-methylpyridinium iodide). Similar cholinesterase reactivators such as P2S and TMB-4 can be given s/c. Wash skin and feathers with weak detergent or soapy water solution. In skilled hands, soapy enemas may be helpful.	Fowls are especially susceptible to parathion toxicity. Diazinon is very toxic for ducks. Lethal doses range from 0.5 mg to 500 mg/kg body wt. and may be as low as 5 p.p.m. of foodstuffs.
Usually found dead. No specific antidote.	

Toxic substance/source or use	Signs of poisoning
Metaldehyde; Slug bait	Excitement, tremor, muscle spasms, rapid laboured breathing, blueness (cyanosis). Lung hemorrhage and brain degeneration.

DISINFESTANTS AND DISINFECTANTS

Aldehydes: Formaldehyde as a fumigant	Abdominal pain, collapse and death.
Sulphur: Burning as fumigating candles.	Sulphur dioxide produced and forms sulphurous acid on reaction with water. Causes conjunctivitis, rhinitis, choking, asthma-like attacks due to respiratory and circulatory disturbances.

MISCELLANEOUS

Halogen Compounds: Carbon tetrachloride. Chloroform, Tetrachlorethylene (Solvents, cleaners, anaesthetics, anthelmintics).	Potent anaesthetics toxic to heart and liver. Heart failure (early) or digestive failure (days later), kidney failure and autointoxication.
Sodium Chloride (Common Salt)	Excessive thirst, respiratory distress, fluid exudes from beak, sloppy droppings, weak legs. On necropsy dark, congested liver, oedema of tissues and congestion of lungs, liver and kidney.
Tar derivatives: Phenol as a caustic, Cresol in Creosote and as disinfectants and in oil pollution.	Absorbed via skin, causing local destruction of tissue if concentrated. Convulsions, signs of shock, rapid respiration, depression and general oedema in chickens.

PLANT TOXINS

Atropine and related substances. Sources: Deadly nightshade (*Atropa belladonna*), Henbane (*Hyoscyamus niger*), Thorn-apple (*Datura stramonium*), Woody nightshade (*Solanum dulcamara*), Black or Garden nightshade (*Solanum nigrum*), Egg-plant (*Solanum melongena*).	Birds are very sensitive. They may exhibit: increased pulse rate and respiration rate; papillary dilatation, blindness, staggering, restlessness, tremors, convulsions, respiratory depression with shallow fluttering breathing.

Treatment/antidote	Comments
No specific treatment. Remove source.	Toxic level in ducks is 0.3 g/kg body wt.
Aromatic spirit of Ammonia orally.	
Nothing very effective. Try Sodium bicarbonate wash, and as drink; inhalation of Ammonia. Much fresh air.	Birds should not be returned to fumigated cages until they are well ventilated.
Calcium borogluconate i/v may help. Free supply of air or oxygen if possible.	Liable to occur in confined premises with poor ventilation.
Diuretic drugs. Ample clean water to drink, remove source of salt.	Inadvertent use of salt or saline in mash foods. Brackish water (0.5% solution) is sufficient to cause signs; birds unable to taste small amounts.
Wash skin thoroughly with soap and water or detergent. No effective treatment exists for tar products which have been swallowed.	
Keep birds warm and active. Stimulants of the central nervous system such as aminophylline and amphetamines.	Variations in sensitivity occur among different species, e.g. hens can eat up to 15 g of Stramonium seed without illness.

Toxic substance/source or use	Signs of poisoning
Glycosides and Cyanogenetic glycosides: Cherry stones *Prunus* spp. *Pyrus* spp. *Sorghum* spp. *Panicum* spp. *Eucalyptus* spp. *Linum* spp. and many more, contain dangerous levels of hydrocyanic acid.	Excitement, convulsions, head pulled back and tail vertical. Jerky eyeball movement, deep rapid respiration. Death within the hour—possibly without earlier signs. Congestion of blood vessels. Suffusion of skin and appendages.
Nicotine and Nicotine-like Group: Tobacco plant (*Nicotiana tabacum*), Wild Tobacco (*N. glauca*). An Australian shrub *Duboisia hopwoodii*. Yellow jessamine (*Gelsemine sempervirens*). Hemlock (*Conium maculatum*).	The alkaloid is absorbed through intact skin. Early signs: excitement, rapid respiration and diarrhoea. Inco-ordination, increased heart rate, but decreased respiratory rate and depth leading to general flaccid paralysis, coma and death from respiratory paralysis.
Boxwood (*Buxus sempervirens*), Oleander (*Nerium oleander*), Yew (*Taxus baccata*), Azalea, Juniper (*Juniperus* spp.), *Daphne* spp., Privet (*Ligustrum vulgare*), other evergreens.	Resins affect C.N.S., kidneys, heart and liver. Excitement to depression. Panting.
Legumes: Rosary peas (*Abrus precatorius*), Black locust (*Robinias* spp.), Wistaria (*Wistaria chinensis*), Locoweed (*Oxytropis* spp.), Java beans and Horsebeans (*Phaseolus* spp.), *Crotalaria* spp., Laburnum (*Laburnum anagyroides*).	Severe gastroenteritis, cardiac and nervous depression. Damage to liver; experimentally found to have cancer-producing qualities. Crotalaria seeds toxic to quail, doves, chicken.
Strychnine: alkaloid from seed of *Strychnos nux vomica* and other members of Loganiaceae.	Apprehension, restlessness, twitches, throwing back the head, extended stiff limbs, voiding of droppings after abdominal contraction. Spasms of several seconds triggered by sounds, vibration, handling, or spontaneously. Respiration becomes difficult, cyanosis and death in a few minutes to 1 hour. Awareness of pain and anxiety appear greatly increased.
Some species of Blue-green algae: *e.g. Microcystis aeruginosa*.	Muscle tremors, convulsions, inco-ordination, paralysis, prostration, death.

PAINTS

Lead paint. Lead also found in fruit spray and petrol additives. Exhaust car gases contaminate grass verges; mine workings contaminate growing herbage.	Depression, loss of appetite, emaciation, excessive thirst, weak muscles, falling over, green diarrhoea.

Treatment/antidote	Comments
1% Sodium nitrate per 25 mg/kg body wt. i/v followed by sodium thiosulphate 25% per 1.25 g/kg body wt. Vitamin B12a (hydrococobalamin) will reverse the toxicity in mice. Chlorpromazine neutralises cyanide effects in pigeons.	Hydrocyanic acid or Prussic acid produced in rotten fruit and in animals stomachs has characteristic smell of bitter almonds. Minimal lethal body wt. dose is 2 mg/kg in many species. A dose of 4 mg/kg body wt. eaten rapidly is generally fatal.
Try caffeine subcutaneously, tea orally. Strychnine tonic in minute doses may help in early stages only. Morphine stated to be an antidote for *Gelsemine* poisoning.	Still used for treatment of premises for redmite. Also for agricultural purposes. Stock solution sold in a strength of 40% w/v. The alkaloids gelsemine from jessamine and coniine from hemlock have a similar action to nicotine.
Symptomatic treatment. Remove bird from source. Check stomach contents of any dead birds.	Berries particularly attractive to hungry young, birds. Bitterness not necessarily deterrent. Yew leaves poisonous to gallinaceous and probably other birds; all parts (especially seed) toxic.
None of value. Symptomatic treatment may help in mild cases only.	
Oral potassium permanganate to oxidise, or tannic acid to precipitate strychnine. In later stages anaesthesia (ether with oxygen) or for convulsions, Pentobarbitone in repeated doses is sufficient to relax muscular spasms and ease respirations, but may take several hours. Strychnine is eliminated from the body fairly rapidly.	Much less opportunity nowadays for ingesting this poison since general use as a rodenticide prohibited. Still obtainable in the U.K. as a bait for moles.
No effective treatment.	Occurs in stagnant water, particularly at temperatures above 20°C, where much soluble organic residue—sewage, fish and duck ponds. Easily confused with botulism.
Sodium and magnesium sulphate, milk, egg-white, Dimercaprol (British Anti-Lewisite), Calcium Versenate.	Levels of lead in the liver above 10 p.p.m. indicate probable lead poisoning.

CLINICAL HISTORY QUESTIONNAIRE

COMMON NAME:

SCIENTIFIC NAME IF KNOWN:

SEX:

RING NUMBER OR OTHER MEANS OF IDENTIFICATION:

OWNER'S NAME AND ADDRESS:

COUNTRY OF ORIGIN AND DATE OF IMPORTATION IF IMPORTED:

SOURCE:

DATE HATCHED OR APPROXIMATE AGE:

DATE ACQUIRED:

DATE OF DEATH:

HOW MANY BIRDS IN AFFECTED GROUP?

HOW MANY BIRDS HAVE DIED?

Diet
Give precise details

Breeding record
(*Tick where appropriate*)
This bird has been the parent of young:
Hatched alive ☐
Died within 48 hours of hatching ☐
Dead in shell ☐

Social status
(*Tick where appropriate*)
Kept alone ☐
Kept with same sex only ☐
One of a true pair ☐
One of a pair, sex not sure ☐
Kept in collection, same species ☐
Kept in collection, mixed species ☐

Information on recently hatched birds
(*Tick where appropriate*)
Hatching was normal ☐
Hatching was difficult ☐
Assistance with hatching was given ☐
Youngsters were fed by parents ☐
Youngsters were abandoned by parents ☐
Parents attacked young ☐
Other birds attacked young ☐

Housing
(*Tick where appropriate*)
Inside only ☐
Outside only ☐
Combination of both ☐
In an aviary ☐
In a cage ☐
In any other artificial enclosure ☐
In fenced park or woodland ☐

How many days before death did any of the following occur?
(Insert figures 0 = day of death, 1 = day before death, etc.)

Chilling ☐
Over-heating ☐
Diet changed ☐
Deterioration in quality of food ☐
Overcrowding ☐
Quarters changed ☐
Courtship display observed ☐
Mating ☐
Nest building ☐
Incubating ☐
Hatching ☐
Rearing young in nest ☐
Fighting ☐
Attacked by companions ☐

How many days before death did you see any of these signs:

Feather loss ☐   Inactivity ☐
Loss of weight ☐   General weakness ☐
Loss of condition ☐   Loss of appetite ☐
Injuries to head ☐   Difficulty in eating ☐
Injuries to body ☐   Unusual aggression ☐
Injuries to limbs ☐   Lameness right leg ☐
Swelling on head ☐   Lameness left leg ☐
Swelling on body ☐   Ruffled feathers ☐
Swelling on limbs ☐   Soiling of vent feathers with excreta ☐

Has the bird ever been sick previously and recovered?
If answer is "Yes" was the illness similar to the present one?
Was any treatment given during previous illness and if so what was it?

Birds kept in contact with sick or dead bird:
(Indicate following where appropriate)
Appear fit and well
Feather loss, etc. (see above list).
Vet. surgeon has previously been consulted (name and address):

Details of any treatment given by owner:
Details of any treatment given by veterinary surgeon:

Further Information
Give any further details which seem relevant:

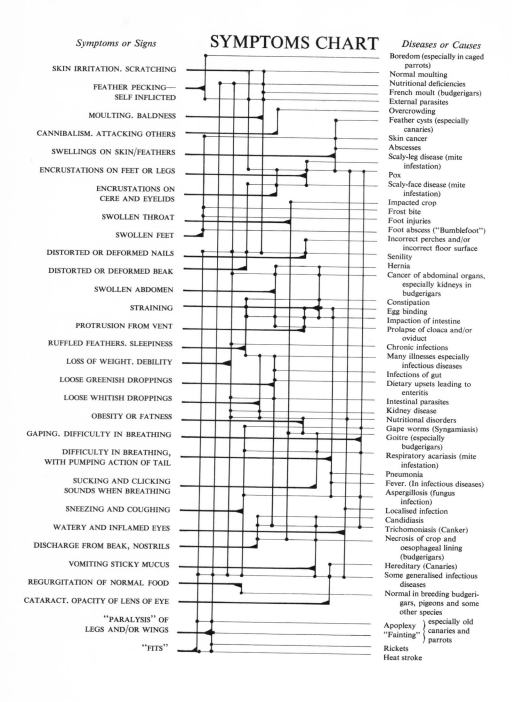

Symptoms or Signs   **SYMPTOMS CHART**   *Diseases or Causes*

Symptoms or Signs:

SKIN IRRITATION. SCRATCHING

FEATHER PECKING—
SELF INFLICTED

MOULTING. BALDNESS

CANNIBALISM. ATTACKING OTHERS

SWELLINGS ON SKIN/FEATHERS

ENCRUSTATIONS ON FEET OR LEGS

ENCRUSTATIONS ON
CERE AND EYELIDS

SWOLLEN THROAT

SWOLLEN FEET

DISTORTED OR DEFORMED NAILS

DISTORTED OR DEFORMED BEAK

SWOLLEN ABDOMEN

STRAINING

PROTRUSION FROM VENT

RUFFLED FEATHERS. SLEEPINESS

LOSS OF WEIGHT. DEBILITY

LOOSE GREENISH DROPPINGS

LOOSE WHITISH DROPPINGS

OBESITY OR FATNESS

GAPING. DIFFICULTY IN BREATHING

DIFFICULTY IN BREATHING,
WITH PUMPING ACTION OF TAIL

SUCKING AND CLICKING
SOUNDS WHEN BREATHING

SNEEZING AND COUGHING

WATERY AND INFLAMED EYES

DISCHARGE FROM BEAK, NOSTRILS

VOMITING STICKY MUCUS

REGURGITATION OF NORMAL FOOD

CATARACT. OPACITY OF LENS OF EYE

"PARALYSIS" OF
LEGS AND/OR WINGS

"FITS"

Diseases or Causes:

Boredom (especially in caged parrots)
Normal moulting
Nutritional deficiencies
French moult (budgerigars)
External parasites
Overcrowding
Feather cysts (especially canaries)
Skin cancer
Abscesses
Scaly-leg disease (mite infestation)
Pox
Scaly-face disease (mite infestation)
Impacted crop
Frost bite
Foot injuries
Foot abscess ("Bumblefoot")
Incorrect perches and/or incorrect floor surface
Senility
Hernia
Cancer of abdominal organs, especially kidneys in budgerigars
Constipation
Egg binding
Impaction of intestine
Prolapse of cloaca and/or oviduct
Chronic infections
Many illnesses especially infectious diseases
Infections of gut
Dietary upsets leading to enteritis
Intestinal parasites
Kidney disease
Nutritional disorders
Gape worms (Syngamiasis)
Goitre (especially budgerigars)
Respiratory acariasis (mite infestation)
Pneumonia
Fever. (In infectious diseases)
Aspergillosis (fungus infection)
Localised infection
Candidiasis
Trichomoniasis (Canker)
Necrosis of crop and oesophageal lining (budgerigars)
Hereditary (Canaries)
Some generalised infectious diseases
Normal in breeding budgerigars, pigeons and some other species
Apoplexy ⎫ especially old
"Fainting" ⎬ canaries and
       ⎭ parrots
Rickets
Heat stroke

518

INDEX

Pages printed in **bold** face refer to illustrations or photographs.

Crop, **44**, 45
  diseases, 225
  impaction, 225, 341
  impaction, relief of, 421, 424-425
"Crop milk", 45, 62
Crossed mandibles, **190**
Cuculiformes, 458
Culex, 148
Culicoides, 148, 149, 196, 198
  spp., 158
Cyanocobalamin (Vitamin B12), 74
Cyclopropane, 398
Cystic fluids, 444
Cystic neoplasm, **372**
Cystic oviducts, 272-273
Cysts, 360, 361, 445
Cytodites nudus, 168

D
DDT, 329
Dead-in-shell chicks, 383
Deformities, skeletal, 371, 374
Depigmentation of feathers, **274**
Dermanyssus, 201
  gallinae, 150, 159
Dermatitis, 201, 336
Dermoglyphus, 168
Deviated mandible, **190**
Diabetes mellitus, 63
Diaphragm, 42
Diarrhoea, 237
Diethyl thiambutene hydrochloride,
  397-398
Diets, 78-81
Digestive system, diseases of, 223-252
Digital examination, 88-89
Dilepis, 173
Diphtheria, 144
Diplotriaena, 196
Dipterous flies, 158-159
Discharges, nasal and ocular, 445
Diseases with signs of the pox, 97
Disinfectants, 327, 490-491, 512-513
Disinfestants, 327, 512-513
Dislocation, 215, 320
Disorientation and depression, **294**
Dominant factor, 17
Dorisella, 151
Double-yolked egg, 273
Dressings, 403
Droppings, 444
Dropsy, 281, 363
Drugs, 327, 329
Drugs and dosages, 483
Dry gangreen, **426**
Duodenum, 45
  diseases of, 237-244
Dystrophy, muscle, 222

E
Ear, 66-67, 305

structure of the, **68**
Eagle, **69**
Edwardsiella tarda, 136
Egg, 21, 27
  abnormalities, 273, 275
  binding, 272
  peritonitis, **251**, 262, 270-271, **369**
  structure of, **21**
  yolk, 270
Eggs, 382-383
  addled, 383
  different bird species, **23-26**
  infertile, 382
Eimeria, 141
  life cycle, **142**
Elizabethan collar, 403
Embarrassment, blood circulation, 280-282
Embolus, 280
Embryo, chick, **28-31**
Embryology, 27, 31
Emphysema, **179**, **318**
Encephalomacia, 335
Endocrine system, 61, 293, 296-297,
  300-301, 304
Enteritis, 113, 116-117, 120-121, 237
Enterobacteriaceae, 113
Enzyme, 68
Epidermoptes, 168
Epidymis, 52, 267
Epignathism, **191**, 204
Epilepsy, 287-288
Epitheliomas, 349
Equipment, surgical, anaesthetic, 403
"Equithesin", 399
Ergot, 325
Erysipelas, 131-132
Erysipelothrix, 258
Erysipelothrix insidiosa, 131
  rhusiopathiae, 131-132
Erythrocytes, 55
Escherichia coli, 96, 121, 248, 258, 270
Ether, 378
Eustachian tube, 66
Excretory system, 50-52
Exocrine glands, 69
Eye, 64
"Eye colds", 109
Eye, disease of, 305
Eyes, 371
  types of, **67**
Excreta, 444
Exostoses, 285

F
Faculifer rostratus, 168
Fainting, 289
Falconiformes, 455
Fats, 71
Fats and oils, 324
Favus, 97, 138-139
Feather mite, 168